# Tissue Nutrition and Viability

# Tissue Nutrition and Viability

Edited by Alan R. Hargens

With 138 Figures

Springer-Verlag
New York Berlin Heidelberg Tokyo

Alan R. Hargens
Professor of Surgery
Division of Orthopaedics
   and Rehabilitation
University of California, San Diego
La Jolla, California 92093
USA

Library of Congress Cataloging-in-Publication Data
Main entry under title:
Tissue nutrition and viability.
   Includes bibliographies and index.
   1. Stress (Physiology)   2. Tissues.   3. Nutrition.
I. Hargens, Alan R. [DNLM:   1. Histology.   2. Stress,
Mechanical. QS 532 T616]
QP82.2.S8T57   1985      611′.018      85-17256

Typeset by Bi-Comp, Inc., York, Pennsylvania.
Printed and bound by Halliday Lithograph, West Hanover, Massachusetts.
Printed in the United States of America.

9 8 7 6 5 4 3 2 1

ISBN 0-387-96202-6   Springer-Verlag New York Berlin Heidelberg Tokyo
ISBN 3-540-96202-6   Springer-Verlag Berlin Heidelberg New York Tokyo

# Preface

Recent research, especially in fields of orthopaedic surgery and rehabilitation, point to the importance of periodic, moderate stress for maintaining normal structure and function of tissues. Moreover, growth and healing of load-bearing tissues such as bone, cartilage, and intervertebral disc are especially dependent upon stress-related stimuli. Extreme levels of stress, however, are usually detrimental to tissue integrity, and most treatment regimens today address problems related to trauma and other conditions of abnormally high stress. Therefore, the purpose of this book is to bring together experts in fields of tissue nutrition and growth in order to review previous work and examine new ideas and results concerning the importance of mechanical stress in tissues.

This book is unique in that the topic of tissue nutrition and growth, especially related to possible benefits of periodic moderate stress, has never been addressed comprehensively, drawing together experts on various tissues and organs. One objective is to focus attention on tissue nutrition where controversy still exists regarding basic mechanisms of metabolite transport and fluid homeostasis within the interstitium. Another objective is to examine the pathophysiology of tissue compression and discuss strategies to improve viability. Tissues which are treated in this book include bone, cartilage, intervertebral disc, lung, nerve, skeletal muscle, umbilical cord, synovium, skin, and subcutaneous tissues. Based upon these objectives, this book is primarily addressed to students, investigators, and teachers in fields of physiology, biochemistry, biomechanics, exercise, orthopaedic surgery, rehabilitation, and sports medicine. Other groups interested in hypokinetic states (bedrest and weightlessness) and mechanisms of healing will find the text of interest. Overall, the chapters provide summaries of recent findings and critical reviews of important issues in the nutrition, growth, and viability of tissues. Directions for future research and clinical applications are also presented.

Alan R. Hargens

# Acknowledgments

Along with the chapter authors, many individuals contributed to this endeavor. Manuscript preparation was aided by the skills of Dyan Williams and Jean Robison. Many of the figures and drawings were prepared by Kurt Smolen. Some of the clinical and experimental research in this book was supported by the Veterans Administration, USPHS/NIH grants AM-25501, AM-26344, my Research Career Development Award AM-00602, GM-24901, National Aeronautics and Space Administration, and by the Division of Orthopaedics and Rehabilitation at UCSD. A generous grant from the Kroc Foundation provided partial travel support for authors to attend a symposium, "Effects of Mechanical Stress on Tissue Transport and Viability," which was a part of the XII European Conference for Microcirculation in Jerusalem. This symposium laid the groundwork for subsequent preparation and revision of manuscripts. Finally, I wish to thank Professor Alexander Silberberg, Polymer Department, Weizmann Institute of Science, and his co-workers for their assistance and wonderful hospitality during the Jerusalem meeting.

# Contents

# Contributors

Wayne H. Akeson, M.D., Professor and Head, Division of Orthopaedics and Rehabilitation, University of California Medical Center, San Diego, California, USA

Itzhak Binderman, D.M.D., Associate Professor of Dentistry, Tel-Aviv University School of Dental Medicine; Head, Dental Unit and Hard Tissues Lab, Medical Center of Tel-Aviv, Israel

Lars B. Dahlin, M.D., Postdoctoral Fellow, Laboratory of Experimental Biology, Department of Anatomy, University of Göteborg, Göteborg, Sweden

Richard H. Gelberman, M.D., Associate Professor of Surgery, Division of Orthopaedics and Rehabilitation, University of California Medical Center, San Diego, California, USA

David H. Gershuni, M.D., F.R.C.S. (England), F.R.C.S. (Edinberg), Associate Professor of Surgery, Division of Orthopaedics and Rehabilitation, University of California, San Diego, California, USA

Alan R. Hargens, Ph.D., Professor of Surgery, Department of Surgery/Orthopaedics, VA and University of California Medical Centers, San Diego, California, USA

George B. Hart, M.D., Assistant Clinical Professor of Surgery, University of California, Irvine, California; Director, Baromedical Department, Memorial Hospital Medical Center of Long Beach, Long Beach, California, USA

Sten H. Holm, Ph.D., Associate Professor of Experimental Orthopaedics, Department of Orthopaedic Surgery I, Sahlgren Hospital, University of Göteborg, Göteborg, Sweden

Mark H. Holmes, Ph.D., Associate Professor of Mathematics, Department of Mathematical Sciences, Rensselaer Polytechnic Institute, Troy, New York, USA

W. Michael Lai, Ph.D., Professor of Mechanics, Department of Mechanical Engineering, Rensselaer Polytechnic Institute, Troy, New York, USA

Göran Lundborg, M.D., Ph.D., Associate Professor, Division of Hand Surgery, Department of Orthopaedic Surgery, University Hospital, Lund, Sweden

Alice Maroudas, Ph.D., Professor, Department of Bio-Medical Engineering, Technion, Israel Institute of Technology, Haifa, Israel

Frank A. Meyer, Ph.D., Senior Scientist, Polymer Department, Weizmann Institute of Science, Rehovot, Israel

Van C. Mow, Ph.D., Clark and Crossan Professor of Engineering, Department of Mechanical Engineering, Rensselaer Polytechnic Institute, Troy, New York, USA

James C. Parker, Ph.D., Associate Professor, Department of Physiology, College of Medicine, University of South Alabama, Mobile, Alabama, USA

Narender P. Reddy, Ph.D., Associate Professor, Institute for Biomedical Engineering Research, University of Akron, Ohio, USA

Bengt Rippe, M.D., Ph.D., Associate Professor, Department of Physiology, Faculty of Medicine, University of Göteborg, Göteborg, Sweden

Björn Rydevik, M.D., Ph.D., Associate Professor, Department of Orthopaedic Surgery I, Sahlgren Hospital, University of Göteborg, Göteborg, Sweden

Geert W. Schmid-Schönbein, Ph.D., Associate Professor of Bioengineering, Department of Applied Mechanics and Engineering Sciences, University of California, San Diego, California, USA

Ole M. Sejersted, M.D., Ph.D., Director, Institute of Muscle Physiology, Oslo, Norway

Zvi Shimshoni, D.M.D., Hard Tissues Unit, Tel-Aviv Medical Center, Tel-Aviv, Israel

Thomas C. Skalak, Ph.D., Postgraduate Research Bioengineer, Department of Applied Mechanics and Engineering Sciences, University of California, San Diego, California, USA

Dalia Somjen, Ph.D., Hard Tissues Unit, Tel-Aviv Medical Center, Tel-Aviv, Israel

Michael B. Strauss, M.D., Clinical Assistant Professor, Orthopaedic Surgery, Harbor-UCLA, Torrance, California; Associate Director, Baromedical Department, Memorial Hospital Medical Center of Long Beach, Long Beach, California, USA

Robert M. Szabo, M.D., Assistant Professor and Chief of Hand Surgery Service, Department of Orthopaedic Surgery, University of California, Davis; Sacramento Medical Center, Sacramento, California, USA

Aubrey E. Taylor, Ph.D., Professor and Chairman, Department of Physiology, College of Medicine, University of South Alabama, Mobile, Alabama, USA

Jill P.G. Urban, Ph.D., Bone and Joint Research Unit, London Hospital Medical College, London, England; University Laboratory of Physiology, University of Oxford, Oxford, England

Benjamin W. Zweifach, Ph.D., Professor of Bioengineering, Department of Applied Mechanics and Engineering Sciences, University of California, San Diego, California, USA

# CHAPTER 1

# Stress Effects on Tissue Nutrition and Viability

Alan R. Hargens and Wayne H. Akeson

## Introduction

An early theory of cellular adaptation to altered mechanical force was proposed by Wolff (1892) and states that tissue architecture is strengthened by increased activity. Wolff emphasized clinical studies of pathological specimens. Although Wolff's Law originally treated adaptations of the hip joint, femur and vertebrae to alterations of externally applied mechanical loads, it is evident that this principle is more general and applies to many other tissues as well. For example, joint contractures due to immobilization (Akeson et al., 1980) are often prevented by early passive joint motion (Frank et al., 1984). Continuous passive motion also aids clearance of hemarthrosis from synovial fluid (O'Driscoll et al., 1983). Ligaments (Tipton et al., 1975; Amiel et al., 1983, Akeson et al., 1985), tendons (Tipton et al., 1975; Gelberman et al., 1981), bone (Woo et al., 1981) and skeletal muscle (Booth and Gollnick, 1983) benefit from early mechanical stress in terms of healing and hypertrophy as compared to immobilized tissues. However, as pointed out by Brickley-Parsons and Glimcher (1984), tissue adaptations to increased mechanical loads may be favorable or unfavorable, depending on the specific tissue and magnitude of mechanical stress as depicted in Figure 1.1.

Tissues, particularly those facilitating motion and load bearing, undergo periodic stress and deformation that may promote nutrition, growth and viability of these tissues. Recent reviews of the effects of continuous passive motion on healing (Frank et al., 1984; Gelberman and Manske, 1985) and tissue deformation on nutrition (Mow et al., 1984) provide strong evidence that periodic, moderate stress is essential for tissue viability. On the other hand, extraordinary levels of stress traumatize tissue and are detrimental to long-term viability (Fig. 1.1). Relatively avascular tissues, which absorb high and variable loads, may be particularly dependent on benefits of periodic moderate stress, possibly for mediation of cellular metabolic rate and for pumping interstitial fluid into and out of the

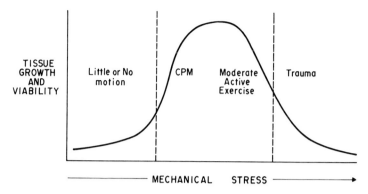

**Figure 1.1.** Qualitative effects of low, moderate and high mechanical stress on tissue growth and viability. CPM is continuous passive motion.

tissue. Such tissues include articular cartilage (probably the most studied in this regard), intervertebral disc, meniscus, ligament and tendon.

## Transport Mechanisms in Tissue

An understanding of stress effects on tissue nutrition must consider tissue structure and its effect on nutrient transport and waste removal during motion. Tissue nutrition depends on the transport of metabolic substrates from blood to cells, whereas tissue viability and growth are often limited by transport of waste products and structural elements from cells to interstitium, lymphatic vessels and blood.

### Anatomy and Function of Interstitium

Tissue nutrition depends greatly on transport of nutrients and waste products between blood, interstitium and cells. Therefore, it is important to examine interstitial anatomy before embarking on possible transport mechanisms for tissue nutrition. The interstitium consists of structural components [collagen fibrils and glycosaminoglycans (GAGs)] and fluid components (water, proteins, ions and other metabolic substrates and endproducts) that surround single cells or clusters of cells. These components comprise the so-called ground substance of the connective tissue that forms the milieu around which all cells and microcirculatory elements function (Fig. 1.2). Collagen fibrils and GAGs interpenetrate each other to provide elasticity, to oppose interstitial deformation and to maintain interstitial volume (Laurent, 1970, 1972). Fibroblasts synthesize collagen precursors (procollagen) that move into the interstitium to form tropocolla-

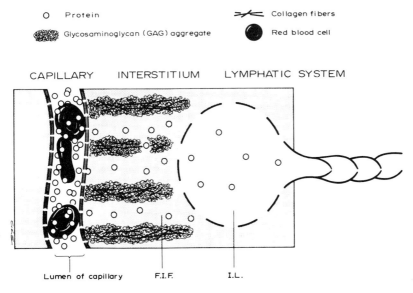

O   Protein

Glycosaminoglycan (GAG) aggregate

Collagen fibers

Red blood cell

CAPILLARY     INTERSTITIUM     LYMPHATIC SYSTEM

Lumen of capillary     F.I.F.     I.L.

**Figure 1.2.** Structure and flow dynamics of tissue fluid. Ultrafiltration of plasma across the capillary wall yields a gradient of plasma protein and hydrostatic pressure from the blood to interstitial fluid. Capillaries have a high protein reflection coefficient and retain most protein in the blood. Tissue can be considered a three-phase system with cells (not shown) surrounded by collagen–GAG aggregates and microscopic channels of free interstitial fluid (F.I.F.). As fluid moves from blood through the interstitium and into the initial lymphatic (I.L.), its composition is altered by exclusion phenomena and chromatography effects. Structural elements are not drawn to scale (refer to text for dimensions). (From AR Hargens, 1986.)

gen polymers which, in turn, polymerize into collagen fibrils (Fig. 1.3). Similarly, hyaluronic acid and proteoglycans are transported extracellularly and constrained by collagen fibrils, thus forming an interstitial matrix.

The volume of interstitial fluid, based on equilibration of various extracellular and intravascular isotopes, ranges from 12% to 20% of body weight (Aukland and Nicolaysen, 1981). Certain tissues contain larger reservoirs of interstitial fluid, and thus these organs are relatively more important in overall fluid balance within the body. Interstitial fluid volume is about 4× plasma volume (2–3× blood volume with hematocrit of 40). Although interstitial structures are well-defined and relatively uniform biochemically, interstitial anatomy varies greatly from one tissue to another and even within a given tissue. For example, some regions are devoid of collagen fibrils, GAGs, or both (Merker and Günther, 1972). As depicted in Figure 1.2, large macromolecules such as globulins are transported preferentially and rapidly within channels of free fluid so that large protein molecules experience a "chromatography effect" as they are

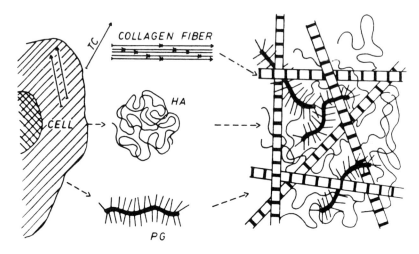

**Figure 1.3.** Interstitial matrix components are formed intracellularly, transported to interstitial spaces, and polymerized to form a framework of interpenetrating macromolecules. Collagen fibers are formed from tropocollagen (TC), whereas glycosaminoglycans form from hyaluronic acid (HA) and proteoglycan (PG). (From TC Laurent, 1972.)

transported from the blood to peripheral lymph (Laurent, 1972; Granger, 1981). Free fluid channels are estimated to range between 2 and 10 $\mu$m in diameter, based on Brownian motion studies (Wiederhielm, 1969). More recently, however, Casley-Smith and Vincent (1978) determined that these tissue fluid channels are 100 to 200 nm in diameter for various tissues.

As indicated earlier, the interstitium consists of a gel-like matrix of collagen fibrils and GAGs that interpenetrate and attract one another by covalent, hydrogen and electrostatic bonds. Whereas collagen fibrils function as structural support for the matrix, aggregated GAGs and hyaluronate macromolecules importantly function to imbibe interstitial fluid and to exclude proteins and other large molecules. Thus, the transport of fluid and solutes from blood to lymph is primarily confined within the interstitial channels of free fluid and represents a complex biorheological phenomenon (Katz, 1980; Johnson and Bloom, 1981; Silberberg, 1982).

Hyaluronate is an unbranched macromolecule with a diameter, length and molecular weight of 10 Å, 3 $\mu$m, and $10^6$ to $10^7$ atomic mass units, respectively. When placed in solution, it assumes a random coil configuration with 5000 Å diameter and imbibes a great deal of saline by virtue of its high density of negative charge. For example, when human umbilical connective tissue (a structure rich in hyaluronate) is placed in Tyrode's solution in the absence of external compression, it swells to twice its usual volume (Granger et al., 1975). At a normal water/dry weight ratio of

10, umbilical cord has an imbibition pressure of $-12$ mm Hg. During dehydration, this imbibition pressure increases as a power-series expansion so that at a water/dry weight ratio of 5, the imbibition pressure reaches $-80$ mm Hg. Repulsive forces within a matrix of high anionic charge density cause the tissue to exert large negative fluid pressures (Hargens, 1981). When water or proteinaceous fluid is available for entry into the tissue, fluid is imbibed and the tissue swells. Granger and co-workers (1975) conclude that the swelling behavior of the interstitial matrix is characterized by: (1) a low compliance ($dV/dP$) state at normal dehydration and (2) a nonlinear compliance decrease to very low levels with dehydration.

On the basis of studies of imbibition pressure in isolated samples of umbilical tissue, elastic recoil or electrostatic expansion forces primarily cause the interstitial matrix to swell when excess fluid is available. With elimination of electrostatic and associated Donnan effects between anionic charges in the matrix (by placing the tissue in a solution with high salt concentration), only a small shift of the volume–pressure relationship occurs. This suggests that electrostatic expansion (swelling) of GAG macromolecules within the interstitial matrix provides the primary mechanism for imbibition (Fig. 1.4). In an unstressed tissue matrix (Fig. 1.4B), the imbibition pressure of these macromolecules is balanced by the external loading pressure so that there is no fluid pressure gradient across the tissue boundary. Normally, therefore, GAG tends to swell and imbibe fluid whereas this tendency is prevented by constraining properties of collagen and external loading pressures. If external loading pressure increases or imbibition pressure decreases by GAG loss (Fig. 1.4A), the matrix is compressed and fluid is lost. On the other hand, if external pressure decreases or imbibition pressure increases, fluid is absorbed (Fig. 1.4C). The intervertebral disc may be a tissue in which these fluid pressure–volume relationships apply. For example, Figure 1.4A could explain water loss from the nucleus pulposus during weight lifting (increased load) and Figure 1.4C could explain the swelling of the nucleus pulposus during sleep (decreased load). During abnormal conditions of severe dehydration or edema, any tissue can assume a compacted or expanded state, respectively. Not all investigators, however, agree with this mechanism of tissue swelling. For example, Meyer and Silberberg (1974) suggest that during normal in vivo conditions, the collagen framework assumes an unstressed state and that dehydration or swelling is opposed by the network of collagen fibrils which tends to restore the tissue to its steady state.

GAG and hyaluronate macromolecules, which interpenetrate the framework of collagen fibrils in the interstitium, will diffuse out of the tissue (e.g., articular cartilage, umbilical tissue) over relatively long time periods. This process is considerably more rapid if the collagen fibrils are digested away by collagenase (Meyer and Silberberg, 1974). Recently,

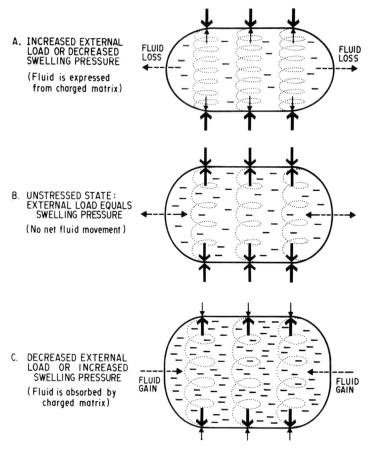

**Figure 1.4.** Relationship between external loading pressure, expansion pressure (swelling due to imbibition or osmosis), and tissue fluid pressure during compression (**A**), unstressed state (**B**), and expansion (**C**) of tissue matrix.

lymph was found to contain detectable hyaluronate concentrations (Laurent and Laurent, 1981), which suggests that this large mucopolysaccharide passes across the interstitial–lymph barrier. Apparently, however, this is a very slow process since hyaluronate and GAG macromolecules are much more highly concentrated in tissue spaces than in lymph (Ogston and Phelps, 1961; Comper and Laurent, 1978; Wiederhielm, 1979).

## Diffusive Transport

In the absence of external force fields, nutrients are transported from regions of high to low solute concentration by random thermal motion.

The tendency of a solute to reach uniform distribution in the presence of a concentration gradient is termed diffusion. A net solute flux occurs from a region of high solute concentration to a region of low solute concentration because statistically more solutes move by Brownian motion into the region of low concentration. When the concentration gradient is not maintained by an external source, for example, by blood flow and cellular metabolism, the solute will eventually assume a uniform distribution through its available tissue space.

The flux of a solute in one dimension $x$ ($J_1$) in terms of number $\times$ area$^{-1}$ $\times$ time$^{-1}$ depends on a diffusion coefficient $D$ and the solute's concentration gradient $\partial c_1 / \partial x$ according to Fick's First Law:

$$J_1 = -D \partial c_1 / \partial x, \tag{1}$$

where a negative sign is used by convention to indicate solute movement in the direction of decreasing concentration. The diffusion coefficient $D$ is a specific property of the solute–solvent pair with units of area $\times$ time$^{-1}$. For systems with zero volume flow across a boundary, the Einstein intra-diffusion (self-diffusion) coefficient $D^*$ depends directly on absolute temperature $T$ and inversely on molecular weight and a concentration-dependent frictional factor $f_1$ according to the following equation (Comper, 1984):

$$D^* = RT/f_1. \tag{2}$$

The rate at which $n$ mol of solute accumulates at point $x$ and time $t$ ($\partial n_1 / \partial t$) is represented by:

$$\partial n_1 / \partial t = J_1(x) - J_1(x + dx), \tag{3}$$

which can be rewritten assuming rate of solute accumulation equals rate of divergence of solute flux:

$$-\partial n_1 / \partial t = (\partial J_1 / \partial x) dx. \tag{4}$$

Since $\partial n_1 / \partial x = \partial c_1$, we derive:

$$-\partial J_1 / \partial x = \partial c_1 / \partial t. \tag{5}$$

To solve for $c_1$ as a function of position and time, we substitute $J_1$ from Eq. 1 into Eq. 5 which yields Fick's Second Law:

$$\partial c_1 / \partial t = D(\partial^2 c_1 / \partial x^2). \tag{6}$$

Recently, Comper (1984) provided an expression relating the mutual diffusion coefficient ($D$) to the intradiffusion coefficient ($D^*$) for transport of macromolecules through interstitial fluid:

$$D = [D^*/(1 - c_1 \bar{V}_1)](1 + 2A_2 M_1 c_1 + 3A_3 M_1 c_1^2 + \ldots .), \tag{7}$$

where $\bar{V}_1$ is partial specific volume, $M_1$ is molecular weight of the macromolecule and $A_2$, $A_3$, etc. are virial coefficients. $D^*$ decreases with greater frictional interactions that slow macromolecular diffusion (see Eq. 2) but $D^*$ increases the value of $D$ in good solvents. $D^*$ decreases greatly with concentration of interstitial macromolecules. However, this expression (Eq. 7) has not been applied to proteoglycan aggregates of articular cartilage, and agreement with experimental data is marginal (Comper, 1984).

Recently, Levick (1984) considered the role of diffusion to nourish cartilage in a synovial joint (Fig. 1.5). Applying a modification of Fick's First Law and assuming that glucose isn't metabolized by synovial fluid and disappears in cartilage:

$$J_1 = DA(\partial c_1/\partial r), \tag{8}$$

where $A = 2\pi r w$ (surface area of flux boundary) and where $c_1$ is glucose concentration in synovial fluid, $r$ is radial distance from the center of the joint and $w$ is thickness of synovial fluid film. Pure diffusion of glucose requires that the concentration gradient between the periphery $c_R$ and joint center $c_0$:

$$c_R - c_0 = R^2 x v_g/Dw, \tag{9}$$

where $x$ is cartilage thickness and $v_g$ is glycolysis rate/volume of cartilage. Assuming $w$ ranges between 26 and 500 $\mu$m, Eq. 9 predicts a $C_R - C_0$ range of between 2066 and 108 mg/cm$^3$ over a radial distance of 1.5 cm. Because glucose concentration at the periphery is $<1$ mg/cm$^3$, Levick (1984) concludes that glucose diffusion is far too slow to transport such a nutrient to central regions of cartilage and that convective transport due to joint motion represents the primary nutritional pathway.

Generally, however, diffusive transport of small solutes is probably sufficient for nutrition of most tissues, especially those tissues that contain rich networks of capillary vessels. For example, oxygen, small ions and sugars are transported rapidly from blood to cells by diffusion. Even avascular tissues such as intervertebral disc seem to depend on diffusion as their primary mechanism of nutrient transport (Urban et al., 1982; Holm and Nachemson, 1983). However, as solutes increase in size and interstitial exclusion slows diffusive flux, convective or volume transport of nutrients and tissue macromolecules becomes more important. For example, transport of growth factors and hormones may depend on volume flows induced by hydrostatic pressure gradients rather than diffusive flow. Such gradients are absent in immobilized tissue but may cause great flows of interstitial fluid during motion. Likewise, movements of large structural components of tissue (GAGs and hyaluronate) and metabolic waste products are probably facilitated by convective flows induced by motion and consequent gradients of hydrostatic pressure. Certainly, it is possible that convective flows are important stress-dependent factors in growth and healing mechanisms set forth in Wolff's Law. More rapid

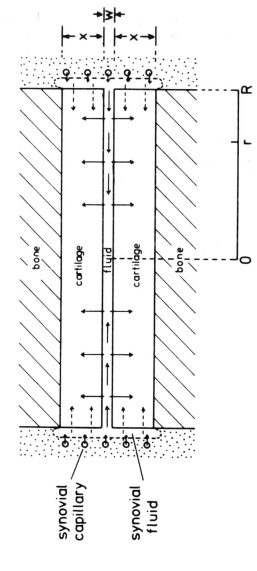

**Figure 1.5.** Simplified synovial joint in section illustrates nutrition of articular cartilage by synovial fluid. Each cartilage plate is of uniform thickness $x$ and radius $R$. Plates are separated in unloaded joint by thin layer of synovial fluid of width $w$. Solid arrows represent passage of nutrient (e.g., glucose) from synovial plasma across blood–joint barrier, through intercartilaginous fluid film, and into two cartilage plates. Theory and experiments indicate flux through intercartilaginous fluid is caused mainly by convection rather than diffusion. *Dashed arrows* represent direct rout by which rim of cartilage plate can be nourished from synovial fluid outside intercartilaginous plane. (From JR Levick, 1984.)

transport of structural macromolecules and waste products from their sites of production may accelerate rates of cellular metabolism.

## Convective Transport

Bulk flow through a porous medium such as the interstitium depends on hydrostatic pressure gradients and sufficiently large channels. This mechanism for solute transport is more rapid than diffusion when criteria regarding magnitudes of pore size, solute size and pressure gradients are satisfied.

In the presence of hydrostatic pressure gradients and sufficiently large tissue pores, solute transport is coupled to the volume of water (saline) flow $J_v$ as follows:

$$J_v = \bar{V}_w J_w, \tag{10}$$

where $\bar{V}_w$ is partial molar volume (18 $cm^3$/mol for water) and $J_w$ is water flow (mol $\times$ $cm^{-2}$ $\times$ $s^{-1}$). Therefore, the coupled flow of solute $J_1'$ to water volume flow $J_v$ is:

$$J_1' = \bar{c}_1 J_v, \tag{11}$$

where $\bar{c}_1$ is the average concentration of the solute in the tissue fluid. Since some solutes are reflected more than other solutes, we must multiply by the fraction of solutes transported with water $(1 - \sigma_s)$, where $\sigma_s$ is the reflection coefficient for a given solute. Therefore, the generalized coupled flux of solute is:

$$J_s' = \bar{c}_s(1 - \sigma_s)J_v. \tag{12}$$

Combining diffusion of solutes with convection yields the well-known Kedem-Katchalsky (1958, 1961) equation:

$$J_s = W\Delta\pi_s + \bar{c}_s(1 - \sigma_s)J_v, \tag{13}$$

in which the first term $W\Delta\pi_s$ represents diffusional transport, where $W$ is tissue permeability ($W = \phi_t D_s/RTr$ where $\phi_t$ is tissue fluid volume fraction, $D_s$ is the diffusion coefficient for a given solute and $r$ is diffusional distance) and the second term represents convective transport as given in Eq. (12).

On the basis of Poiseuille's Law and Darcy's Law, Curry (1984) provides an equation for volume flow per unit area of porous matrix ($J_v/S$):

$$J_v/S = (A/S)(\Delta P/\Delta x)r_h^2/G\eta, \tag{14}$$

where $A/S$ is the fractional surface area available for fluid penetration, $\Delta x$ is matrix thickness, $r_h$ is the hydraulic radius available for flow, $G$ is the Kozeny geometric constant (Carmen, 1937), $\eta$ is viscosity and $\Delta P/\Delta x$ is the pressure gradient. Poiseuille's Law is obeyed when $G = 2$. For a fibrous macromolecular network in Curry's model, volume flow per unit area is:

$$J_v/S = [A_{net}r_f^2E^3/\Delta xS(1 - E)^24G\eta]\Delta P, \qquad (15)$$

where $A_{net}$ is total network area, $r_f$ is fiber radius, $E$ is volume available to water in the network ("fractional void volume") and other terms retain their previous definitions (see Eq. 14). $G$ increases with greater tortuosity within the fiber network (Curry, 1984).

Early studies by Ogston and associates (1961, 1973) demonstrated that GAG and related macromolecules profoundly affect the transport and distribution of proteins and other macromolecules within a tissue matrix. Thus, the interstitial matrix excludes any solute whose diameter is greater than the pore diameter of the entangled matrix of collagen fibrils and GAGs. Recently, Granger (1981) summarized these relationships for the interstitium in quantitative terms. Assuming a tissue matrix of equivalent fibrils, the fraction of fluid space excluded by the matrix is $F_E$:

$$F_E = 1 - e^{-\{(r_p + r_f)/r_f\}^2 \cdot \bar{V}_f c_f}, \qquad (16)$$

where $r_p$ is protein radius, $r_f$ is fibril radius, $\bar{V}_f$ is partial specific volume of fibril polymers and $c_f$ is fibril concentration. This relationship indicates that exclusion increases with protein size and fibrillar density such that dehydration raises $F_E$. In addition to these steric considerations, electrostatic repulsion between the negatively charged proteins and negatively charged GAG matrix at physiological pH values offers further exclusion to protein penetration. High charge densities within articular cartilage, intervertebral disc and meniscus are particularly important for exclusion phenomena in these tissues.

In addition to diffusion and convection of solutes through tissue, Preston and co-workers (1980) propose another extremely rapid transport mechanism for solutes through solutions of polymers. Although unproven in a biological context, this mode of transport is facilitated by formation of ordered structures in polymer solutions, allowing a "microscopic convection mechanism."

## Stress Effects on Connective Tissue: The Importance of Mechanical Factors for Connective Tissue Homeostasis

The profound degree to which mechanical stress affects many specialized musculoskeletal tissues has been evident for many years. The declaration of Wolff's Law of bone in 1892 was the clearest early presentation of this concept although the layman's observations on the effects of work, or the lack of it, on muscle bulk undoubtedly precedes recorded observation. The influence of stress enhancement or deprivation on fibrous connective tissue is less intuitive than the above and has required more sophisticated technical approaches to measure matrix changes for clear documentation of physical influences on the fibroblast. To be sure, early clinicians observed that joint contractures were caused by prolonged immobility, but the nature of the underlying process controlling contracture development was only recently elucidated.

The nature of the signals to which the fibroblast responds can be only a matter for speculation at present. Electrical and direct mechanical inputs to cells are among numerous possibilities for consideration. The mechanism by which the cell responds to a signal is even more speculative at present. Among such mechanisms for consideration are the influence of nutrition on cellular synthetic and/or resorptive activities. Mechanical factors must influence the convective aspects of interstitial fluid movement as previously discussed, and therefore, the rates of ingress of metabolic substrates and egress of degradative products are important factors in tissue growth and healing. These factors undoubtedly influence the maintenance of fibrous connective tissue matrix. It is clear that the mechanisms controlling the response of fibrous connective tissue to stress enhancement or stress deprivation are both numerous and complex. It will be the purpose of this section to discuss the net effect of these two extreme functional states on fibrous connective tissue.

A brief mention of anatomical–biomechanical interactions will be necessary to understand the fundamental changes operating. Soft tissue support structures about joints have an almost uniform biochemical composition despite dissimilar functional roles. The body exhibits wise economy in this solution since a single building block, collagen, can provide both resistance to high tensile forces and at the same time the properties of flexibility that synovial joints require. Two major structural components are found: collagen and ground substance. They exist as composite materials with viscoelastic properties. The ground substance is a material with high water content containing proteoglycans, very large molecules that attract and hold water, restricting its flow. The collagen fiber pattern changes when tension is applied, causing the fibers to straighten. The rate of the straightening is limited by the swelling properties of the tissue displaced. This dampens the mechanical force and gives rise to the properties of viscoelasticity.

The collagen fiber patterns about joints vary greatly in detail, but generally fall into two categories: a relatively straight, parallel waveform and a matrix form commonly called a nylon-hose pattern (Fig. 1.6). The parallel waveform is seen in tendon and ligament. This structure straightens under tension. The degree of elongation is limited to 10% at most. The nylon-hose form is present in flexible structures such as capsule, synovium and skin. The apparent ability of this structure to stretch is well known as the nylon hose fits legs of all sizes and shapes. The individual fibers are inelastic, but the pattern of weave creates apparent elasticity. The ability

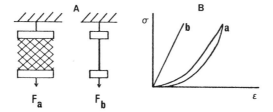

**Figure 1.6. A:** Schematic representation of collagen patterns with applied forces: nylon-hose with $F_a$ (left) and straight with $F_b$ (right). **B:** Nylon-hose model demonstrates nonlinear hysteresis behavior (a) as opposed to linear stress–strain behavior of uniform material (b). $\sigma$ is stress and $\varepsilon$ is strain. (From WH Akeson et al., 1985.)

of this structure to lengthen may be more than 100-fold, depending on the pattern of the mesh weave. Crucial to the change in shape of the nylon mesh is the ability of fibers to glide past one another at intercept points. If intercept points are locked, the mesh loses its ability to stretch. Under these circumstances, the structure will no longer adapt to functional demands that require a change in shape. An example of this concept is the Chinese finger trap. If the two ends are pulled, the small cables glide past one another so that the structure narrows and clamps the finger securely. If a few solder junctions are placed on the intercept points, the gliding is defeated and the clamping function no longer occurs. We will return to this structure later. The pathological and biomechanical events that underlie the stress deprivation and stress augmentation processes will now be described.

## Stress Deprivation

The events of stress deprivation involve all joint structures. Best known are changes in muscle and bone which can be appreciated by clinical exam and radiographs without sophisticated tools. Connective tissue changes are encountered as contractures varying in degree from patient to patient under similar treatment programs, but generally, the severity of the contracture is proportionate to the degree of joint injury and time in cast.

Findings on joints from autopsies of humans and studies on experimental animals generally agree. The proliferation of fibrofatty connective tissue within the joint space has been demonstrated in immobilized human joints by Enneking and Horowitz (1972). A similar process was described in early experimental studies by Evans and co-workers (1960). The fibrofatty connective tissue overgrows the cartilage surfaces, creating a pannus-like membrane. This membrane is firmly fixed to cartilage to the degree that it tears when the joint is manipulated and may produce cartilage damage. Further damage to cartilage is caused by persistence of the fibrofatty tissue overgrowth on the cartilage surfaces, probably interfering with the nutritional mechanisms and causing enzymatic degradation of the matrix. Additional damage to cartilage may result from stationary contact of cartilage–cartilage interfaces during cast immobilization. Pressure at the surface accelerates the process and creates an ulcer-like damage as noted in early works of Salter and Field (1960), Trias (1961) and Thaxter and associates (1965). With time, gross adhesions are noted between synovial folds, a particular problem in joints such as the shoulder where redundant folds are useful in achieving a wide range of motion.

Further, ligament attachment sites are subject to significant weakening due to localized osteoporosis. Osteoclasts resorb both bone and Sharpey's fibers passing into bone from the ligament. These changes, first described by Laros and collaborators (1971), obviously greatly weaken the ligament functionally.

The processes operative at the cellular level are also dramatic, though not as easily appreciated. They lead to altered mechanical and structural properties of the tissue that have important clinical implications. Cell pattern changes are dramatic comparing the anterior cruciate ligament from an immobilized rabbit joint to a paired control (Fig. 1.7). The

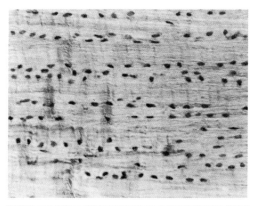

A

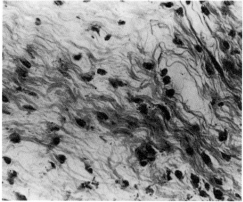

B

Figure 1.7. A: Anterior cruciate ligament from cage activity rabbit knee (×310). B: Anterior cruciate ligament from 9-week immobilized rabbit knee showing matrix disorganization (×310). (From WH Akeson et al., 1980.)

changes from an ordered to a more disorganized pattern are clearly evident.

## Biochemical Events

The biochemical events following stress deprivation include the following:

1. Small decrease in size of ligament
2. Small loss of collagen mass
3. Loss of water content of matrix
4. Loss of content of GAGs
5. Large increase in reducible chemical cross-linkages
6. Large increase in collagen turnover
7. Large increase in collagen synthesis
8. Large increases in collagen resorption

The resorption rate exceeds the synthesis rate. The meaning of these changes is best understood in the context of altered mechanical and structural properties and will be discussed later.

Gross mechanical properties of experimental models of joint contracture generally parallel observations on human joint contracture. One experimental model is a rabbit knee joint that had been previously immobilized for 9 weeks. The muscle tissue has been trimmed away. The joint was tested in a device called an arthrograph to characterize its stiffness quantitatively. Typical curves of the immobilized and normal joints are presented (Figs. 1.8 and 1.9). Changes in mechanical and structural properties of individual ligaments can be appreciated from these curves of load deformation and stress strain. Both mechanical and structural properties are reduced to about one-third of normal in rabbit knees immobilized 9 to

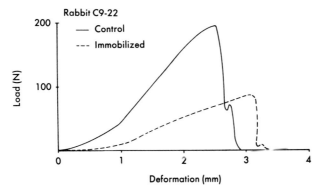

**Figure 1.8.** Typical load-deformation curves of lateral collateral ligaments of normal and immobilized knees of same rabbit. (From D Amiel et al., 1982.)

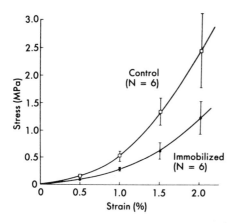

**Figure 1.9.** Stress–strain relationship of normal and immobilized rabbit lateral-collateral ligaments. (From D Amiel et al., 1982.)

12 weeks. Noyes and co-workers (1974) showed similar changes in the primate knee immobilized for 8 weeks.

How can these data be integrated into a meaningful whole? Contradictions are apparent. It is paradoxical that the whole joint composite presents a contracture whereas individual ligament structures are weakened within their substance and at their insertion sites. We believe that the contracture is best explained by the process of randomness of the synthesis and resorption of collagen fibers that occurs in the absence of the control signals which are somehow generated by physical activity. Evidence has been presented showing piezoelectric phenomena in fibrous connective tissue as well as bone. It is possible that such signals or even direct mechanical force signals represent the mediators of the changes observed. Whatever the mechanism, the net effect of random collagen turnover is a disturbance of free gliding in the nylon mesh system. It is most unlikely that the process results from a chemical bond at the intercept point. Distances are too great and the forces required are too large. More likely, we believe, are fiber–fiber crossovers created by the insertion of new fibers into the meshwork so as to impede gliding, much as gliding is impeded by the solder junctions in the finger trap problem. The process is favored by loss of ground substance noted earlier which removes a space buffer and lubricating factors between adjacent collagen bundles. These changes are clearly time-dependent, but reversible by remodeling if the new fibers are not too numerous and do not enlarge beyond some average critical size as yet undefined.

Structural properties of ligaments are weakened, we believe, by the same random events. Here the increased collagen turnover is operative on the parallel arrays of ligaments. The disorganization of the fibers is again secondary to the lack of the organizing signals usually provided by normal mechanical events. Because the stiffness properties of normal ligaments result from the highly ordered arrays, any loss in the orderly parallel pattern will produce a less stiff structure. Simultaneously, bone resorption at the ligament insertion site greatly weakens that structure, so that the ligament is in double jeopardy. It becomes structurally weaker both within its substance *and* at its point of attachment.

It is clear that the influences of stress deprivation are profound and wide-ranging and that the clinical concepts of early motion are well founded in what is at present known about normal joint physiology and mechanics. Time does not permit a thorough review of the effects of exercise and rehabilitation on articular fractures. However, three points are of such importance as to deserve summary mention.

## Exercise Effects

Exercise effects on joint supporting structures are detected in animal models in which the exercise activity is sufficient to increase cardiac output. In an exercising swine model, our laboratory demonstrated an increase in flexor and extensor tendon structural properties. The effect, however, was small (about 10%) and a full year was required to develop a significant increase. Hence, the available evidence supports the concept that hypertrophy of fibrous connective tissue can occur, but requires a large expenditure of effort and a long period of time to achieve a small increment of change.

## Tendon Healing

Salter and colleagues (1980) pioneered the concept of cartilage healing enhanced by continuous passive motion (CPM). Superior repair of small drill-hole defects in rabbit femoral condyles was obtained in animals exposed to CPM. In our laboratory at UCSD, Gelberman and co-workers (1980) have demonstrated significant benefits also in flexor tendon healing by the expedient of controlled intermittent passive motion in the early postoperative period. However, only brief periods of passive motion were used as compared to CPM for fear of rupture of the suture line. In the model chosen (a laceration of tendon with the flexor tendon sheath, the so-called "no-man's land"), controlled intermittent passive motion inhibited ingrowth of granulation tissue from the tendon sheath. Furthermore, intrinsic healing was stimulated to such an extent that the rate and strength of healing in the motion group far exceeded that of the immobilized group. Intrinsic healing was achieved more rapidly with greater strength as well as greater tendon and joint mobility. These were clear bonuses for the controlled intermittent passive motion group. Efforts at several research labs are underway on ligament healing under conditions of passive motion and preliminary results are similarly encouraging.

## Rehabilitation

Rehabilitation of stress-deprived connective tissue appears to be a slow process (Fig. 1.10). The data points on the recovery curve were derived from the limited literature available. Noyes and colleagues (1974) found that the primate knee immobilized 8 weeks had a loss in ultimate strength of the anterior cruciate ligament to about one-third of normal. One year later, ligament strength was still only 80% of normal on ultimate load testing of a bone ligament bone preparation. This created serious conceptual problems in the rehabilitation of joints following a period of cast treatment. It seemed as if the recovery curve of ligament strength was much slower than the onset of the changes (an abrupt deterioration slope).

Since that time, Savio Woo and colleagues working in our lab at UCSD have made an important observation on this process. Using video dimension analysis, preliminary data suggest that recovery of mechanical and structural properties of ligament in a canine knee experimental model immobilized for 9 to 12 weeks occurs within about 12 weeks. However, the ligament insertion site weakness persists. Therefore, the structural failure of the model is as Noyes and associates described for the primates with incomplete recovery at 1 year. The difference is that with more sophisticated testing, these properties recover in a nonuniform process. The structural weakness of the ligament insertion site is more vulnerable, at least in the experimental model, so that the recovery curve must be divided into two events: (1) ligament substance events requiring weeks for recovery and (2) ligament insertion site events requiring months for recovery. Unfortunately, if this analysis holds, the bottom line remains the

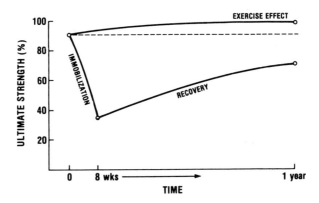

**Figure 1.10.** Schematic representation of ultimate strength of connective tissue (% of maximum) as decreased by immobilization and partially restored with subsequent recovery, and separately, as increased by exercise to a maximal level. Note qualitative patterns of deviation from normal (*dashed line*) and periods of time involved.

same with respect to the difficulty of reestablishing prior conditions after a period of cast immobilization. The chain is only as strong as the weakest link and for practical terms, whether the vulnerable point is ligament substance or insertion site, the implications for rehabilitation programs are the same.

This problem is clearly important with respect to potential clinical applications and implications. This area invites more work because the information base is much too sparse and generalizations must be drawn on this limited data base. The NIH Musculoskeletal Diseases Program Analysis Task Force recommends that priority be given to work in this area in the coming decade–a hopeful sign for young investigators interested in orthopedic research.

## Stress Effects on Muscle and Nerve

### Adaptations to Low and Moderate States of Stress

Observed changes in mass and fiber size with altered activity are well-documented for skeletal muscle of animals and humans (Booth, 1977; Saltin and Gollnick, 1983). Most studies agree that as opposed to affecting muscle fiber, reduced and increased activity levels primarily decrease and increase, respectively, the cross-sectional area of fibers. The great adaptability of skeletal muscle to environmental perturbations (chronic exercise, chronic electrical stimulation, cross-innervation, denervation, immobilization, mechanical overload, reinnervation, motor neuron lesion, and tenotomy) are well known (Pette, 1980; Saltin and Gollnick, 1983) and space limitations prevent an examination of this immense body of knowledge. However, it should be mentioned that muscles are not completely "plastic" in that fiber composition within a muscle of a given individual is genetically determined so that, for example, long-distance elite runners and cross-country skiers have predominantly slow-twitch fibers in their leg muscles. Research concerning muscle adaptations to activity and electrical stimulation is gaining greater emphasis today among investigators of exercise physiology, gravitation physiology, sports medicine and rehabilitation medicine. For example, recent results concerning intramuscular pressure distribution during contraction (Chapter 13) and possible mechanisms of lymph transport in skeletal muscle (Chapter 12) are examined in this book. Relatively little is known of the effects of low and moderate stress on the physiology and function of nerves, although there does appear to be some effect (Herbison et al., 1980).

### Responses to High States of Stress

Muscle and nerve tissues are particularly susceptible to pressure-induced ischemia and degeneration. For example, trauma or prolonged compression may swell muscles and increase tissue pressure in compartments that are confined in noncomplaint osseofascial boundaries (Hargens et al., 1984). If the muscle tamponade is sufficiently severe to cause ischemia in the affected muscle compartment, a compartment syndrome exists. Emergency decompression is usually performed by fasciotomy to prevent Volkmann's contracture. Nerve entrapment syndromes, for example, carpal tunnel syndrome, and "mini-compartment syndromes" are well-documented phenomena that cause pain and loss of function in nerves of the back, hand and foot (see Chapters 7 and 8). Similarly, compression of skin and subcutaneous tissues may induce pressure sores (Chapter 11).

## Healing of Muscle and Nerve

The capacity of myoneural tissues to regenerate and heal is poorly appreciated. Fiber degeneration and regeneration continuously occur in muscle exposed to exercise (Carlson, 1973; Allbrook, 1981). Historically, orthopedic practice has emphasized management of bone fractures with only limited consideration of treatment regimens to maintain soft tissue integrity and function. However, gathering evidence indicates that early motion and possibly electrical stimulation of the injured musculoskeletal unit are desirable to optimize recovery.

Recent knowledge and technical advances provide important insights into promoting myoneural regeneration. Often, neurotic muscle fibers are the loci of viable myoblastic cells, and therefore massive debridement of apparently nonviable tissue may be counterproductive (Allbrook, 1981). Advances in microsurgical techniques with replants and autogenous implants allow restitution of normal function after loss of entire muscles. Exposure of injured tissue to hyperbaric oxygen may be important for maintaining muscle viability and promoting regeneration (see Chapter 14). Connective tissue within a regenerating muscle may require longitudinal tension to regain normal function. Finally, new techniques for promoting nerve growth factors and anastomoses are developing rapidly and show great future potential (Lundborg, in press).

## Summary

Much emphasis is now placed on strategies for improving healing and maintaining viability of tissue. It is apparent that transport of metabolites to and from cells is an important rate-limiting step that sometimes depends on stressed-induced, convective flows of tissue fluid. Certainly there's abundant evidence that periodic, moderate stress (exercise, continuous passive motion, intermittent passive motion, electrical stimulation) improves tissue nutrition, viability and healing. The present chapter as well as others concerning cartilage, intervertebral disc, bone, nerve, skin, and skeletal muscle in this book provide strong evidence of stress effects on tissue physiology. Presumably, there is an important adaptation and dependence of load-bearing and motion-producing tissues on moderate stress in evolutionary terms. Thus, investigators of tissue nutrition and function should consider the fact that tissues are usually not stationary even during sleep and that anesthetized, immobilized animals may be poor experimental subjects in some instances. Whenever possible, one should try to maintain normal periodic motion of the tissue during experiments in which function depends on motion. However, too much pressure or stress is detrimental to tissue transport as well as integrity and viability (cartilage tears, fractures, nerve compression, disc degeneration, muscle compression, decubitus ulcer). New treatment modalities such as continuous passive motion, electrical stimulation and hyperbaric oxygen will play important roles for improving nutrition and viability of tissue in the future. Intelligent application of the fundamental relationship between physical forces and tissue health will improve rehabilitation techniques for the injured and disabled.

## Acknowledgments

These studies were supported by the Veterans Administration and by USPHS/NIH grants AM-25501, AM-26344, AM-14918 and a Research Career Development Award to ARH (AM-00602).

## References

Akeson WH, Amiel D and Woo SL-Y (1980). Immobility effects on synovial joints: the pathomechanics of joint contracture. *Biorheology* 17:95–110.

Akeson WH, Frank CB, Amiel D and Woo SL-Y (1985). Ligament biology and biomechanics. In: *Symposium on Sports Medicine, The Knee,* G Finerman, (ed.). St. Louis: Mosby, pp. 111–151.

Allbrook D (1981). Skeletal muscle regeneration. *Muscle Nerve* 4:234–245.

Amiel D, Akeson WH, Harwood FL and Frank CB (1983). Stress deprivation effect on metabolic turnover of the medial collateral ligament collagen: a comparison between nine and 12 week immobilization. *Clin Orthop* 172:265–270.

Amiel D, Woo SL-Y, Harwood F and Akeson WH (1982). The effect of immobilization on collagen turnover in connective tissue: a biochemical-biomechanical correlation. *Acta Orthop Scand* 53:325–332.

Aukland K and Nicolaysen G (1981). Interstitial fluid volume: local regulatory mechanisms. *Physiol Rev* 61:556–643.

Booth FW (1977). Time course of muscle atrophy during immobilization of hindlimbs in rats. *J Appl Physiol: Respir Environ Exercise Physiol* 43:656–661.

Booth FW and Gollnick PD (1983). Effects of disuse on the structure and function of skeletal muscle. *Med Sci Sports Exerc* 15:415–420.

Brickley-Parsons D and Glimcher M (1984). Is the chemistry of collagen in intervertebral discs an expression of Wolff's Law? A study of the human lumbar
spine. *Spine* 9:148–163.
Carlson BM (1973). The regeneration of skeletal muscle—a review. *Am J Anat*
137:119–150.
Carmen PC (1937). Fluid low through granular beds. *Trans Inst Chem Eng Lond*
15:150–166.
Casley-Smith JR and Vincent AH (1978). The quantitative morphology of intersti-
tial channels in some tissues of the rat and rabbit. *Tissue Cell* 10:571–584.
Comper WD (1984). Interstitium. In: *Edema*, NC Staub and AE Taylor (eds.).
New York: Raven Press, pp. 229–262.
Comper WD and Laurent TC (1978). Physiological function of connective tissue
polysaccharides. *Physiol Rev* 58:255–315.
Curry F-RE (1984). Mechanics and thermodynamics of transcapillary exchange.
In: *Handbook of Physiology, IV. Microcirculation*, EM Renkin and CC Michel
(eds.), Bethesda, MD: American Physiological Society, pp. 309–374.
Enneking WF and Horowitz M (1972). The intra-articular effects of immobiliza-
tion on the human knee. *J Bone Joint Surg* 54A:973–985.
Evans EB, Eggers GWN, Butler JK and Blumel J (1960). Experimental immobilization and remobilization of rat knee joints. *J Bone Joint Surg* 42A:737–758.
Frank C, Akeson WH, Woo SL-Y, Amiel D and Coutts RD (1984). Physiology
and therapeutic value of passive joint motion. *Clin Orthop* 185:113–125.
Fraser JRE, Laurent TC, Pertoft H and Baxter E (1981). Plasma clearance, tissue
distribution and metabolism of hyaluronic acid injected intravenously in the
rabbit. *Biochem J* 200:415–424.
Gelberman RH, Amiel D, Gonsalves M, Woo SL-Y and Akeson WH (1981). The
influence of protected passive mobilization on the healing of flexor tendons: a
biochemical and microangiographic study. *Hand* 13:120–128.
Gelberman RH and Manske PR (1985). Flexor tendon repair. Kappa Delta Award
Paper, 52nd Annual Meeting, American Academy of Orthopaedic Surgeons, p.
32, J Orthop Res, in press.
Gelberman RH, Menon J, Gonsalves M and Akeson WH (1980). The effects of
mobilization on the vascularization of healing flexor tendons in dogs. *Clin
Orthop* 153:283–289.
Granger HJ (1981). Physiochemical properties of the extracellular matrix. In:
*Tissue Fluid Pressure and Composition*, AR Hargens (ed.). Baltimore: Wil-
liams and Wilkins, pp. 43–61.
Granger HJ, Dhar J and Chen HI (1975). Structure and function of the intersti-
tium. In: *Proceedings of the NIH Symposium on Albumin*, JT Sgouris and A
Rene (eds.). Bethesda: NIH, pp. 114–124.
Hargens AR (1981). Interstitial osmotic pressure associated with Donnan equilib-
ria. In: *Tissue Fluid Pressure and Composition*, AR Hargens (ed.). Baltimore:
Williams and Wilkins, pp. 77–85.
Hargens AR (1986). Interstitial fluid pressure and lymph flow. In: *Handbook of
Bioengineering*, R Skalak and S Chien (eds.). New York: McGraw-Hill, in
press.
Hargens AR, Akeson WH, Garfin SR, Gelberman RH and Gershuni DH (1984).
Compartment syndromes. In: *Practice of Surgery*, J. Denton (ed.) Philadelphia:
Lippincott, V. 1, Ch. 7, pp. 1–18.

Herbison GJ, Jaweed MM and Ditunno JF (1980). Effect of activity and inactivity on reinnervating rat skeletal muscle contractility. *Exp Neurol* 70:498–506.

Holm S and Nachemson A (1983). Variations in the nutrition of the canine intervertebral disc induced by motion. *Spine* 8:866–874.

Johnson JA and Bloom G (1981). Permeability and reflection coefficients from osmotic transients—extravascular factors. *Microvasc Res* 22:80–92.

Katz MA (1980). Interstitial space—the forgotten organ. *Med Hypotheses* 6:885–898.

Kedem O and Katchalsky A (1958). Thermodynamic analysis of the permeability of biological membranes to non-electrolytes. *Biochim Biophys Acta* 27:229–246.

Kedem O and Katchalsky A (1961). A physical interpretation of the phenomenological coefficients of membrane permeability. *J Gen Physiol* 45:143–179.

Laros GS, Tipton CM and Cooper RR (1971). Influence of physical activity on ligament insertions in the knees of dogs. *J Bone Joint Surg* 53A:275–286.

Laurent TC (1970). The structure and function of the intercellular polysaccharides in connective tissues. In: *Capillary Permeability,* C Crone and NA Lassen (eds.). Copenhagen: Munksgaard, pp. 261–277.

Laurent TC (1972). The ultrastructure and physical-chemical properties of interstitial connective tissue. In: *Capillary Exchange and the Interstitial Space,* OH Gauer et al. (eds.). *Pflügers Arch* 336 (Suppl): 21–42.

Laurent UBG and Laurent TC (1981). On the origin of hyaluronate in blood. *Biochem Int* 2:195–199.

Laurent TC and Ogston AG (1963). The interaction between polysaccharides and other macromolecules, 4. The osmotic pressure of mixtures of serum albumin and hyaluronic acid. *Biochem J* 89:249–253.

Levick JR (1984). Blood flow and mass transport in synovial joints. In: *Handbook of Physiology, IV. Microcirculation,* EM Renkin and CC Michel (eds.). Bethesda, MD: American Physiological Society, pp. 917–947.

Lundborg G (1986). *Nerve Injury and Repair.* London: Churchill Livingstone, (in press).

Merker HJ and Günther T (1972). Morphologic observations. In: *Capillary Exchange and the Interstitial Space,* OH Gauer et al. (eds.). *Pflügers Arch* 336: (Suppl) 33–34.

Meyer FA and Silberberg A (1974). *In vitro* study of the influence of some factors important for any physicochemical characterization of loose connective tissue in the microcirculation. *Microvasc Res* 8:263–273.

Mow VC, Holmes MH and Lai WM (1984). Fluid transport and mechanical properties of articular cartilage: a review. *J Biomechanics* 17:377–394.

Noyes FR, Torvik PJ, Hyde WB and DeLucas JL (1974). Biomechanics of ligament failure. II. An analysis of immobilization, exercise, and reconditioning effects in primates. *J Bone Joint Surg* 56A:1406–1418.

O'Driscoll SW, Kumar A and Salter RB (1983). The effect of continuous passive motion on the clearance of a hemarthrosis from a synovial joint: an experimental investigation in the rabbit. *Clin Orthop* 176:305–310.

Ogston AG and Phelps CF (1961). The partition of solutes between buffer solutions containing hyaluronic acid. *Biochem J* 78:827–833.

Ogston AG and Sherman TF (1961). Effects of hyaluronic acid upon diffusion of solutes and flow of solvent. *J Physiol Lond* 156:67–74.

Ogston AG, Preston BN and Wells JD (1973). On the transport of compact particles through solutions of chain polymers. *Proc R Soc (Lond) Ser A* 333:297–316.

Pette D (1980). *Plasticity of Muscle*. New York: de Gruyter.

Preston BN, Laurent TC., Comper WD and Checkley GJ (1980). Rapid polymer transport in concentrated solutions through the formation of ordered structures. *Nature* 287:499–503.

Salter RB and Field P (1960). The effects of continuous compression on living articular cartilage: an experimental investigation. *J Bone Joint Surg* 42A:31–49.

Salter RB, Simmonds DF, Malcolm BW, Rumble EJ, MacMichael D and Clements ND (1980). The biological effect of continuous passive motion on the healing of full-thickness defects in articular cartilage. *J Bone Joint Surg* 62A:1232–1251.

Saltin B and Gollnick PD (1983). Skeletal muscle adaptability: significance for metabolism and performance. In: *Handbook of Physiology Section 10: Skeletal Muscle*. Bethesda, MD: American Physiological Society, pp. 555–631.

Silberberg A (1982). The mechanics and thermodynamics of separation flow through porous molecularly disperse, solid media—the Poiseuille Lecture 1981: *Biorheology* 19:111–127.

Thaxter TH, Mann RA and Anderson CE (1965). Degeneration of immobilized knee joints in rats: histological and autoradiographic study. *J Bone Joint Surg* 47A:567–585.

Tipton CM, Matthes RD, Maynard JA and Carey RA (1975). The influence of physical activity on ligament and tendons. *Med Sci Sports* 7:165–175.

Trias A (1961). Effect of persistent pressure on the articular cartilage: an experimental study. *J Bone Joint Surg* 43B:376–386.

Urban JPG, Holm S, Maroudas A and Nachemson A (1982). Nutrition of the intervertebral disc: effect of fluid flow in solute transport. *Clin Orthop* 170:296–302.

Wiederhielm CA (1969). The interstitial space and lymphatic pressures in the bat wing. In: *The Pulmonary Circulation and Interstitial Space*, AP Fishman and HH Hecht (eds.), Chicago, IL: University of Chicago Press, pp. 29–41.

Wolff J (1892). *Das Gesetz der Transformation der Knochen*. Berlin: Quarto.

Woo SL-Y, Kuei SC, Amiel D, Gomez MA, Hayes WC, White FC and Akeson WH (1981). The effect of prolonged physical training on the properties of long bone: a study of Wolff's Law. *J Bone Joint Surg* 63A:780–787.

Woo SL-Y, Matthews JV, Akeson WH, Amiel D and Convery FR (1975). Connective tissue response to immobility: correlative study of biomechanical measurements of normal and immobilized rabbit knees. *Arthritis Rheum* 18:257–264.

CHAPTER 2

# Distribution and Transport of Fluid as Related to Tissue Structure

Frank A. Meyer

## Introduction

Because there is continuous exchange of fluid between the interstitial space and the vascular compartments (blood and lymph), the distribution and flow of fluid in the interstitium can generally be maintained within narrow limits (Granger and Shepherd, 1979; Silberberg, 1979; Wiederhielm, 1979; Zweifach and Silberberg, 1979). Control so exercised serves to stabilize tissue volume (largely determined by its water content) and to maintain a physicochemically stable environment in which cells can function normally. The conditions that arise are part of the steady state that exists in tissue in contact with the circulation of blood and lymph.

The fluid involved in this exchange (the interstitial fluid) can be regarded as composed essentially of two distinguishable components, the dissolved proteins and the support fluid which I will call "water." "Water" refers to all the low-molecular-weight components that cross the endothelial wall in a nonselective fashion and in addition to water also include salts and low-molecular-weight metabolites. The dissolved proteins are diffusible macromolecular components, mainly albumin, and are representative of the plasma proteins selectively filtered through the endothelial wall. This major difference with respect to the capillary wall makes it necessary to consider these two classes separately. In the case of "water," steady-state conditions are achieved by a balance between filtration from capillary blood into tissue on the arterial side and a return flow either by reabsorption on the venous side or by drainage via the lymphatics. Protein flux, on the other hand, is from blood into interstitium with a return flow via lymph. The chemical potential gradient for "water" is produced by gradients of hydrostatic and osmotic pressures and that for protein is produced by gradients of hydrostatic pressure and protein concentration (activity). In the interstitium there are practically no measurable gradients for "water" and protein (Zweifach and Silberberg, 1979), and in steady state their chemical potentials are those required for the normal physiological functions of the tissue. The structure of tissue, therefore, must selectively adjust these chemical potentials and establish the appropriate gradients with blood and lymph.

This chapter discusses tissue composition and features of tissue structure that determine the chemical potential of "water" along with the activity and diffusion of protein in the interstitium. It is based on previous studies (Meyer and Silberberg, 1974, 1976; Klein and Meyer, 1983; Meyer, 1983; Meyer et al., 1983) in which the composition and arrangement of interstitial space and the effect of removal of specific structural components on tissue properties were investigated. Experiments involve mostly human umbilical cord which is largely composed of a relatively simple loose connective tissue, the Wharton's jelly.

## Tissue Structure

The structure of Wharton's jelly (Meyer et al., 1983) is probably similar to that of other stromal connective tissues. Wharton's jelly contains soluble open-coil polysaccharides, held within an insoluble three-dimensional fibrillar network system that consists of collagen fibrils and some glycoprotein microfibrils (Table 2.1). The soluble polysaccharides are mainly hyaluronic acid together with some proteoglycans. Elastin is not found in the tissue.

The fibrillar network within a tissue slice can be freed quantitatively from the polysaccharides by prior digestion with hyaluronidase (Fig. 2.1A). The collagen fibrils are banded and have an average diameter of $39 \pm 6$ nm whereas the glycoprotein microfibrils have a nonbanded, thinner and beaded appearance. Subsequent treatment of the tissue slice with collagenase quantitatively removes collagen and leaves behind the microfibrils which are mostly 13 nm in diameter (Fig. 2.1B). The tissue at this stage becomes translucent and fragile, but remains physically intact, indicating that the microfibrils are present as a separate network. The collagen fibrils are also present as a network, as break-up of the glycoprotein

**Table 2.1.** Structural components and their amounts (means $\pm$ SD) in Wharton's jelly

|  | Relative weight (g/g collagen) |
| --- | --- |
| Insoluble fibril network phase |  |
|   Collagen | 1.00 |
|   Glycoprotein microfibrils | $0.08 \pm 0.01$ |
| Interfibrillar soluble phase |  |
|   Hyaluronic acid | $0.105 \pm 0.009$ |
|   Proteoglycans | $0.045 \pm 0.004$ |

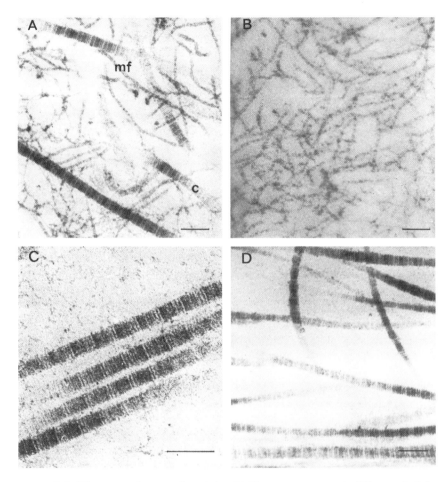

**Figure 2.1.** Electron micrographs of the fibrillar components in Wharton's jelly after removal of polysaccharides with testicular hyaluronidase. **A:** The fibrillar components include collagen fibrils (c) and glycoprotein microfibrils (mf). **B:** Glycoprotein microfibril network after removal of collagen by exhaustive digestion with bacterial collagenase. **C:** Break-up of the microfibrillar network on limited protease digestion with trypsin. **D:** Collagen network left behind after extensive digestion of the microfibril network with Pronase. Each bar indicates 100 nm. (From FA Meyer et al., 1983.)

microfibrillar system by proteases (e.g., trypsin or Pronase) instead of collagenase does not visibly affect the integrity of the tissue slice (Fig. 2.1C and D). The action of proteases on the fibrillar network is selective. There is no release of collagen from the preparation as judged by hydroxyproline analysis, and the collagen fibrils appear unaffected ultrastructurally (Fig. 2.1C and D). The insoluble fibrillar network of tissue, therefore, involves two independent mutually interpenetrated networks. Available evidence (discussed later) indicates that these networks are coupled mechanically such that the collagen network is under a constraint imposed by the glycoprotein microfibrillar network.

The nature and organization of the soluble polysaccharides in tissue has been studied in some detail in the case of hyaluronic acid, the major polysaccharide in Wharton's jelly (Klein and Meyer, 1983). Hyaluronic acid is not chemically linked within tissue, as it can be readily extracted on physical disruption of the fibrillar network (Fessler, 1960). Hyaluronic acid, obtained by extraction of finely milled frozen tissue with a physiological buffer, has a high molecular weight of approximately $15 \times 10^6$ atomic mass units and a coil diameter of about 600 nm (Klein and Meyer, 1983). In its random coil configuration each molecule encompasses a volume so large that at normal tissue concentrations, individual molecular coils of hyaluronic acid interpenetrate each other and form a fine meshwork (Comper and Laurent, 1978). On the other hand, the molecular characteristics of proteoglycan in Wharton's jelly are not known. Proteoglycans from other tissues, however, have a lower molecular weight than hyaluronic acid (Comper and Laurent, 1978). They are highly branched (glycosaminoglycan chains are linked to a protein backbone in a "bottle brush" structure) (Mathews and Lozaitye, 1958) and their molecular structure is more compact than the linear chain hyaluronic acid molecule.

How effectively hyaluronic acid is held within tissue is indicated in studies (Klein and Meyer, 1983) in which structural modification of tissue affects the elution rate of endogenous hyaluronic acid (Fig. 2.2). Elution is monitored from thin tissue slices maintained at their in vivo volume and shape. The elution obeys Fick's diffusion kinetics. The diffusion of hyaluronic acid through intact tissue is approximately two orders of magnitude lower than that in free solution. This reduction may be compared with the approximately one order of magnitude decrease in diffusion rate through a collagen network alone. In the latter case, hyaluronic acid elution is monitored from tissue slices that have been protease-digested by trypsin. In addition to degrading the glycoprotein microfibril network, such treatment breaks up proteoglycans by digesting their protein core. This removes proteoglycans from the tissue. Hyaluronic acid, on the other hand, is unaffected by proteases and remains behind in the collagen fibril network. Hyaluronic acid is thus held in tissue both by the collagen network and by the microfibrillar network and/or proteoglycans.

Reduced mobility of hyaluronic acid in a collagen network of protease-treated tissue can be attributed largely to entanglement of the flexible hyaluronic acid molecular coils with the fixed fibril network (Klein and Meyer, 1983). The coil diameter of hyaluronic acid is about three times larger than the mean pore size of the collagen network (estimated from molecular exclusion studies). Translational movement is, therefore, re-

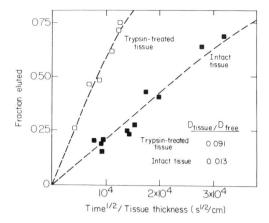

**Figure 2.2.** Fraction of hyaluronic acid eluted as a function of time from intact tissue and from trypsin-treated tissue. The data points are used to calculate diffusion coefficients ($D_{tissue}$) from which theoretical elution profiles for Fick's diffusion (*dashed lines*) are generated. $D_{tissue}$ is expressed relative to the diffusion coefficient of hyaluronic acid in free solution ($D_{free}$). (From J Klein and FA Meyer, 1983.)

stricted to reptational motion (De Gennes, 1971) which involves the flexible hyaluronic acid molecular chain threading its way through the network. Calculations of the reduced mobility expected for this type of movement (based on the flexibility and size of the hyaluronic acid molecule and the pore size of the collagen network) agree quantitatively with the experimental result. For intact tissue a similar calculation (based on the effective pore size of the network system as reduced by the additional presence of glycoprotein microfibrils) indicates that mobility should be reduced only by a factor of about 20 relative to its free diffusion value. Since the mobility of hyaluronic acid in intact tissue is reduced by a factor of 77 (Fig. 2.2), other effects in addition to entanglement must be involved. These effects may involve chemical (secondary bond) interactions between hyaluronic acid and perhaps the proteoglycan present in the intact tissue. Such binding between hyaluronic acid and proteoglycan may form a larger branched complex that is more restricted in its passage through the fibrillar network system. Such complexes are reported in cartilaginous tissues (Hardingham and Muir, 1972; Hascall, 1977) and may also occur in loose connective tissues (Gardell et al., 1980). Indeed, preliminary experiments indicate that the rate of elution of proteoglycan from umbilical cord slices is comparable to that of hyaluronic acid (unpublished results), suggesting that these polysaccharides are present in the tissue as a complex. The relatively small size of the proteoglycan precludes significant entanglement effects with other components, and thus,

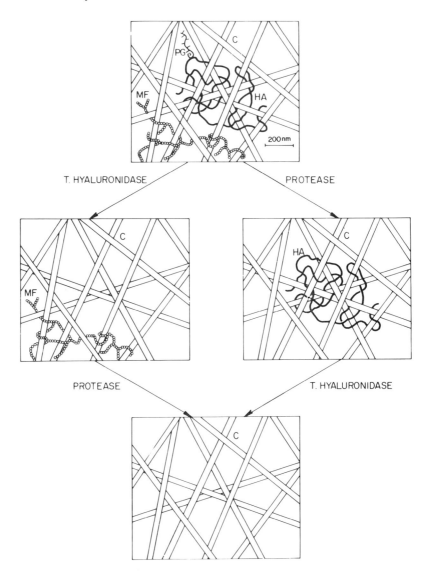

**Figure 2.3.** Schematic illustration (approximately to scale) of intact tissue structure modified by treatment either with testicular hyaluronidase or protease, or in combination. The components indicated are collagen (C), glycoprotein microfibrils (MF), hyaluronic acid (HA) and proteoglycan (PG). For clarity, only part of the microfibril network and a single polysaccharide molecule are shown.

an energetic interaction that ties proteoglycan to hyaluronic acid is strongly suggested.

These intact and enzymatically modified tissues (Fig. 2.3) are used to investigate the respective contributions of the structural components to the physicochemical behavior of tissue. These contributions are described in the following sections.

## Protein Activity and Steric Exclusion

The structural components of tissue will influence the activity of plasma proteins dispersed in it. For steric reasons macromolecular solutes will be excluded from domains of the matrix occupied by tissue components and from spaces whose dimensions are smaller than that of the macromolecule (Ogston, 1958; Laurent, 1964; Maroudas, 1975; Wiederhielm and Black, 1976; Granger, 1981; Bert et al., 1982). The volume excluded is a function of macromolecular size, as with increasing size there will be fewer holes available in the meshwork to accommodate the macromolecule. As a result of exclusion, the available volume within which the macromolecules can distribute is reduced and their effective concentration and hence activity is increased.

The structural basis of exclusion by tissue has been investigated using compact globular macromolecules comparable in shape and size to the major plasma proteins. Exclusion is measured in tissue slices, maintained at their in vivo volume, by incubation in solutions containing the molecules whose exclusion behavior are under investigation. At equilibrium the concentration of the molecule in tissue and in the external solution is determined either by considering material balance or by using radioactively labeled molecules. The ratio of these concentrations gives the partition coefficient $K$, which is $<1$ if the molecules are noninteracting. In this case $K$ is related to the excluded volume fraction $V_{exc}/V_T$ by:

$$K = V_{av}/V_T = 1 - V_{exc}/V_T, \tag{1}$$

where $V_{av}$ and $V_{exc}$ are available and excluded volumes for the molecule in the tissue, respectively, and $V_T$ is total tissue volume.

The exclusion behavior of intact and hyaluronidase-treated tissue for spherical molecules is a function of their hydrodynamic radius, $r_s$ (Fig. 2.4). The molecules studied include: sorbitol ($r_s = 0.36$ nm), the plasma protein albumin ($r_s = 3.55$ nm) and globular proteins up to $r_s = 8.17$ nm. In the case of the hyaluronidase-treated tissue, larger open-coil dextran molecules are also used (Meyer et al., 1977; Meyer, 1983). Since these molecules have diameters less than or comparable with that of the excluding elements, mutual interpenetration will not occur and the dextran coils are expected to behave as hard spheres with respect to the fibrillar network system in the hyaluronidase-treated tissue case. This expectation is borne

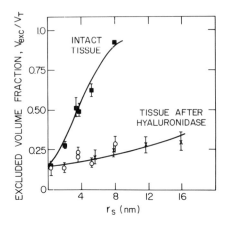

**Figure 2.4.** Excluded volume fraction ($\pm$ SD) in intact and hyaluronidase-treated tissues for spherical molecules of hydrodynamic radius, $r_s$. both compact ($\blacksquare$, $\bigcirc$) and open-coil (x) molecules are used. The former are sorbitol ($r_s = 0.36$ nm), myoglobin ($r_s = 1.98$ nm), albumin ($r_s = 3.55$ nm), transferrin ($r_s = 3.82$ nm), catalase ($r_s = 5.20$ nm) and thyroglobulin ($r_s = 8.17$ nm) whereas the latter are dextran fractions having $r_s$ values of 8.0 nm, 11.7 nm and 16.0 nm. (Redrawn from FA Meyer, 1983.)

out by the comparable exclusion behavior found for dextrans and globular proteins of similar radii (Fig. 2.4). Exclusion is produced both by polysaccharides (the difference between the intact and hyaluronidase-treated tissues) and by insoluble components of the tissue (Fig. 2.4). The relative contribution of each is dependent on solute molecular size. With increasing solute size, exclusion by the polysaccharides rapidly becomes dominant such that the largest protein tested (thyroglobulin) is almost completely excluded by the tissue.

Steric exclusion is due partly to the actual volume occupied by the tissue elements and partly to the surrounding domain of closest approach of the center of mass of the spherical molecule to the surface of the excluding element. The relative contribution of the latter becomes very important if the radius of the spherical molecule is large compared to the radius of the excluding element. However, as the size of the spherical molecule increases, excluded regions are likely to overlap wherever the excluding elements are closely spaced. This produces an excluded volume that is less than that for widely spaced excluding elements. These concepts form the basis of the relation derived by Ogston (1958) for the exclusion of hard spherical molecules by a random network of fibers:

$$V_{exc}/V_T = 1 - e^{-cv(1 + r_s/r_f)^2}, \qquad (2)$$

where $c$ is the concentration of network fibers, $v$ is the self-volume of the fibers and $r_f$ is the fiber radius. Since collagen and the glycoprotein microfibrils are present in tissue as fibrillar networks, the Ogston relation describes their exclusion behavior. This relation also applies to exclusion by polysaccharides, as exclusion by hyaluronic acid solutions, for example (Laurent, 1964), is accounted for if the entangled hyaluronic acid coils are regarded as a random meshwork of fibrils of molecular chain dimensions $r_f = 0.35$ nm with a self-volume per gram given by the partial specific volume of hyaluronic acid.

Exclusion by the various macromolecules in tissue is, therefore, calculated using the Ogston equation and compared with experimentally derived exclusion data. In such calculations we assume that exclusion by the polysaccharides is similar to that of a solution of hyaluronic acid at a concentration equivalent to that of the polysaccharides in tissue. Since polysaccharides are confined to the extrafibrillar, extracellular spaces of tissue, their exclusion effects occur in these regions and their concentration will be correspondingly higher than that estimated from total tissue volume. Exclusion by the collagen fibril network and by the glycoprotein microfibril network is calculated using the fibrillar radii found by electron microscopy ($r_f = 19.5$ nm and 6.5 nm, respectively), by their concentrations in tissue and by their self-volumes, assuming these to be 1.89 ml/g as found for collagen fibrils (Katz and Li, 1973; Meyer et al., 1977). In this instance, the self-volume of the fibrils differs from the partial specific volume because it also includes the inaccessible intrafibrillar voids that arise when polypeptide chains are organized into fibrillar structures.

Exclusion behavior predicted by the Ogston equation for the individual tissue components at the in vivo volume of tissue is shown (Fig. 2.5A). Also included in Figure 2.5A is the exclusion due to the presence of cells. Since their size is so large, exclusion by cells is essentially represented by the volume of cells (about 10% of the total tissue volume of human umbilical cord). Summation of the exclusion curves for the polysaccharides, collagen, microfibrils and cells and for collagen, microfibrils and cells gives the exclusion predicted for the intact and hyaluronidase-treated tissues, respectively (Fig. 2.5B). Comparison of these curves with the experimental exclusion data points (Fig. 2.5B) indicates that the latter lie reasonably well on the predicted curves. It is evident that albumin ($r_s = 3.65$ nm), the major plasma protein entering tissue, is influenced by exclusion, primarily by effects of the polysaccharides, although considerable exclusion effects by the fibrillar components and cells are also apparent. Other plasma proteins (which are larger than albumin) are excluded to a greater extent mainly due to the effect of the polysaccharides. The curves in Figure 2.5B are extrapolated to infer the upper size limit for molecular entry, and hence, effective pore size. In intact tissue, effective pore size is about 18 nm and is clearly determined by the polysaccharides. This pore size is much smaller than that estimated for the fibrillar network or collagen network, which are approximately 110 nm and 180 nm, respectively.

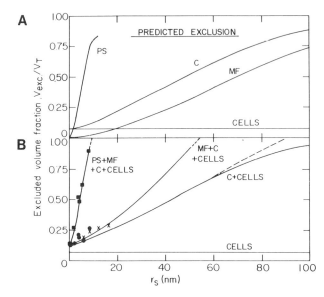

**Figure 2.5. A:** Exclusion predicted for spherical molecules by the individual components in umbilical cord tissue. **B:** Comparison of the exclusion determined experimentally (Fig. 2.4) for intact and hyaluronidase-treated tissues with that predicted by summation of the individual curves in (A). Exclusion relationships for polysaccharides (PS), collagen (C) and microfibrils (MF) were predicted from their respective concentrations in tissue and physical characteristics using Eq. (2). The *dashed line* extrapolations in (B) were used to obtain effective pore radii. (From FA Meyer, 1983.)

## Protein Diffusion

The influence of tissue structure on protein diffusion has been studied for albumin (Klein and Meyer, 1983). Diffusion was determined by monitoring elution from tissue slices preequilibrated with labeled albumin. Tissue slices were relatively thick so that only a small loss of polysaccharides (~6%) occurred during the course of the experiment. For intact tissue held close to the in vivo volume, the diffusion coefficient of albumin was reduced by some 30% as compared with its value in free solution (Table 2.2). The influence of tissue composition on this reduction was investigated by considering separately the effects of the fibrillar network and the polysaccharides on diffusion.

The effect of the fibrillar network system on the diffusion coefficient was studied by determining albumin diffusion through hyaluronidase-treated tissue. In this case $D_{tissue}/D_{free}$ is given by the available volume fraction for albumin. This result is expected for a simple two-phase model (Klein, 1977) where one phase (the network) consists of impenetrable, fixed obstacles whose separation distances and dimensions are large com-

**Table 2.2.** Percent reduction in protein diffusion ($\pm$ SD) relative to free diffusion $(1 - D_{\text{tissue}}/D_{\text{free}}) \times 100$, in intact tissue[a]

| Diffusant | Percent reduction predicted from tissue composition | | | Percent reduction from experiment |
| | Polysaccharide-free tissue matrix[b] | Tissue polysaccharides[c] | Intact tissue | |
|---|---|---|---|---|
| [125]I-Albumin | 16 $\pm$ 9 | 24 $\pm$ 2 | 40 $\pm$ 11 | 28 $\pm$ 4 |
| Endogenous diffusible proteins | 14 $\pm$ 6 | 27 $\pm$ 2 | 41 $\pm$ 8 | 45 $\pm$ 10 |

[a] From Klein and Meyer, 1983.
[b] From available volume fraction.
[c] From diffusion in polysaccharide solution (Ogston et al., 1973).

pared with the size of albumin, and the other (the interobstacle space) is a fluid in which albumin can freely diffuse.

The effect of polysaccharides on the diffusion coefficient is assessed by considering albumin diffusion in a solution of hyaluronic acid at a concentration equivalent to that of the polysaccharides in tissue. Replacing the polysaccharides by hyaluronic acid is justified since the rate of diffusion of albumin in solutions of hyaluronic acid is very similar to that in solutions of proteoglycan (Ogston et al., 1973).

The reduction in diffusion predicted for albumin and for endogenous diffusible proteins in tissue (represented essentially as a 4:1 mixture of albumin and $\gamma$-globulin), based on the above considerations, is compared with the experimental result for intact tissue close to its in vivo volume (Table 2.2). Semiquantitative estimates of $D_{\text{tissue}}/D_{\text{free}}$ predicted for tissue agree reasonably well with the measured values. Therefore, estimates based on a tissue model consisting of a network of well-separated impenetrable obstacles of large dimensions (compared to the diffusant) and polysaccharide components, agree well with values for the diffusional behavior of protein in tissue. The results also indicate that the reduction of diffusion is primarily caused by polysaccharides (approximately two-thirds of the reduction) as compared to the reduction by impenetrable matrix components (approximately one-third).

## "Water" Chemical Potential (Tissue Swelling Pressure)

Structural macromolecules may influence the chemical potential of "water" in tissue (and hence tissue swelling pressure) by osmotic forces produced by the effects of macromolecular solutes on "water" activity and/or by hydrostatic forces arising from structural components held in a state of strain.

The influence of the various structural components can be separated by using excised tissue (Meyer and Silberberg, 1974; Meyer, 1983; Meyer et al., 1983). Human umbilical cord slices placed in open contact with a physiological buffer (Ringer's solution or phosphate-buffered saline) will take up the buffer solution and swell to twice their in vivo volume (Fig. 2.6). Swelling is not dependent on the diffusible plasma proteins initially in the tissue, as they rapidly diffuse out and their concentration drops to near zero if the buffer volume is large. Polysaccharides, on the other hand, remain in the tissue, as their rate of diffusion is much lower than the rate of swelling. Therefore, swelling can be considered as an effect of the structural macromolecules on the chemical potential of "water" in tissue. Initially the chemical potential is less than that outside so that buffer flows into the tissue. As swelling proceeds, the chemical potential increases until at swelling equilibrium it is equal to that of the buffer.

The structural macromolecules primarily responsible for the chemical potential of "water" at the in vivo volume of tissue are the polysaccharides (Meyer and Silberberg, 1974; Meyer et al., 1983). Their removal by hyaluronidase leaves the tissue in equilibrium with buffer at its in vivo volume (Fig. 2.6), indicating that the chemical potential of buffer or "water" in the fibrillar network system at this volume is zero. Therefore, at the in vivo volume of tissue, the fibrillar system exerts neither a hydrostatic pressure affecting chemical potential nor, as expected in view of its small surface/bulk ratio, an osmotic pressure. Polysaccharides provide the driving force for the swelling of intact tissue seen in vitro by affecting the chemical potential of "water." As swelling proceeds, this driving force decreases due to dilution of the polysaccharides. At the same time elastic stresses that oppose swelling build-up in the network as fibrils untwist and straighten out. At swelling equilibrium both forces are equal and the net pressure of the tissue is that of the buffer. Once tissue has swelled to equilibrium, polysaccharide removal leaves the elastic stresses

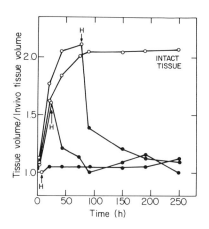

**Figure 2.6.** Time dependence of swelling in physiological buffer of intact tissue (O), and of tissue treated with hyaluronidase (H) at time zero and at two subsequent times during the experiment. (Redrawn from FA Meyer and A Silberberg, 1974.)

unopposed and these return the network to the configuration associated with zero stress. As was shown, this configuration is that of the tissue at its in vivo volume (Fig. 2.6). In this configuration, the network is in a thermodynamic state of minimum energy. An elastic return to this configuration also occurs when partially swollen tissue is treated with hyaluronidase (Fig. 2.6).

The above findings suggest that the unstressed configuration of the fibrillar network system provides the basic skeletal shape and volume of tissue in vivo while the polysaccharides (together with the plasma proteins) adjust "water" chemical potential so that steady-state balance with blood and lymph is achieved. Polysaccharides are presumably synthesized in sufficient amounts so that the chemical potential of "water" matches a steady-state volume given by the zero-stress configuration of the fibrillar system. A similar functional division between the fibrillar network and the polysaccharides may apply to other tissues as well. This is suggested by the finding that the swelling pressures of heart valve tissue (Meyer, 1971), skin (Wiederhielm, 1981) and cartilages (Mathews and Decker, 1977; Maroudas and Bannon, 1981) are essentially accounted for by the molecularly disperse components. Therefore, in these cases as well, the latter components provide the change in chemical potential of "water," while the fibrillar system is essentially in its stress-free zero pressure configuration.

The minimum energy configuration of the fibrillar network in the case of Wharton's jelly is determined by an interaction between the interpenetrated networks of collagen fibrils and glycoprotein microfibrils in which the former is held in compression by the latter (Meyer et al., 1983). This conclusion is based on the swelling behavior of hyaluronidase-treated tissue in buffer after selective enzymic attack on the individual fibrillar networks (Fig. 2.7). Treatment with proteases breaks up the glycoprotein microfibril network and relieves constraint on the collagen network which now expands and adopts its zero stress configuration at approximately twice its volume in vivo (Fig. 2.7). On the other hand, if the collagen network instead of the microfibrillar network is subjected to digestion using collagenase, no swelling results. Collagenase solubilizes 46% of the collagen as judged by hydroxyproline released into the medium. The collagenase attack is uniform (since the enzyme is allowed to diffuse into tissue before commencement of digestion) and corresponds to the loss of the outer three molecular layers from the collagen fibrils. The decrease in fibril diameter lowers the stresses generated on bending and, therefore, collagenase digestion, if anything, causes shrinkage. The weakened elasticity of the collagen network may explain its diminished capability to expand after the microfibrillar constraint is removed (Fig. 2.7).

The zero stress configuration of the collagen fibrillar network, like that of the combined fibrillar network, is a thermodynamic minimum energy state, as the network will return to this configuration after forces causing

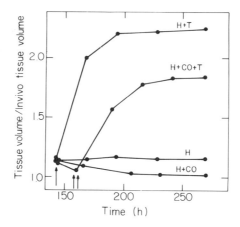

**Figure 2.7.** Time-dependent swelling in physiological buffer of hyaluronidase-digested tissue treated either singly with trypsin (T) or bacterial collagenase (CO) or in combination. Hyaluronidase (H) was added to all tissues at zero time. Addition of test enzyme is indicated by the single arrow and by the double arrow where a second test enzyme was employed. The effects of trypsin on swelling also occur after use of other proteases, for example chymotrypsin, elastase and Pronase. (From FA Meyer et al., 1983).

expansion or contraction are relieved. Thus, this configuration is obtained when the collagen network (expanded by hyaluronic acid after treatment with a protease to break up the microfibrils and proteoglycan) is treated with hyaluronidase, and when the compressed collagen network in tissue (after polysaccharide removal) is treated with a protease to remove the microfibrillar constraint (Fig. 2.8).

Interaction between the collagen and microfibril networks is probably physical rather than chemical in nature, because independent, interpenetrated networks with relatively bulky fibrils are involved. A physical interaction is also suggested by the findings with collagenase where interaction is little affected despite removal of the outer molecular layers of the collagen fibrils and hence disruption of any chemical links between interacting fibrillar surfaces.

Glycoprotein microfibrils constrain the collagen network in Wharton's jelly in a manner similar to that of elastin in other tissues (Karlinsky et al., 1976; Hoffman et al., 1977; Missirlis, 1977; Oakes and Bialkower, 1977). Indeed, elastin is, in general, intimately associated with the microfibrils (Ross and Bornstein, 1969). In tissues that function over an entire lifetime and not just for a short period as in the case of the umbilical cord and/or tissues subjected to considerable mechanical stress (for example, the intima and media of blood vessels), the role of the microfibrils is largely taken over by elastin. Indeed, the robust character and general inertness of elastin is better suited to the task in these cases, as compared with the

**Figure 2.8.** Time dependence of swelling in physiological buffer of tissue treated singly either with trypsin (T) or hyaluronidase (H) or in combination. In the latter case the *arrows* indicate when the second enzyme was added; the first enzyme was added at the outset of the experiment. (Redrawn from FA Meyer and A Silberberg, 1974.)

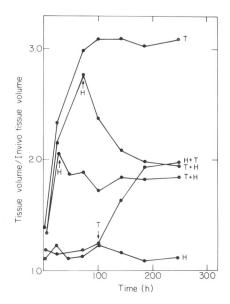

more delicate and labile structure of the microfibrils. Therefore, glycoprotein microfibrils, as part of the elastic fibers, influence tissue shape by affecting the collagen network. Moreover, their early synthesis during development allows the glycoprotein microfibrils to influence uniquely the organization of the elastin and collagen fibrils which appear only at a later stage (Robert et al., 1976).

The nature and magnitude of pressure generated by the polysaccharides have been investigated in experiments where tissue sections (freed of diffusible plasma proteins) were allowed to equilibrate by swelling or shrinking against an external pressure (Meyer, 1983). Shrinkage is provided by buffered solutions of hyaluronic acid of known concentration and osmotic pressure (Silpananta et al., 1968). Since buffer equilibration time is very much faster than the time required for outside hyaluronic acid to penetrate tissue or tissue polysaccharides to diffuse out, the osmotic pressure of the outside hyaluronic acid solution at swelling equilibrium is a measure of the swelling pressure of the tissue.

A plot of the polysaccharide concentration (in the extrafibrillar, extracellular space of tissue) against external hyaluronic acid concentration at swelling equilibrium is presented (Fig. 2.9). The arrow corresponds to the tissue volume where the fibers are at zero pressure (essentially the in vivo volume of tissue). At this point, therefore, the swelling pressure is due only to the polysaccharides. For the swelling pressure to be balanced by the osmotic pressure of the external hyaluronic acid solution, a concentration of hyaluronic acid 1.26 times higher than that of the tissue polysaccharide is required. This value is consistent with the osmotic activity

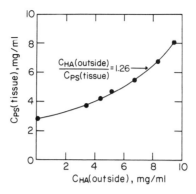

**Figure 2.9.** Plot of polysaccharide concentration $C_{PS}$ in the extrafibrillar, extracellular space of intact tissue against outside hyaluronic acid concentration $C_{HA}$ at swelling equilibrium. The *arrow* corresponds to the volume of tissue at which the overall fibrillar system is in its relaxed zero-stress configuration. (From FA Meyer, 1983.)

expected from the hyaluronic acid/proteoglycan mixture that constitutes the tissue polysaccharides. The osmotic pressures of hyaluronic acid and proteoglycan solutions are predominantly due to Donnan counter-ion effects (Comper and Preston, 1974; Brace and Guyton, 1979; Maroudas and Urban, 1980). For the concentrations involved in tissue, ideal Donnan behavior applies, as the fixed charge density of the polysaccharides (approximately 0.019 $M$) is very much smaller than the physiological microion concentration (approximately 0.15 $M$) of the buffer. Therefore, proteoglycan, which carries two charges per disaccharide, has an osmotic pressure approximately twice that of hyaluronic acid, which carries only one charge per disaccharide. Hence the osmotic pressure for the 70% hyaluronic acid/30% proteoglycan mixture of polysaccharides in tissue is equivalent to that of a hyaluronic acid solution at 1.30 times higher concentration, consistent with experimental findings. This result indicates that the polysaccharides influence swelling pressure essentially through their osmotic effects and, therefore, that polysaccharides affect "water" chemical potential in tissue by their influence on "water" activity.

By equilibrating intact and enzymatically modified tissues (after removal of diffusible plasma proteins) against hyaluronic acid solutions, swelling pressures as a function of tissue volume and macromolecular composition are obtained (Fig. 2.10). The results show that tissue swelling pressure over much of the volume range is negative and is due mainly to the osmotic pressure of the polysaccharides which tend to imbibe "water." There also is a net pressure contribution from the insoluble fibrillar system when tissue is swollen or shrunken relative to its in vivo volume (at which the fibrillar system is essentially in its zero-pressure configuration). When the fibrillar system is in a strained configuration, elastic stresses are generated. These produce a positive hydrostatic pressure for an expanded configuration (Fig. 2.10) that tends to expel "water" and a negative hydrostatic pressure for a contracted configuration (Fig. 2.10) that tends to imbibe "water."

The pressure contribution of the fibrillar network consists of the individual contributions of the collagen and microfibril networks. The collagen network is in compression over the entire range of tissue volumes studied while the microfibril network crosses over from compression to tension (Fig. 2.10). As a consequence, a transition point is also seen for the combined fibrillar network. This occurs close to the in vivo volume of tissue and represents the state where the combined fibrillar network produces a net overall pressure of zero.

At the in vivo volume of tissue, the swelling pressure is given essentially by the polysaccharides and is some −4 mm Hg (Fig. 2.10). The role of the polysaccharides in providing this internal pressure in tissue is indi-

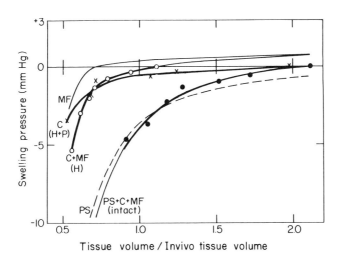

**Figure 2.10.** Swelling pressure of intact tissue and individual contributions of polysaccharides (PS), collagen (C) and microfibrils (MF) as a function of tissue volume. Experiments were performed using tissues from which diffusible proteins were removed. The pressure is given in mm Hg, above or below atmospheric pressure (regarded as zero pressure) and corresponds respectively to a tendency of tissue to shrink or swell. The curve (PS + C + MF) represents intact tissue, the curve (C + MF) represents hyaluronidase-digested tissue (H) and the curve C represents tissue after hyaluronidase and Pronase digestion (H + P). The curve for PS was calculated (*dashed line*) assuming its contribution is given by the osmotic pressure of a solution of hyaluronic acid at a concentration 1.26 times that of the polysaccharides in the extrafibrillar, extracellular space (Fig. 2.9). The *solid curves* were constructed from experimental data (*thick lines*) and by difference using the experimental and PS curves (*thin lines*). (From FA Meyer, 1983.)

cated by considering the case where the pressure is generated by the fibrillar system alone. Figure 2.10 shows that for this to occur, tissue volume has to collapse to approximately 50% of its in vivo volume.

In addition to the swelling pressure due to the structural components of tissue, there is an osmotic contribution from diffusible interstitial proteins. At the in vivo volume of tissue, their concentration is about 12 mg/ml (Klein and Meyer, 1983). For albumin, an osmotic pressure of $-7$ mm Hg is expected (Laurent and Ogston, 1963; Meyer, 1983) after accounting for exclusion effects (Fig. 2.4), if albumin in tissue is separated from blood by an "ideal" semipermeable membrane, which is selective for protein but not for "water." However, in vivo this is not the case as there is a membrane (the endothelial lining) that is only partially selective for proteins. As a consequence, the contribution of diffusible proteins to the effective swelling pressure of tissue is considerably less than $-7$ mm Hg and the major contribution is probably due mainly to the polysaccharides.

The curves in Figure 2.10 provide a basis for understanding the decrease in water content generally seen for tissues with age (Meyer and Silberberg, 1976; Maroudas et al., 1980; Maroudas and Urban, 1980). This is illustrated in the case of bovine heart valves (Table 2.3). With age there is a decrease in the net polysaccharide content relative to collagen, causing a decrease in charge content and hence a decreased osmotic contribution by the polysaccharide. Despite this the swelling pressure of the tissue need not change if tissue were to adopt a smaller volume (Fig. 2.10). In this way, the chemical potential of "water" in tissue could be maintained at a similar level with age, allowing tissue to function under essentially the same steady-state conditions. For tissue swelling pressure to remain constant with age, the fixed charge density of the polysaccharides, which

**Table 2.3.** Bovine heart valve composition and polysaccharide charge ($\pm$ SD) at different ages[a]

| Relative weight (g/g collagen) | Fetus | Calf (0.5–2 years) | Adult (7–9 years) |
|---|---|---|---|
| Water | 20.2 ± 0.4 | 12.4 ± 0.2 | 8.9 ± 0.2 |
| Hyaluronic acid | 0.014 ± 0.001 | 0.011 ± 0.001 | 0.006 ± 0.001 |
| Proteoglycan[b] | 0.049 ± 0.004 | 0.027 ± 0.002 | 0.024 ± 0.002 |
| Polysaccharide charge[c] per gram collagen (mEq/g) | 0.250 ± 0.019 | 0.147 ± 0.010 | 0.120 ± 0.011 |
| Fixed charge density (polysaccharide charge[c] per gram water) (mEq/g) | 0.0124 ± 0.0012 | 0.0119 ± 0.0010 | 0.0135 ± 0.0015 |

[a] Based in part on data from Meyer and Silberberg, 1976.
[b] Taken to be the sum of the chondroitin sulfate and dermatan sulfate contents.
[c] Calculated from composition.

determines their osmotic pressure, should remain constant. The contribution of the fibers is not considered, as these may be in their unstressed configuration at physiological tissue volumes. Table 2.3 shows that a relatively constant fixed charge density is indeed seen with age, suggesting that it is the relative decrease in polysaccharide charge in the tissue with age that is responsible for the decrease in tissue water content.

## Summary

The findings on Wharton's jelly suggest a rather distinct assignment of function to the structural components of connective tissue. Of the matrix components, the fibrillar network provides the skeletal shape while the entrapped polysaccharides confer to it the means whereby it is in steady state with the vascular circulation and at the same time allows flow of extravascular fluid ("water" and plasma proteins).

The basic structural shape of tissue is determined by an interaction between interpenetrating networks of collagen fibrils and glycoprotein microfibrils, involving the accommodation of a mutual constraint. The fibrillar components, however, do not strongly affect the chemical potential and transport rates of "water" and diffusible proteins in interstitial fluid. These are mainly influenced by the polysaccharides which affect the chemical potential of "water" through Donnan effects primarily. Since the net stress in the fiber networks is close to zero at in vivo tissue volumes, tissue hydrostatic pressure approximates zero and "water" chemical potential is influenced only by osmotic effects. Protein activity is also modulated by the polysaccharides through the effect of molecular exclusion. Polysaccharides create a fine-pore molecular meshwork in the tissue interstitium that modulates diffusible protein penetration and diffusion rates. This meshwork is also the main source of hydrodynamic resistance to convective transport of "water" and protein. Our findings for the behavior of the polysaccharides in tissue accord well with their physicochemical behavior in solution if the polysaccharides are assumed to be uniformly distributed in the extrafibrillar, extracellular regions of the tissue. Although the presence of some channels of low convective resistance (Watson and Grodins, 1978; Földi, 1982) are not excluded if these are in only a small part of the polysaccharide space, the work of Granger (1981) showing the absence of a "chromatography effect" indicates that at least in umbilical tissue, such "channels" do not exist.

Finally, it is concluded that the physicochemical properties of Wharton's jelly (and perhaps of other tissues) relevant to understanding the physiological distribution and transport of fluid are based on tissue composition and the physicochemical nature of the component structural macromolecules.

# References

Bert JL, Mathieson JM and Pearce RH (1982). The exclusion of human serum albumin by dermal collagenous fibres and within human dermis. *Biochem J* 201:395–403.

Brace RA and Guyton AC (1979). Interstitial fluid pressure: capsule, free fluid, gel fluid, and gel absorption pressure in subcutaneous tissue. *Microvasc Res* 18:217–228.

Comper WD and Laurent TC (1978). Physiological function of connective tissue polysaccharides. *Physiol Rev* 58:255–315.

Comper WD and Preston BN (1974). Model connective tissue systems. A study of polyion-mobile ion and of excluded volume interactions of proteoglycans. *Biochem J* 143:1–9.

De Gennes PG (1971). Reptation of a polymer chain in the presence of fixed obstacles. *J Chem Phys* 55:572–579.

Fessler JH (1960). A structural function of mucopolysaccharides in connective tissue. *Biochem J* 76:124–132.

Földi M (1982). Tissue channels, prelymphatics and lymphatics. *Experientia* 38:1120–1124.

Gardell S, Baker JR, Caterson B, Heinegard DK and Roden L (1980). Link protein and a hyaluronic acid-binding region as components of aorta proteoglycan. *Biochem Biophys Res Commun* 95:1823–1831.

Granger HJ (1981). Physicochemical properties of the extracellular matrix. In: *Tissue Fluid Pressure and Composition*, AR Hargens (ed.). Baltimore: Williams & Wilkens, pp. 43–61.

Granger HJ and Shepherd AP (1979). Dynamics and control of the microcirculation. *Adv Biomed Eng* 7:1–63.

Hardingham TE and Muir H (1972). The specific interaction of hyaluronic acid with cartilage proteoglycan. *Biochim Biophys Acta* 279:401–405.

Hascall VC (1977). Interaction of cartilage proteoglycans with hyaluronic acid. *J Supramol Struct* 7:101–120.

Hoffman AS, Grande LA and Park JB (1977). Sequential enzymolysis of human aorta and resultant stress-strain behavior. *Biomater Med Devices Artif Organs* 5:121–145.

Karlinsky JB, Snider GL, Franzblau C, Stone PJ and Hoppin FG (1976). In vitro effects of elastase and collagenase on mechanical properties of hamster lungs. *Am Rev Respir Dis* 113:769–777.

Katz EP and Li ST (1973). The intermolecular space of reconstituted collagen fibrils. *J Mol Biol* 73:351–369.

Klein J (1977). Diffusion of long molecules through solid polyethylene. 1. Topological constraints, *J Polym Sci Polym Phys Ed* 15:2057–2064.

Klein J and Meyer FA (1983). Tissue structure and macromolecular diffusion in umbilical cord. Immobilization of endogenous hyaluronic acid, *Biochim Biophys Acta* 755:400–411.

Laurent TC (1964). The interaction between polysaccharides and other macromolecules. 9. The exclusion of molecules from hyaluronic acid gels and solutions. *Biochem J* 93:106–112.

Laurent TC and Ogston AG (1963). The interaction between polysaccharides and other macromolecules. 4. The osmotic pressure of mixtures of serum albumin and hyaluronic acid. *Biochem J* 89:249–253.

Maroudas A (1975). Biophysical chemistry of cartilaginous tissues with special reference to solute and fluid transport. *Biorheology* 12:233–248.

Maroudas A and Bannon C (1981). Measurement of swelling pressure in cartilage and comparison with the osmotic pressure of constituent proteoglycans. *Biorheology* 18:619–632.

Maroudas A, Bayliss MT and Venn MF (1980). Further studies on the composition of human femoral head cartilage. *Ann Rheum Dis* 39:514–523.

Maroudas A and Urban JPG (1980). Swelling pressures of cartilaginous tissues. In: *Studies in Joint Disease I,* A Maroudas and EJ Holborow (eds.). Tunbridge Wells, Kent: Pitman Medical, pp. 87–116.

Mathews MB and Decker L (1977). Comparative studies of water sorption of hyaline cartilage. *Biochim Biophys Acta* 497:151–159.

Mathews MB and Lozaitye I (1958). Sodium chondroitin sulfate-protein complexes of cartilage. I. Molecular weight and shape. *Arch Biochem Biophys* 74:158–174.

Meyer FA (1971). *A Biochemical and Biophysical Approach to the Structure of Heart Valves.* Ph.D. Thesis, Monash University, Clayton, Australia.

Meyer FA (1983). Macromolecular basis of globular protein exclusion and of swelling pressure in loose connective tissue (umbilical cord). *Biochim Biophys Acta* 755:388–399.

Meyer FA, Koblentz M and Silberberg A (1977). Structural investigation of loose connective tissue by using a series of dextran fractions as non-interacting macromolecular probes. *Biochem J* 161:285–291.

Meyer FA, Laver-Rudich Z and Tanenbaum R (1983). Evidence for a mechanical coupling of glycoprotein microfibrils with collagen fibrils in Wharton's jelly. *Biochim Biophys Acta* 755:376–387.

Meyer FA and Silberberg A (1974). Invitro study of the influence of some factors important for any physicochemical characterization of loose connective tissue in the microcirculation. *Microvasc Res* 8:263–273.

Meyer FA and Silberberg A (1976). Aging and the interstitial content of loose connective tissue. A brief note. *Mech Aging Dev* 5:437–442.

Missirlis YF (1977). Use of enzymolysis techniques in studying the mechanical properties of connective tissue components. *J Bioeng* 1:215–222.

Oakes BW and Bialkower B (1977). Biomechanical and ultrastructural studies on the elastic wing tendon from the domestic fowl. *J Anat* 123:369–387.

Ogston AG (1958). The spaces in a uniform random suspension of fibers. *Trans Faraday Soc* 54:1754–1757.

Ogston AG, Preston BN and Wells JD (1973). On the transport of compact particles through solutions of chain polymers. *Proc R Soc Lond Ser A* 333:297–309.

Robert L, Junqua S and Moczar M (1976). Structural glycoproteins of the intercellular matrix. *Front Matrix Biol* 3:113–142.

Ross R and Bornstein P (1969). The elastic fiber. The separation and partial characterization of its macromolecular components. *J Cell Biol* 40:366–381.

Silberberg A (1979). Microcirculation and the extravascular space. In: *Microcirculation in Inflammation,* G Hauck and JW Irwin (eds.). Basel: Karger, pp. 54–65.

Silpananta P, Dunstone JR and Ogston AG (1968). Fractionation of a hyaluronic acid preparation in a density gradient. *Biochem J* 109:43–50.

Watson PD and Grodins FS (1978). An analysis of the effects of the interstitial matrix on plasma-lymph transport. *Microvasc Res* 16:19–41.

Wiederhielm CA (1979). Dynamics of capillary fluid exchange. A non-linear computer simulation. *Microvasc Res* 18:48–82.

Wiederhielm CA (1981). The tissue pressure controversy, a semantic dilemma. In: *Tissue Fluid Pressure and Composition,* AR Hargens (ed.). Baltimore: Williams & Wilkins, pp. 21–33.

Wiederhielm CA and Black LL (1976). Osmotic interaction of plasma proteins with interstitial macromolecules. *Am J Physiol* 231:638–641.

Zweifach BW and Silberberg A (1979). The interstitial-lymphatic flow system. In: *Intentional Review of Physiology. Vol. 18. Cardiovascular Physiology III,* AC Guyton and DB Young (eds.). Baltimore: University Park Press, pp. 215–260.

# CHAPTER 3

# Mechanisms of Fluid Transport in Cartilaginous Tissues

## Alice Maroudas

## Introduction

Cartilaginous tissues, such as articular cartilage and the intervertebral disc, consist of a network of collagen fibrils. These fibrils, capable of resisting tension but not compression, are embedded in an aqueous concentrated proteoglycan gel. The proteoglycans endow the matrix with a high osmotic pressure and a low hydraulic permeability, and hence constitute the compression-resisting component of these tissues.

When an external compressive stress is applied to cartilage or the disc, the tissue deforms due to a combination of two effects: (1) the rearrangement of the polymer network, which leads to a change in the *shape* of the specimen *at constant volume* and (2) creep associated with the *loss of fluid* from the matrix, which causes a decrease in the total volume of the tissue and hence a closer packing of the solid constituents (Fig. 3.1). The so-called instantaneous deflection (effect 1) is thought to be associated with the very rapid *bulk movement* of the proteoglycan-water gel, which is resisted by the collagen fiber network (Weightman and Kempson, 1979). Effect (2) is much slower than effect (1) since it involves the movement of fluid relative to the very fine pores formed by the proteoglycans molecules. In the present chapter we will concern ourselves with the basic mechanism of fluid flow in cartilaginous tissues, induced by changes in the external pressure. We will also deal with the question of whether the expression of fluid from the tissue and the subsequent reabsorption of fresh fluid constitutes an important contribution to cartilage and/or disc nutrition.

Although 60 years ago Benninghoff (1924) theorized that the deformation and recovery of cartilage were dependent on extracellular fluid expression and imbibition, respectively, it was not until the 1960s that systematic studies on this subject were undertaken. McCutchen (1962) measured the permeability of cartilage to water and observed that it decreased with distance from the articular surface. He also attempted to describe mathematically the compression and the recovery of a cylindri-

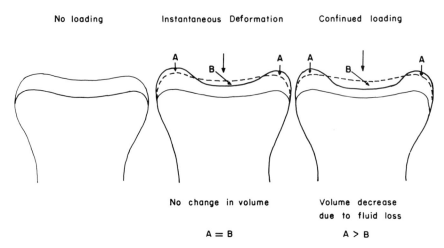

**Figure 3.1.** Schematic representation of the instantaneous deformation of cartilage compared with creep due to fluid loss. **A**: initial volume of cartilage. **B**: deformed volume of cartilage.

cal plug of cartilage using both fluid flow and matrix stiffness terms. Linn and Sokoloff (1965) and Sokoloff (1966) showed that there was a close parallelism between the creep behavior of different types of cartilage (human articular and costal cartilage) and the amount of fluid that could be expressed from them. Elmore and co-workers (1963) demonstrated experimentally that the ability to be indented of cartilage was dependent on the concentration of the outside equilibrating solution. They found that, for a given load, the equilibrium deformation was increased in a hypertonic (3.4%) NaCl solution as compared with an isotonic solution, whereas it was decreased if distilled water was used. Linn and Sokoloff (1965) showed that both the total amount of water expressed under a given load and the rate at which it was being expressed were affected by the concentration of the equilibrating solution. These results were attributed by the authors to the operation of osmotic forces resulting from the Gibbs-Donnan equilibrium involving the anionic charges of the glycosaminoglycans. Contemporary with the above work on cartilage, research was carried out along similar lines by investigators studying fluid transport and swelling behavior of the cornea.

In the late 1970s a number of papers appeared, particularly by Mow and colleagues (e.g., Mow & Lai, 1979; Mow et al., 1980) analyzing the mechanical response of cartilage in terms of a biphasic model that treats cartilage as a mixture of a linear elastic solid and an incompressible liquid. Mow and colleagues particularly focused their attention on relating stress, strain and fluid flow during uniaxial, confined transient creep and stress relaxation. The equations that they developed to relate the above parameters to one another are similar in form to those of Fatt and Goldstick (1965) to describe corneal swelling. The latter equations were adapted by Urban (1977) and by Urban and Maroudas (1980a) to analyze the course of fluid flow and reimbibition in articular cartilage and intervertebral disc. The main difference between the approach of Mow and colleagues and our own is that they do not identify swelling pressure as an explicit variable in the system but use an aggregate elastic modulus of the solid phase to characterise the final equilibrium. Unlike the tissue's swelling pressure, which varies nonlinearly with hydration, the modulus is usually treated as a constant. The nonlinearity of the system is thus attributed to that of the hydraulic permeability alone.

Our studies describe the mechanism of fluid flow in cartilage and the disc in terms of two basic properties of the matrix: swelling pressure and hydraulic permeability (Maroudas, 1968, 1975a,b, 1976, 1979; Urban et al., 1979; Maroudas and Urban, 1980; Urban and Maroudas, 1980a,b). It is the author's belief that a description of fluid flow, the major component of creep, should be based explicitly on the above two parameters, which in turn can be directly related to the chemical composition and structure of the matrix.

## Matrix Composition and Structure

The matrix of articular cartilage and intervertebral disc consist principally of collagen fibers embedded in a gel of proteoglycan and saline. Collagen fibers range between 250 and 2000 Å in diameter (depending on the location and age) with gaps in between the fibers in the range 500 to 4000 Å (Byers et al., 1983). Thus, the proteoglycan–saline gel fills these relatively large gaps and determines the fine structure of the matrix. Table 3.1 shows a typical size of the pores in cartilage, obtained from three

**Table 3.1.** Pore size in normal human articular cartilage from the femoral head (middle zone) estimated from different types of measurement

| Type of measurement | Pore size (Å) |
| --- | --- |
| Globular protein exclusion | 21 |
| GAG concentration (total tissue basis) | 42 |
| GAG concentration (extrafibrillar space only) | 32 |
| Hydraulic permeability (total tissue basis) | 40 |

independent types of measurement. All three methods indicate a size range of 20 to 40 Å. The size differences obtained by the three methods are not large, considering each procedure uses a different set of simplifications. Partition data yield a smaller pore size than the other two methods because they are based on minimum pore dimensions (pore "necks") rather than on average dimensions. Also contained within this matrix are cells, the chondrocytes, that maintain and repair the cartilage. The cell content of the cartilage is small, occupying about 2% to 5% of cartilage volume (Stockwell and Meachim, 1973).

The structure of cartilage proteoglycans is described in detail in a number of reviews (for example, see Rosenberg, 1974). In brief, proteoglycan is the name given to the macromolecule composed of a central protein core to which are attached the glycosaminoglycan (GAG) side chains. In cartilage and disc, proteoglycans exist, to a varying extent, in the form of aggregates formed by attachment of the subunits to a hyaluronate backbone. The GAG side chains consist of polymers of chondroitin sulfate (CS) and keratan sulfate (KS). Both molecules contain acidic groups, $OSO_3^-$ and $COO^-$, which give the matrix a high negative fixed charge. The fixed charge density is a measure of the GAG concentration alone, as the collagen fibrils exhibit no net charge at physiological pH (Freeman and Maroudas, 1975; Venn and Maroudas, 1977). The fixed charged groups are responsible for the high swelling pressure of the tissue (Urban et al., 1979; Maroudas and Bannon, 1981). This swelling pressure together with the low hydraulic permeability of the matrix maintains the hydration of the tissue under external load and so enables the tissue to fulfill its physiological role. The fixed charge also determines ionic equilibria between cartilage and synovial fluid and between intervertebral disc and surrounding plasma (Maroudas, 1968; Urban et al., 1978).

The presence of fixed negatively charged groups on CS and KS have made it possible to develop rapid methods for the estimation of the total GAG content both in articular cartilage (Maroudas et al., 1969; Maroudas and Thomas, 1970) and disc (Urban and Maroudas, 1979). The GAG concentration and hence the fixed charge density (FCD) vary from joint to joint and also with position in the joint. The highest mean concentrations occur in the nucleus pulposus where the FCD can rise to 0.3 mEq/g wet tissue. In articular cartilage the highest FCDs are found in the femoral head, where values reach 0.2 mEq/g (Maroudas, 1979). In other joints, such as the patella, FCD is somewhat lower (Ficat and Maroudas, 1975). FCD also varies with the condition of the joint, being lower in degenerate cartilage. In osteoarthrotic areas of the knee and femoral head, FCD is sometimes as low as 0.05 mEq/g (Ficat and Maroudas, 1975; Venn and Maroudas, 1977; Brocklehurst et al., 1983). Water content, collagen and FCD (and hence the GAG content) vary with depth of cartilage below the articular surface for the superior surface of the femoral head (Fig.

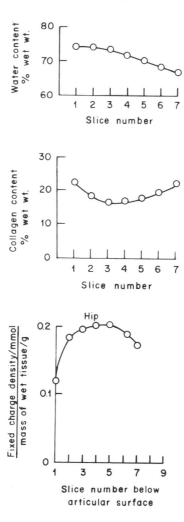

**Figure 3.2. A**: Variation in water content, collagen content and fixed charge density with depth in cartilage from the superior surface of a normal adult human femoral head. *Abscissa:* slices counted from articular surface (slice thickness: approx. 250 $\mu$m).

3.2A). Regional differences also exist between FCD profiles within a single joint (femoral condyles) and also from one joint to another (Fig. 3.2B). Similar nonuniformity occurs in the intervertebral disc (Fig. 3.2C). Figure 3.2C presents typical curves of FCD and water content across both a young and aged disc.

It is of interest to note that in the disc the water content parallels the fixed charge density, both being at a minimum in the outer annulus and

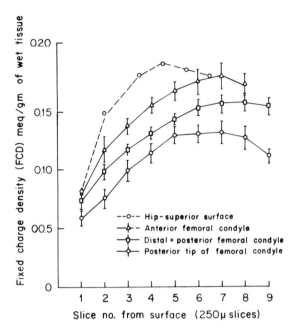

**Figure 3.2. B**: Variation in fixed charge density with depth for different sites of the normal adult human femoral condyles. The curve for femoral head cartilage is also shown for comparison.

increasing to a maximum in the nucleus. By contrast, although FCD increases from the articular surface to the middle zone in cartilage, decreasing again slightly in the deep zone, water content decreases uniformly with depth. This difference must be related to the difference between the relative extensibilities of the collagen network in cartilage and disc, since the actual tendency to imbibe water is due in both tissues to the same mechanism, i.e., the Donnan osmotic pressure arising from the presence of high concentrations of fixed negatively charged groups of the GAG (Urban et al., 1979).

Although in cartilage the collagen network is so tight that the normal tissue hardly swells even when the GAG osmotic pressure is substantially increased (Maroudas, 1976), the disc swells under the influence of its normal osmotic pressure as soon as the external constraining load is lifted (Urban and Maroudas, 1980a,b). This difference is probably due to the considerable cross-linking of cartilage collagen. Teleologically, cartilage must have a very tight collagen net to prevent its proteoglycans from unrestricted swelling when a joint is unloaded. The disc, on the other hand, is always subjected to a residual external compressive stress (provided by muscles and ligaments), which controls the tissue's hydration;

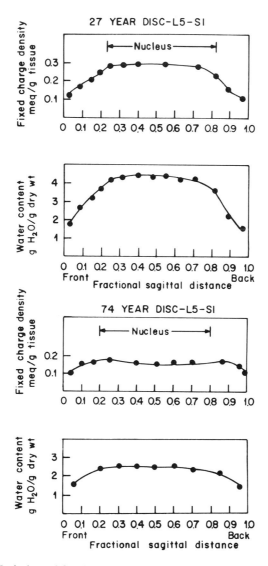

**Figure 3.2. C**: Variation of fixed charge density and water content with position for a young and an old human lumbar intervertebral disc.

hence its collagen network need not be so stiff. On the contrary, for the disc to function in torsion, bending, etc. flexibility is a very desirable characteristic.

Articular cartilage is avascular in the adult, and the bone–cartilage junction is virtually impermeable to solutes and fluid (Maroudas et al.,

1968; McKibbin and Maroudas, 1979). Accordingly, most nutrient and fluid exchange occurs across the interface between cartilage and synovial fluid whereas, within the tissue, the transport of nutrients and metabolites takes place through the matrix, and thus depends on its structure and composition. The latter is also true of the intervertebral disc. However, because the disc is so large an avascular structure, the bone–disc interface is at least partially permeable to solute and fluid flow as transport from the peripheral blood vessels alone could noₜ provide nutrients for the nucleus or the inner annulus (Urban et al., 1978; Holm et al., 1981).

## Flow of Fluid in Cartilage and Disc

When cartilage is not under an external load, the swelling tendency of proteoglycan gel is exactly balanced by elastic resistance of the collagen network. If a load is suddenly applied, the cartilage instantaneously deforms due to bulk movement of the matrix (Weightman and Kempson, 1979). This is followed by a creep phase (Fig. 3.3), which is due mainly to the expression of fluid from the matrix (Maroudas, 1975a). Fluid loss leads to a higher GAG concentration per tissue volume, and hence a higher swelling pressure. Outward flow continues until the swelling pressure increases enough to balance the applied load. Thus the equilibrium amount of fluid lost under a given load will depend on the composition of the tissue. The rate at which fluid is expressed depends on both swelling pressure and hydraulic permeability. The same holds true of fluid imbibition when the external load is removed. To describe fluid transport in cartilage, the relationship of both swelling pressure and hydraulic permeability to tissue composition must be understood.

### Swelling Pressure

The net swelling pressure of cartilage $P_{Sw}$ results from the difference between the swelling tendency of the proteoglycans due to their osmotic pressure $\Pi$ and the resisting force of the collagen network $P_C$. The applied external pressure $P_A$ required to balance the difference between $\Pi$ and $P_C$ is defined as the net swelling pressure of the tissue $P_{Sw}*$ and characterizes the swelling tendency of the latter at a given hydration:

$$P_A = P_{Sw} = \Pi - P_C. \tag{1}$$

$\Pi$ consists of two components, which are simply additive (Wells, 1973; Maroudas, 1975a). These components are the Donnan swelling pressure

---

* $P_{Sw}$ is determined by measuring the applied pressure $P_A$ which is required to stop the tissue from gaining or losing water. For a given tissue specimen, it varies with the hydration of the specimen.

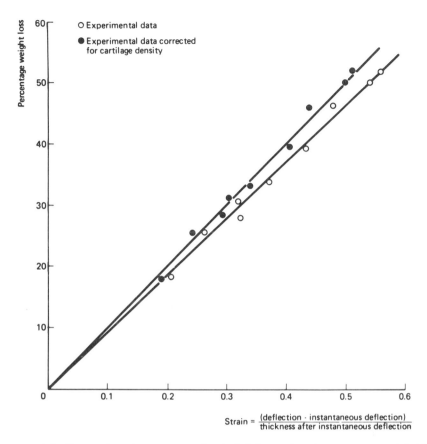

**Figure 3.3.** Comparison between mechanical deformation due to creep and fluid loss from a plug of cartilage. (From A Maroudas, 1975a.)

$P_{Don}$ which results from the excess of positive ions in the tissue due to the polyanionic nature of the GAGs and $P_{Excl}$, which is an entropic contribution resulting from the steric exclusion that the polymer chains exert on one another:

$$\Pi = P_{Don} + P_{Excl}. \tag{2}$$

Both components depend on GAG concentration; however, at GAG concentrations normally present in cartilaginous tissues, $P_{Don}$ is the dominant term, being responsible for approximately 85% of the total osmotic pressure developed by the proteoglycans (Urban et al., 1979).

Once the osmotic pressure of the constituent proteoglycans is known, it is possible to calculate the tensile contribution ($P_C$) of the collagen network at a given hydration from the measurement of the net swelling pressure of the tissue at that hydration. However, to use osmotic pressure curves obtained from isolated proteoglycans for the purpose of predicting their response in the tissue quantitatively, it is necessary to know their actual concentration in the extrafibrillar tissue water since, because of their actual size, they are excluded from the intrafibrillar space.

In articular cartilage, intrafibrillar water is approximately 0.7 g/g of dry collagen, (Maroudas and Bannon, 1981).† Using this figure, fixed charge density is calculated on the basis of the extrafibrillar water alone (in what follows, this parameter is referred to as the *effective* fixed charge density, in contrast to the *overall* fixed charge density, based on the total water content). Experimentally obtained net swelling pressures of a cartilage slice are plotted versus the overall fixed charge density on the one hand, and the effective fixed charge density on the other hand (Fig. 3.4). The curve of the osmotic pressure of isolated proteoglycans $\Pi_{PG}$ versus fixed charge density is also given in Figure 3.4.

Bearing in mind Eq. 1, $P_C$ can be calculated from the difference between the net swelling pressure of the tissue slice and the osmotic pressure of the isolated proteoglycans at the same concentration (or fixed charge density). If one uses results such as those in Figure 3.4, based on the overall fixed charge density, one obtains negative values of $P_C$, which become larger with decreasing cartilage volume. This does not make physical sense, since tension in the collagen network must oppose and not enhance the osmotic pressure of the proteoglycans, and since the tension must decrease and not increase as the tissue shrinks. On the other hand, if the effective fixed charge density is used, $P_C$ is initially positive and gradually decreases as the fixed charge density increases. This is entirely consistent with the physical picture: in fully hydrated cartilage, tensile stresses are sufficient to counterbalance the osmotic pressure of the proteoglycans; as the fluid is squeezed out, the tissue shrinks and tensile stresses in the collagen network are relieved. In fact, at hydrations below about 90% to 95% the curves for $P_A$ and $\Pi$ coincide, which means that $P_C = 0$.

In intervertebral disc, the nucleus pulposus contains very little collagen—about 3% by wet weight only as compared to 15% to 20% in articular cartilage. Since the total water in the nucleus accounts for about 80% of the tissue's wet weight, the fraction accounted for by the intrafibrillar collagen water is rather small and the error introduced by expressing

---

† Although this figure for the intrafibrillar water gave a reasonably good agreement with experimental results, it was only a rough approximation. In particular, it has recently become apparent (Katz et al., 1985) that the average intermolecular (lateral) collagen spacing in cartilage is not a constant, but is dependent on the osmotic pressure prevailing in the extrafibrillar space and hence on the proteoglycan concentration. The fraction of water present in the intrafibrillar space thus varies from the surface to the deep zone and is also dependent on the applied pressure. It is also likely to change in osteoarthritic cartilage.

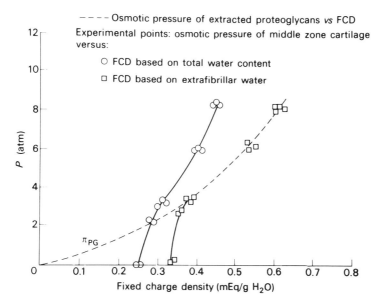

**Figure 3.4.** Comparison between the swelling pressure of femoral head cartilage (*solid lines*) and the osmotic pressure of extracted proteoglycans (*dashed line*) at equivalent fixed charge densities. (From A Maroudas and Bannon, 1981.)

proteoglycan concentration on a total water basis rather than on extrafibrillar water alone is not significant ($<5\%$). Thus, it is not surprising to find that the swelling pressure of a normal nucleus slice corresponds reasonably closely to the osmotic pressure of the isolated proteoglycans at the same fixed charge density (see typical result in Fig. 3.5); however, with increasing collagen coutent in the nucleus, a correction for the intrafibrillar space must be made (Urban and McMullin, 1985).

At present, swelling pressures in different regions of the annulus cannot yet be directly related to the osmotic pressure of their proteoglycans because of uncertainties as to the proportion of the intrafibrillar water. Depending on the area, collagen constitutes as much as 20% to 35% of total wet tissue weight and the fraction of water present in the intrafibrillar spaces, which so far has not yet been accurately determined, cannot be ignored. Therefore, it is not possible at present to use measurements of $P_A$ and $\Pi$ for the quantitative estimation of the collagen tension $P_C$. However, it is possible to discuss the effect of the collagen network in a qualitative manner for different regions of the disc.

Typical graphs of applied pressure versus equilibrium hydration for articular cartilage as well as the nucleus and different parts of the annulus in disc are presented (Fig. 3.6). It should be noted that at equilibrium, applied pressure is equal to net swelling pressure of the tissue slice. At a given hydration, swelling pressure of the nucleus is considerably greater

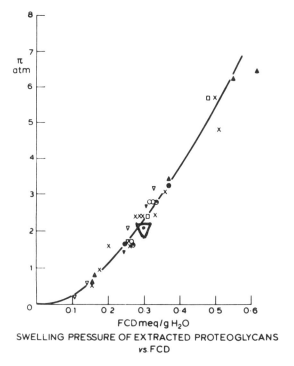

SWELLING PRESSURE OF EXTRACTED PROTEOGLYCANS
*vs.* FCD

**Figure 3.5.** Comparison between the swelling pressure of a young disc nucleus at physiological hydration and fixed charge density ($\nabla$) with the osmotic pressures of extracted proteoglycans. The different symbols correspond to different forms of extracted proteoglycans. (Reproduced in part from JPG Urban et al., 1979.)

than that of the outer annulus. Across the annulus itself, for the same water content, there is a gradual increase in swelling pressure as one passes from the outer periphery to the region adjacent to the nucleus. This variation arises partly from the variation in proteoglycan content across the disc (see Fig. 3.2C) and partly from differences in extensibility of the collagen network. Collagen in the nucleus, apart from being present in very small amounts, is arranged in a loose random network, whereas in the annulus the collagen fibers run as tight lamellae between adjoining vertebral bodies. Osmotic pressure of proteoglycans in the nucleus is greater than that in the annulus whereas, in contrast, tension in the collagen network $P_C$ is greater in annulus than in nucleus. With a decrease in hydration (as the tissue shrinks), the collagen network relaxes, $P_C$ becomes relatively unimportant and the value of $P_{Sw}$ approaches that of $\Delta\Pi$ alone. As far as degenerate discs are concerned, their swelling pressure is lower than that of normal discs at equivalent hydrations (Maroudas & Urban, 1983; Urban & McMullin, 1985; Ziv and Maroudas, unpublished results). This is consistent with the fact that degenerate discs have a lower

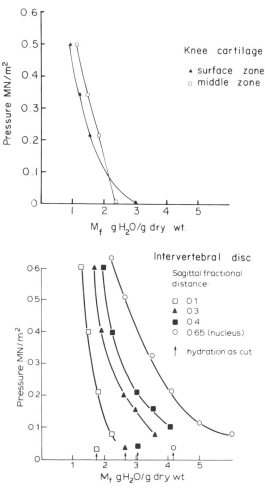

**Figure 3.6.** Typical curves of swelling pressure versus equilibrium hydration $M_f$ for slices from the superficial and middle zones of human knee cartilage and for different regions of a human lumbar disc.

proteoglycan content than normal discs. The same holds true for degenerate articular cartilage (Maroudas et al., 1985).

Water contents of different parts of the disc, as excised from the spine (i.e., without drying or exposure to any solution) correspond for all parts of the disc to a swelling pressure of about 0.2 MN/m². This pressure is approximately equal to that measured in vivo in the nucleus of lumbar discs with the subject lying prone (Nachemson and Elfstrom, 1970). Thus, although the disc in effect contacts a physiological saline solution in vivo, it is prevented from swelling beyond a certain limit by the residual load that it must bear. In this regard, it is noteworthy that the Skylab astronauts, who were weightless for 85 days, increased about 5 cm in height (Thornton et al., 1974). This may be due in part to swelling of intervertebral discs under decreased load. On the other hand, a large increase in applied pressure will lead to only a small decrease in hydration. Thus, the normal disc is able to maintain a relatively constant composition over large changes in applied load, a highly desirable functional feature.

As discussed earlier, in contrast to the disc, the net swelling pressures at hydrations characteristic of unloaded cartilage are zero since the collagen network exactly balances the osmotic pressure of the proteoglycans (see Fig. 3.6). Tensile stresses in the collagen network are released as soon as the cartilage begins to decrease in volume under the effect of an applied load. As in the case of the disc, the curves are steep so that increased applied pressure does not lead to severe dehydration. Over most of the range, for a given applied pressure, the cartilage from the surface zone has a lower water content than the cartilage from the middle zone. This is because the GAG concentration is lower near the articular surface, increasing gradually with depth (see Fig. 3.2A and B). In the region of hydrations close to those in unloaded tissue (i.e., when stresses in the collagen network come into play), curves for the two zones cross over (see Fig. 3.6). The swelling pressure curves for articular cartilage are similar to the curve for the outer annulus. Although the annulus has a lower overall FCD, it has a much higher collagen content than articular cartilage and therefore, their effective FCDs and hence osmotic pressures are approximately similar.

## Hydraulic Permeability $k$

Virtually all treatments of fluid flow through connective tissue such as cartilage use models in which tissue contains interconnecting water-filled "pores" through which flow takes place. The flow is assumed to follow Poiseuille's law. This means that a constant hydraulic permeability $k$ can describe water flow, and that this $k$ is independent of flow rate or driving force, but is a property of the tissue only and therefore will be a function of tissue composition. If a pressure gradient is applied across a slice of connective tissue, the ensuing flow of liquid at any point can be described by Darcy's law:

$$q = -kA \frac{dP}{dx},\qquad(3)$$

where $q$ = flow rate
$k$ = hydraulic permeability
$A$ = cross-sectional area of the tissue
$\frac{dP}{dx}$ = pressure gradient across the segment.

## Steady-State Measurement of $k$

If a tissue slice of thickness $2L$ separates two fluid-filled compartments, fluid will flow through the tissue if the compartments are not at the same hydrostatic or osmotic pressure. At steady state, Darcy's law becomes:

$$q = -kA \frac{\Delta P}{2L}. \tag{4}$$

Thus, by applying a constant pressure gradient $\Delta P$‡ across a tissue slice and measuring the flow rate, $k$ is calculated directly. This method for measuring $k$ in articular cartilage was first used by McCutchen (1962), who measured the normal component of $k$. He found that the average value of $k$ for the cow's ankle was $5.8 \times 10^{-13}$ cm$^3$s $\cdot$ g$^{-1}$ and that $k$ varied with distance from the articular surface. The present author measured $k$ in human cartilage and showed that permeability varied with FCD and that this accounts for most of its variation with depth. However, collagen content and fibril size influence $k$ to a slight extent as well (Muir et al., 1970; Maroudas, 1979).

The tangential permeability of cartilage has also been measured (Maroudas, 1974; Mulholland et al., 1975). Mulholland and co-workers (1975) measured tangential hydraulic permeabilities as well as permeabilities normal to the surface and found that the former were approximately 2.5 times greater than the latter. However, they did not consider possible variations of FCD across their cartilage specimen which must have included several zones of cartilage. When this is taken into account, permeabilities in both directions are found to be equal (Maroudas, 1974, 1975a), a result that is expected for flow through an isotropic gel.

Maroudas (1975a, see Fig. 3.7) and Mansour and Mow (1976) also studied $k$ as a function of strain or hydration, by measuring steady-state flow through cartilage slices subjected to known deformation. In both studies it was found that $k$ decreases sharply with decreased hydration (or increased strain). This is consistent with the idea that fluid flow occurs through "pores" of the proteoglycan gel and that higher proteoglycan concentration caused by a decrease in water content must lead to a smaller pore size and hence a lower $k$. This variation of hydraulic permeability with proteoglycan concentration has important physiological implications, since it means that in cartilage or disc depleted of proteoglycans there will be a faster loss of fluid under normal compressive loads. The hydraulic permeability of the disc tissue will be discussed in the section on transport coefficients since it is obtained from measurements of these coefficients.

---

‡ This pressure gradient must be small compared to that which produces tissue compaction; otherwise there will not be a linear relationship between $q$ and $\Delta P$, and there will be an apparent variation of $k$ with $\Delta P$ (this effect is discussed by Holmes et al., in the next chapter).

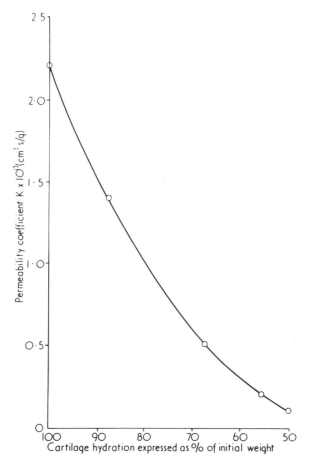

**Figure 3.7.** Typical curve of hydraulic permeability versus equilibrium hydration for a slice of femoral head cartilage. (From A Maroudas, 1975*a*.)

## Fluid Transport under Unsteady-State Conditions

Although in vitro it is possible to arrange experiments in which fluid flows *through* a tissue slice under steady-state conditions (with pressure gradients and hydration remaining constant) in vivo changes in the applied load to which articular cartilage and intervertebral disc are subjected in the course of a normal day's activity induce fluid flow *out of* or *into* the tissues. This, in turn, alters hydration and hence, changes both swelling pressure and hydraulic permeability. During the process of tissue compression, the driving force for fluid outflow is the difference between the externally applied pressure $P_A$ and the tissue's swelling pressure $P_{sw}$ (Maroudas, 1975a; Maroudas, 1979). Thus, Eq. (3) has to be rewritten in the following form:

$$q = -kA \frac{d(P_a - P_{sw})}{dx}.$$  (5)

During fluid imbibition, the driving force for fluid flow is provided by the tissue's net swelling pressure $P_{sw}$. The following procedure, based on the work of Fatt and Goldstick, who studied flow in the cornea, was used in the quantitative treatment.

Fatt and Goldstick (1965) considered a confined slice of tissue of total thickness $L$, unit cross-sectional area ($A = 1$) and water content (hydration) $M$, to which a pressure $P_A$ was applied through permeable plates. As the slice creeps, water is expressed from the tissue. Thus, $L$ and $M$ are obviously functions of time. However the total "dry" thickness of the material $z$ remains constant during the compression of the slice. If the volumes of water and dry material are additive,

$$z = L \left[ \frac{\alpha}{\alpha + M} \right],$$  (6)

where $[\alpha/(\alpha + M)]$ is the fractional volume of dry material and $\alpha$ is the ratio of the specific volume of dry material $V_s$ to the specific volume of water $V_w$, i.e., $\alpha = V_s/V_w$, and the water content $M$ is expressed as mass water/mass dry material.

Using Darcy's law (Eq. 5) and the continuity equation for water flow, Fatt and Goldstick derived Eq. (7), which is analogous to the diffusion equation:

$$\frac{\partial M}{\partial t} = \frac{\partial}{\partial z} \left[ D(H) \frac{dM}{dz} \right],$$  (7)

where $M$ is the hydration

$t$ is time

$z$ is the distance based on dry tissue volume (Eq. 6), assuming net flow is in the direction $z$ only

$D(H)$, the so-called transport coefficient, is defined by Eq. (8) below:

$$D(H) = k \frac{\alpha^2}{\alpha + M} \cdot \frac{dP_{sw}}{dM},$$  (8)

where $k$ is the hydraulic permeability coefficient and $dP_{sw}/dM$ is the slope of the curve of swelling pressure versus hydration. It should be noted that $P_{sw}$ (net swelling pressure of the tissue) is a monotonic function of the tissue hydration. Similarly, the hydraulic permeability $k$ can be expressed as a function of hydration. Therefore, $D(H)$ is a function of tissue hydration only.

Since $D(H)$ varies with hydration, Eq. (7) is nonlinear and has no general solution. It has the form of a diffusion equation with $D(H)$ being equivalent to a diffusion coefficient, which is a function of solute concentration. Accordingly, methods described by Crank (1975) for handling diffusion equations with concentration-dependent diffusion coefficients can be used to solve Eq. (7).

Fatt and Goldstick solved Eq. (7) by assuming that $D(H)$ remains at some mean value $\bar{D}(H)$ if the equation applies only to small changes in hydration. The resulting change in overall hydration with time then has an analytical solution:

$$\bar{H} = 2 \left(\frac{\overline{D(H)}t}{z^2}\right)^{1/2}\left(\frac{1}{\sqrt{\pi}} + 2 \sum_{n=1}^{\infty} (-1)^n \text{ ierfc} \left(\frac{n^2 z^2}{\overline{D(H)}t}\right)^{1/2}\right), \qquad (9)$$

where $M_0$ is the initial hydration

$M_f$ is the final equilibrium hydration under the applied load, $P_a$

$M$ is the hydration at time $t$

$2z$ is the total "dry" thickness of the tissue

$\bar{H}$ is the mean relative hydration and is defined as:

$$\bar{H} = \frac{M - M_0}{M_f - M_0}. \qquad (10)$$

## The Mean Transport Coefficient $\overline{D(H)}$ and its Relationship to $D(H)$

Crank (1975) demonstrated that for solute transport by diffusion, the amount absorbed is directly proportional to the square root of time for the period during which diffusion is taking place into a semi-infinite medium (even if the diffusion coefficient is concentration-dependent). Therefore, by analogy, the same applies to the transport of fluid such as described by Eq. (7) during the period when hydration at point $z = 0$, i.e., the center of the slice (or the contact with an impermeable surface) remains equal to the initial hydration. Thus, during compression from $M = M_0$ to $M = M_f$, fluid loss from the tissue is described by Eq. (9) for times such that ierfc $n^2 z^2/D(H)t \simeq 0$, even over large changes in hydration. If $M - M_0/M_f - M_0$ is plotted versus $\sqrt{t}$, the initial slope is given by $2(\overline{D(H)}/z^2)^{1/2}$ (see Eq. 9). $\overline{D(H)}$ is thus determined as a function of $M_0$ and $M_f$.

To be able to predict the complete creep behavior of a specimen one needs to know $D(H)$ over the entire hydration range of interest. Several methods of using the experimental coefficient $\overline{D(H)}$ to obtain $D(H)$ as a function of hydration $M$ are discussed by Crank (1975). Once this is done, Eq. (7) is solved numerically to give creep rate. Alternatively $\overline{D(H)}$ is calculated from experimental values of $D(H)$ for each particular hydration range and used together with Eq. (9) to calculate creep or swelling rate over this range. Also, from experimental values of $D(H)$ the hydraulic permeability $k$ is determined from Eq. (8) provided the variation of swelling pressure $P_{sw}$ with hydration $M$ is known. $\overline{D(H)}$ does not, generally, have the same value for compression from $M_1$ to $M_2$, as for reabsorption from $M_2$ to $M_1$. In the disc creep is slower than recovery because the flow coefficient $D(H)$, defined by Eq. (9), increases with increasing hydration over the physiological range. Thus, during recovery (where the driving force for resorption $\Delta P$ is greatest), $D(H)$ is smallest, and as equilibrium is approached, the decrease in $\Delta P$ is compensated for by the increase in $D(H)$. For creep, however, as $\Delta P$ decreases, $D(H)$ also decreases. Therefore, creep rate diminishes rapidly with decreasing hydration.

## Transport Coefficients

The transport coefficients and hydraulic permeability depend highly on tissue hydration (Fig. 3.8). For nucleus slices from a 23-year-old disc, the swelling pressure curve is similar to that from the 54-year-old disc in Figure 3.6. Hydraulic permeability $k$, in particular, decreases 10-fold as the hydration $M$ decreases from $M = 4$ to $M = 2$. With water contents higher than those in vivo ($M \geq 5$), i.e., in the swelling region, the hydraulic permeability is very high. As our understanding of relationships between tissue structure and $D(H)$ becomes more complete, it will be possible to calculate $D(H)$ from a knowledge of tissue composition alone.

## Contribution of Fluid Flow to Solute Transport

Solute transport through cartilaginous matrices is important for the nutrition of chondrocytes and the disposal of their waste products. Since sol-

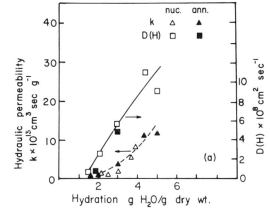

**Figure 3.8.** Dependence of hydraulic permeability and transport coefficient $D(H)$ on tissue hydration. (From JPG Urban and A Maroudas, 1980a.)

utes move both by molecular diffusion and by flowing fluid, it is important to assess whether both mechanisms contribute equally under physiological conditions or whether one transport mode predominates over the other. The present author originally calculated that the contribution of fluid flow to the transport of small solutes is very much smaller than molecular diffusion (Maroudas et al., 1968; Maroudas, 1980). Recently, more data have been obtained, relevant to this question and these will now be briefly reviewed.

By defining the mean transport coefficient $\bar{D}(H)$ see previous section) and determining it under given physiological conditions, its value can be compared to that of the diffusion coefficient and this will yield a measure of the relative contributions of fluid flow and molecular diffusion to the transport of various solutes. Since the diffusivities of common small solutes range between $3 \times 10^{-6}$ and $6 \times 10^{-6}$ cm$^2 \cdot$ s$^{-1}$ (as summarized by Maroudas, 1980) whereas the transport coefficients range between $2 \times 10^{-8}$ and $2 \times 10^{-7}$ (Urban, 1977; Urban and Maroudas, 1980a,b), it follows that the contribution of fluid flow will be one to two orders of magnitude less than that of molecular diffusion. On the other hand, as far as larger solutes are concerned (such as serum albumin, for instance), the diffusion coefficients are of the order of $10^{-7}$ cm$^2 \cdot$ s$^{-1}$ (Maroudas, 1976) and hence, about the same order of magnitude as the transport coefficients $\overline{D(H)}$. Thus, in the case of the larger solutes, fluid flow may play an important part in their transport through the matrix.

The above predictions were tested experimentally both in vivo and in vitro. In vivo verification involved the following experiments which are described later in more detail in the chapter by Urban and Holm. In essence, radioactively labelled sulfate was injected intravenously a few hours before sacrifice into two groups of dogs: one group was left anesthetized until death whereas the other group was exercised throughout the period between tracer introduction and death. Tracer profiles were then analyzed and compared. Concentration profiles were also calculated on the assumption of one-dimensional diffusion from the periphery of the annulus as well as from the end plate in the region of the nucleus (Urban, 1977). Where the assumption of one-dimensional diffusion was justified, i.e., in the outer annulus (from the periphery of the disc) and in the nucleus (from the bone–disc interface), the experimental points lie close to the predicted profiles for both groups of dogs. Moreover there was no significant difference between the two sets of experimental results in any region of the disc (Fig. 3.9).

Although the load distribution is clearly different in dogs and humans, the stresses on the dog's spine must be larger during load-bearing and exercise than when the dogs are lying anesthetized. The fact that no difference in the distribution of radioactively labelled sulfate was observed between the two groups of dogs implies that load-bearing and

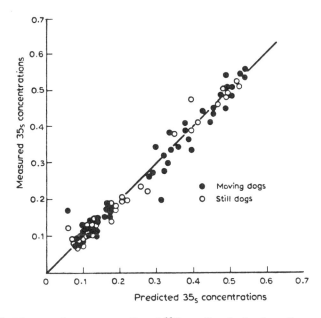

**Figure 3.9.** Measured versus predicted $^{35}$S profiles in lumbar discs of still and moving dogs. (From JPG Urban et al., 1982.)

hence fluid flow has little effect on intradiscal transport of a small solute such as the sulfate ion.

The reason for using discs rather than articular cartilage in in vivo experiments is that the latter is too thin to yield concentration profiles within the minimum practicable time intervals. However, for in vitro experiments, human articular cartilage from the femoral head and femoral condyles were used (O'Hara, Maroudas, Urban, Tomlinson, unpublished observations). Cartilage plugs were subjected to cyclic loading and rates of movement of radioactively labelled serum albumin and potassium iodide were measured by the desorption technique (Maroudas, 1976). Similar experiments were carried out in the absence of loading. When the two sets of results were compared, there was no difference between the rates of desorption with and without cyclic loading of a small solute (potassium iodide), but cyclic loading significantly increased the rate of transport of a large solute, serum albumin (Fig. 3.10). This result was consistent with our theoretical predictions.

In conclusion, transport of small solutes (simple nutrients such as oxygen, glucose, amino acids) is chiefly dependent on diffusion and is practically independent of fluid flow and hence of mechanical compression. On the other hand, fluid flow significantly contributes to the supply of large solutes such as hormones, enzymes and their inhibitors or activators.

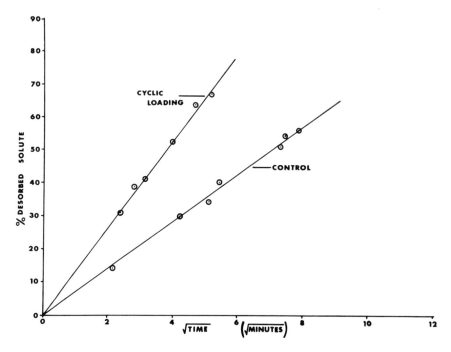

**Figure 3.10.** Rate of movement of radioactively labelled serum albumin in a specimen of cartilage, in the presence and absence of cyclic loading. Rate of transport expressed as percentage of desorbed solute versus square root of time.

## Comparison of the Properties of Cartilage and Disc with Those of Other Connective Tissues

Table 3.2 presents hydration and glycosaminoglycan content of some connective tissues with corresponding swelling pressure, hydraulic permeability and approximate pore size. Cartilage and disc lie at one end of the spectrum with the highest GAG concentration, lowest pore size and hydraulic permeability and highest swelling pressure, whereas the vitreous humor lies at the opposite end, with the lowest GAG content, highest pore size and hydraulic permeability and lowest osmotic pressure. Although the variation in some of the properties from vitreous humor to cartilage spans over several orders of magnitude, these changes correlate with, and are predicted from, the differences in glycosaminoglycan content. It should therefore be stressed that fluid transport in connective tissues (whether they are like Wharton's jelly, or load-bearing and stiff, like articular cartilage) takes place through the pores of the proteoglycan–water gel filling the matrix of the tissue, and should therefore be studied in relation to this porous gel.

**Table 3.2.** Comparison between different connective tissues with respect to hydration, glycosaminoglycan content, swelling pressure, flow characteristics, and pore size

| Tissue | Hydration (wt of water g dry weight$^{-1}$) | Glycosaminoglycan content (% wet weight) | Swelling pressure | Hydraulic permeability (cm$^3$ s · g$^{-1}$) | Pore size (Å) |
|---|---|---|---|---|---|
| Articular cartilage disc [1-4] | 2–4 | 2–6 | 0.5–3 atm | $10^{-13}$–$10^{-12}$ | 20–60[a] |
| Cornea[5-7] | 3.4 | 1–2 | 60 mm Hg | $10^{-12}$–$10^{-11}$ | 150 |
| Wharton's jelly[8] | 5.6 | 0.5 | 4 mm Hg[b] | | 200[c] |
| Vitreous humour[9] | — | 0.05 | of the order of mm $H_2O$ | $10^{-8}$ | 4000 |

[a] Depending on GAG content and method of determining pore size.
[b] This does not include the protein contribution, which is about 6 mm Hg.
[c] From globular protein exclusion data.
Refs: [1] Maroudas, 1979; [2] Maroudas and Bannon, 1981; [3] Byers et al., 1983; [4] Urban and Maroudas, 1980a,b; [5] Hedbys et al., 1963; [6] Fatt, 1968; [7] Friedman and Green, 1971; [8] Meyer, 1983; [9] Fatt, 1977.

## Summary

Creep and swelling of cartilaginous tissues are analyzed in terms of swelling pressure and hydraulic permeability. The latter parameters are closely dependent on the chemical composition of the tissues. Experimental data are given relating the variations in transport properties to hydration and fixed charge density. Properties of cartilage and intervertebral disc are compared with each other and with those of other connective tissues.

## Acknowledgment

This work was partially supported by a grant from the Technion VPR Fund-H. Gutwirth Fund whose help is gratefully acknowledged.

## References

Benninghoff A (1924). Experimentalle Untersuchungen uber den Einfluss verschiedenarung auf den Knorpel, *Verh Anat Ges (Jena)* 33:194–200.
Brocklehurst R, Bayliss MT, Maroudas A, Coysh HL, Obst D, Freeman MR, Revell PA and Ali SY (1984). The composition of normal and osteoarthritic articular cartilage from human knee joints. *J Bone Joint Surg* 66A:95–106.
Byers PD, Bayliss MT, Maroudas A, Urban J and Weightman B (1983). Hypothesising about joints. In: *Studies in Joint Disease, Vol. 2*, A Maroudas and J Holborow (eds.) London: Pitman Medical, pp. 241–276.
Crank J (1975). *Mathematics of Diffusion.* London and New York: Oxford University Press (Clarendon).

Elmore SM, Sokoloff L, Norris G and Carmeci P (1963). Nature of imperfect elasticity of articular cartilage. *J Appl Physiol* 18:393–396.

Fatt I (1968). Dynamics of water transport in the corneal stroma. *Exp Eye Res* 7:402–412.

Fatt I (1977). Hydraulic flow conductivity of the vitreous gel. *Invest Opthalmol* 16:565–568.

Fatt I and Goldstick TK (1965). Dynamics of water transport in swelling membranes. *S Colloid Sci* 20:962–989.

Ficat C and Maroudas A (1975). Cartilage of the patella. *Ann Rheum Dis* 34:515–519.

Freeman WDSC and Maroudas A (1975). Charged group behaviour in cartilage proteoglycans in relation to pH. *Ann Rheum Dis* 34 (Suppl 1): 44–46.

Friedman MH and Green K (1971). Ion binding and Donnan equilibria in rabbit corneal stroma. *Am J Physiol* 221:356–363.

Hedbys BO, Mishima S and Maurice DM (1963). The imbibition pressure of corneal stroma. *Exp Eye Res* 2:99–111.

Holm S, Maroudas A, Urban J, Selstam G and Nachemson A (1981). Nutrition of the intervertebral disc: solute transport and metabolism. Part 1: Oxygen uptake and lactic acid production in the canine disc. Part 2: Oxygen and lactate concentration profiles. *Connect Tissue Res* 8:101–119.

Katz EP, Wachtel EJ and Maroudas A (1985). Extrafibrillar proteoglycans osmotically regulate the molecular packing of collagen in cartilage. *Nature*, submitted.

Linn FC and Sokoloff L (1965). Movement and composition of interstitial fluid of cartilage. *Arthritis Rheum* 8:481–494.

Mansour JM and Mow VC (1976). Permeability of articular cartilage under compressive strain at high pressures. *J Bone Joint Surg (Am)* 58:509–516.

Maroudas A (1968). Physico-chemical properties of cartilage in the light of ion exchange theory. *Biophys J* 8:575–594.

Maroudas A (1974). Transport through articular cartilage and some physiological implications: In: *Normal and Osteoarthrotic Articular Cartilage.* SY Ali, MW Elves and DH Leaback (eds.), London: Institute of Orthopaedics, pp. 33–45.

Maroudas A (1975a). Fluid transport in cartilage. *Ann Rheum Dis* 34 (Suppl. 2): 77–81.

Maroudas A (1975b). Biophysical properties of cartilaginous tissues, with special reference to solute and fluid transport. *Biorheology* 12:233–247.

Maroudas A (1976). Transport of large solutes through cartilage. *J Anat* 122:335–347.

Maroudas A (1979). Physico-chemical properties of articular cartilage. In: *Adult Articular Cartilage,* 2nd ed. MAR Freeman (ed.), London: Pitman Medical, pp. 215–290.

Maroudas A (1980). Physical chemistry of articular cartilage and the intervertebral disc. In: *The Joints and Synovial Fluid II.* L Sokoloff (ed.). New York: Academic Press, pp. 240–293.

Maroudas A and Bannon C (1981). Measurement of swelling pressure in cartilage and comparison with the osmotic pressure of constituent proteoglycans. *Biorheology* 18:619–632.

Maroudas A, Bayliss M and Venn M (1980). Further studies in the chemical composition of femoral head cartilage. *Ann Rheum Dis* 39:514–523.

Maroudas A, Bullough P, Swanson SAV and Freeman MAR (1968). The permeability of articular cartilage. *J Bone Joint Surg (Br)* 50:166–177.

Maroudas A, Muir H and Wingham J (1969). The correlation of fixed negative charge with glycosaminoglycan content of human articular cartilage. *Biochim Biophys Acta* 177:492–500.

Maroudas A and Thomas H (1970). A simple physico-chemical micromethod for determining fixed anionic groups in connective tissue. *Biochim Biophys Acta* 215:214–216.

Maroudas A and Urban JPG (1980). Swelling pressure in articular cartilage and the intervertebral disc. In *Studies in Joint Disease, Vol. 1*. A Maroudas and J Holborow (eds.). London: Pitman Medical, pp. 87–116.

Maroudas A and Urban JPG (1983). Proprietes Biochimiques et Biophysiques du Disque Lombaire Normal et Pathologique. In *Lombalgies et Medecine de Reeducation* L Simon and JP Rabourdin (eds.). Paris: Masson.

Maroudas A, Ziv I, Weisman N and Venn M (1985). Studies of hydration and swelling pressure in normal and osteoarthritic cartilage. *Biorheology* 22:159–169.

McCutchen CW (1962). The frictional properties of animal joints. *Wear* 5:1–17.

McKibbin B and Maroudas A (1979). Nutrition and metabolism. In: *Adult Articular Cartilage*, 2nd ed. MAR Freeman (ed.). London: Pitman Medical, pp. 461–486.

Meyer F (1983). Macromolecular basis of globular protein exclusion and of swelling pressure in loose connective tissue. *Biochim Biophys Acta* 755:388–399.

Mow VC, Kuei SC, Lai WM and Armstrong CG (1980). Biphasic creep and stress relaxation of articular cartilage: theory and experiments. *J Biomech Eng* 102:73–84.

Mow VC and Lai WM (1979). Mechanics of animal joints. *Annu Rev Fluid Mech* 11:247–288.

Muir H, Bullough P and Maroudas A (1970). The distribution of collagen in human articular cartilage with some of its physiological implications. *J Bone Joint Surg* 52B:554–563.

Mulholland R, Millington PF and Manners J (1975). Some aspects on the mechanical behaviour of articular cartilage. *Ann Rheum Dis* 34 (Suppl. 2): 104–107.

Nachemson A and Elfström G (1970). Intravital dynamic pressure measurements in lumbar discs. *Scand J Rehab Med Vols 1 and 2*, (Suppl. 1): pp. 5–40.

Rosenberg L (1974). Structure of cartilage proteoglycans. In: *Dynamics of Connective Tissue Macromolecules*. PMC Burleigh and AR Poole (eds.). Amsterdam: North-Holland. pp. 105–128.

Sokoloff L (1966). Elasticity of aging cartilage. *Fed Proc* 25:1089–1095.

Stockwell RA and Meachim G (1973). The Chondrocytes. In: *Adult Articular Cartilage 1st ed.* MAR Freeman (ed.). London: Pitman Medical. pp. 51–99.

Thornton W, Hoffler GW and Rummel JA (1974). Anthropometric changes and fluid shifts. *Proc. Skylab Life Sciences Symposium*. RS Johnson and LF Dietlein (eds.). Houston, Texas: NASA, pp. 637–658 (TM-58154).

Urban JPG (1977). *Fluid and Solute Transport in the Intervertebral Disc*. Ph.D. Thesis, London University, pp. 159–206.

Urban JPG, Holm S and Maroudas A (1978). Diffusion of small solutes into the intervertebral disc. *Biorheology* 15:203–223.

Urban JPG, Holm S, Maroudas A and Nachemson A (1982). Nutrition of the intervertebral disc—effect of fluid flow on solute transport. *Clin Orthop* 170:296–302.

Urban JPG and Maroudas A (1979). Measurement of fixed charge density in the intervertebral disc. *Biochim Biophys Acta* 586:166–178.

Urban JPG and Maroudas A (1980*a*). Measurement of swelling pressures and fluid flow in the intervertebral disc with reference to creep. In: *Engineering Aspects of the Spine*. Institute of Mechanical Engineers Conference Publications, pp. 63–69.

Urban JPG and Maroudas A (1980*b*). The chemistry of the intervertebral disc in relation to its physiological function and requirements. *Clin Rheum Dis* 6:51–76.

Urban JPG, Maroudas A, Bayliss MT and Dillon J (1979). Swelling pressures of proteoglycans at the concentrations found in cartilaginous tissues. *Biorheology* 16:447–464.

Urban JPG, and McMullin JF (1985) Swelling pressure of the intervertebral disc: influence of proteoglycan and collagen contents. *Biorheology* 22:145–157.

Venn, MF and Maroudas A (1977). Chemical composition and swelling of normal and osteoarthritic femoral head cartilage. I. Chemical Composition. *Ann Rheum Dis* 36:121–129 and II. Swelling. *Ann Rheum Dis* 36:399–406.

Weightman B and Kempson G (1979). Load Carriage. In: *Adult Articular Cartilage*, 2nd ed. MAR Freeman (ed.). London: Pitman Medical. pp. 291–331.

Wells JD (1973). Salt activity and osmotic pressure in connective tissue. *Proc R Soc Lon Ser B* 183:399–419.

CHAPTER 4

# Compression Effects on Cartilage Permeability

Mark H. Holmes, W. Michael Lai, and
Van C. Mow

## Introduction

To be able to understand the mechanics of normal synovial joints and the
dysfunction of articular cartilage during degenerate joint disease, it is
necessary to understand the biomechanical properties of articular cartilage and its normal function within the joint (Sokoloff, 1969; Freeman and
Meachim, 1979; Mow and Lai, 1980). It is for this reason that early investigators—Bär (1926), Göcke (1927), Hirsch (1944), and Sokoloff (1966)—
as well as more recent ones—Kempson and co-workers (1971), Coletti
and co-workers (1972), and Parsons and Black (1977), have studied the in
situ indentability of articular cartilage. These indentation experiments
have led to the general acceptance that the principal deformational character of articular cartilage is viscoelastic (on sudden application of an
indenting load, the tissue exhibits an instantaneous elastic response that is
followed by a slow creep that gradually reaches an equilibrium value).
However, Sokoloff and co-workers showed that after removal of the load
complete recovery of the tissue is obtained only if it is submerged in a
bath of fluid (Elmore et al., 1963; Sokoloff, 1963), and that the ionic
concentration within the bath substantially influences the creep indentability of the tissue (Sokoloff, 1963; Parsons and Black, 1979). Linn and
Sokoloff (1965) showed remarkable similarities between creep deformation
curves and fluid exudation curves for cartilage under static compression.
Further, Hayes and Mockros (1971) observed that the magnitude of the
creep displacement of the tissue in uniaxial confined compression depends on the permeability of the tissue. Motivated by these and other
studies, in recent years we have extensively examined, theoretically and
experimentally, this flow-dependent viscoelastic behavior of various human, bovine and porcine cartilages of nasal and articular tissues (Mow
and Lai, 1980; Mow et al., 1980; Lai et al., 1981; Armstrong and Mow,
1982b). In this study, we present results of our investigation concerning
the influence of the nonlinear permeability function (Lai and Mow, 1980;

Mow and Lai, 1980) on the stress-relaxation behavior of cartilage under compression.

It is evident, even from the earliest studies, that to obtain a viable model to describe the deformational behavior of articular cartilage, it is necessary to account for both the solid and fluid components of the tissue. Accordingly, Mow and co-workers (1980) formulated a biphasic model for articular cartilage which includes the flow of the interstitial fluid as well as the deformation of the solid phase of the tissue. Over the last few years this model and the biphasic concept were used to describe the deformational characteristics of cartilage in a variety of tests, such as in compressive stress relaxation (Lai et al., 1981), compressive creep (Armstrong and Mow, 1982b), and tensile stress relaxation (Grodzinsky et al., 1981). Moreover, because the biphasic theory uncouples the compressional behavior of the solid matrix and fluid flow, it can be used to assess the mechanical properties of the organic solid matrix of articular cartilage ("intrinsic" compressive properties of the organic matrix: Mow and Lai, 1980; Armstrong and Mow, 1982a). Because of these factors, it is now possible to assess the influence of cartilage composition and molecular structure on the deformational behavior of the solid organic matrix. Of course, more general multiphasic theories can be adapted to account for the influence of mobile electrolytes in the interstitial fluid on various observed electromechanical and mechanochemical transduction effects in the organic solid matrix of cartilage.

## Structural and Physicochemical Aspects of Cartilage Deformation

Comprehensive descriptions of the composition and ultrastructure (Sokoloff, 1969; Freeman and Meachim, 1979) and mechanical behavior (Mow and Lai, 1980; Mow et al., 1982) of articular cartilage are available. We shall only mention, rather briefly, how some of the constituents can effect the biomechanical response of the tissue.

In normal articular cartilage, the interactions of collagen and proteoglycans with themselves and with each other provide sufficient cohesiveness to create a composite solid organic matrix. At the same time, the propensity of the hydrophilic proteoglycans to expand and occupy a large solution volume makes this solid matrix a microporous structure filled with fluid (Fig. 4.1). The architecture of the collagen network and proteoglycan aggregates provides the fine meshwork, with a "pore" size range of 10 to 60 Å as estimated by a straight-tube Poiseuille model, through which the interstitial fluid flows (Lai and Mow, 1980). The size of these molecular "pores" is important in the function of the extracellular matrix in that by steric exclusion, they restrict passage of large molecules, for example, infiltration of enzymes into the interior of the tissue (Maroudas, 1979).

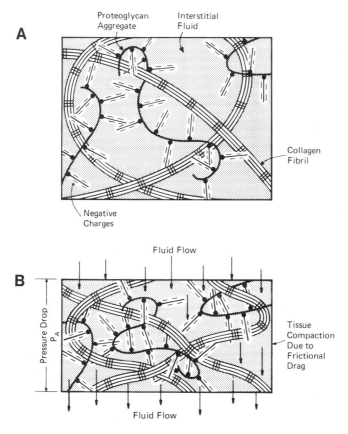

**Figure 4.1. A:** Schematic representation of the microporous proteoglycan–collagen solid matrix filled with interstitial fluid. **B:** The applied pressure gradient $P_A$ caused by fluid flow across the specimen. The frictional drag of permeation exerted by the fluid onto the solid compacts the tissue. (From Lai and Mow, 1980.)

Even though the "pores" are very small, interstitial water makes up 65% to 85% of the total tissue mass by wet weight; collagen makes up 50% to 70% and proteoglycans make up 20% to 30% of the organic matrix by dry weight. Importantly, the relative composition of the tissue plays a dominant role in governing its mechanical deformational properties (Kempson, 1979; Armstrong and Mow, 1982a; Stahurski et al., 1981; Armstrong and Mow, 1982b).

Each constituent of cartilage produces a special set of mechanical properties. The tensile stiffness of the matrix is derived primarily from intrinsic collagen fibril properties and collagen cross-linking strength and, secondarily, from collagen-proteoglycan interactions. The compressive properties arise primarily from the physicochemical properties and structural rigidity of the immobilized proteoglycans within the collagen network, whereas the shear properties of the matrix are believed to be primarily dependent on the collagen content and collagen–proteoglycan interactions within the matrix (Hayes and Bodine, 1978; Mow et al., 1982; Mow et al., 1983).

To support these concepts, we recently reported a number of definitive experimental findings on the relationship of the aggregate equilibrium compressive modulus, $H_A$, and hydraulic permeability of the solid matrix with both the water content and uronic acid content of the tissue (Armstrong and Mow, 1982a,b). These intrinsic matrix properties are predominantly dependent on these two compositional variables. Moreover, recent shear experiments to determine the viscometric properties of proteoglycan monomer and aggregate solutions, in concentrations similar to those found in situ ($\sim$50 mg/ml), reported that the magnitude of the complex shear modulus was $10^4$ times less than that of whole tissue (Armstrong et al., 1981; Mak et al., 1982). Thus, the proteoglycan aggregates apparently do not provide significant shear resistance, but rather interact with the collagen network to produce a solid matrix with significant shear strength. In situ disaggregation, with little or no depletion of proteoglycans, dramatically decreases the magnitude of the complex shear modulus of the matrix as well as the intrinsic compressive Young's modulus (Mow et al., 1983). In other words, proteoglycan and collagen form a fiber-reinforced composite solid whose shear rigidity is maintained by the spatial framework of the collagen ultrastructure that can sustain the tensile strains induced by the shear deformations (Hayes and Bodine, 1978; Mow et al., 1983). Hence, the compressive stiffness of the solid matrix is ultimately derived not only from the closely spaced, negatively charged sulfate and carboxyl groups on the glycosaminoglycans and the associated Donnan osmotic effect, but from the resistance to bulk compression and shear of the neutral composite proteoglycan–collagen solid matrix as well. An appreciation of these structural effects is important because they form the conceptual basis of the biphasic fluid–solid mixture theory for articular cartilage.

The physicochemical characteristics of counter-ions within the interstitial fluid (valency and concentration) also have profound effects on the response of articular cartilage to imposed stresses and strains (Sokoloff, 1963; Maroudas, 1979; Grodzinsky et al., 1981; Mow et al., 1981). For example, an increase of interstitial $Na^+$ concentration causes a charge-shielding effect on the closely spaced ($\sim$5–15 Å) anionic groups of the glycosaminoglycans; that, in turn, causes the proteoglycans to contract from their extended solution volume (Pasternack et al., 1974). Macroscopically, this produces a measurable shrinkage in tissue size and a decrease in tissue mass caused by the decrease in tissue fluid content. Recent experimental and theoretical evidence shows that the modulation of intra- and intermolecular electrostatic repulsion forces, by the proteoglycan charge groups (Grodzinsky et al., 1981) and/or disruption of collagen–proteoglycan electrostatic interactions (Muir, 1979) by changes in the counter-ion environment in the interstitial fluid, affect both tensile (Mow et al., 1981) and compressive (Maroudas, 1979) properties of the tissue. Thus, techniques must be devised that can assess both the movement of interstitial fluid and rates of ion transport in situ. Further, these techniques should be applicable in ranges of pressure and deformation experienced by cartilage in vivo, since it is known that high pressures and compressive strain do dramatically decrease the hydraulic permeability and diffusion coefficients of articular cartilage (Mansour and Mow, 1976; Lai and Mow, 1980; Mow and Lai, 1980; Mow et al., 1980). This chapter is concerned only with the development of a method to assess the nonlinear, strain-dependent permeability parameters by using the observed mechanical, biphasic, stress–relaxation phenomenon that articular cartilage exhibits during compression. Later, these fluid flow phenomena will be coupled with ion diffusion mass transfer effects to develop a comprehensive multiphasic theory for articular cartilage.

## A Biphasic Model of Articular Cartilage

The mechanical behavior of articular cartilage can be understood best by considering it as a multiphasic continuum. The two principal phases are the solid matrix phase, which is composed predominantly of proteoglycan macromolecules and collagen fibrils, and the movable interstitial fluid phase, which is predominantly water (see Fig. 4.1). The deformational behavior of cartilage is strongly dependent not only on the mechanical properties of the deforming solid matrix in the mixture, but also on the flow of the interstitial fluid through the matrix. Therefore, at the very least, cartilage should be modeled as a biphasic material.

The biphasic model for articular cartilage formulated by Mow and co-workers (Mow and Lai, 1980; Mow et al., 1980) is based on the mixture theory of Craine and co-workers (1970) and Bowen (1976). In essence, this model depicts articular cartilage as a soft, porous and permeable, elastic solid that is filled with interstitial fluid. Assuming that both phases are intrinsically incompressible, the continuity equation for this binary mixture is:

$$\text{div } \mathbf{v}^f + \alpha \text{div } \mathbf{v}^s + \alpha(\mathbf{v}^s - \mathbf{v}^f) \cdot \text{grad } \ln \rho^s = 0, \tag{1}$$

where $\mathbf{v}^s$ and $\mathbf{v}^f$ are the velocities of the fluid phase and the solid phase, respectively, and $\rho^s$ is the apparent density of the solid. The coefficient $\alpha$ is defined as the solid content, which is given by the ratio of solidity ($V^s/V^T$) to porosity ($V^f/V^T$) of the tissue. Here $V^s$, $V^f$ and $V^T$ are the solid, fluid and total volume of the tissue, respectively. The momentum balance equations for the two components of the mixture, omitting inertial forces, are:

$$\operatorname{div} \boldsymbol{\sigma}^s - K(\mathbf{v}^s - \mathbf{v}^f) = \mathbf{0}, \tag{2a}$$

and

$$\operatorname{div} \boldsymbol{\sigma}^f + K(\mathbf{v}^s - \mathbf{v}^f) = \mathbf{0}, \tag{2b}$$

where $\boldsymbol{\sigma}^s$ and $\boldsymbol{\sigma}^f$ are the stress tensors for the solid and fluid phases, respectively. The second term in Eqs. (2) represents the diffusive drag arising from the relative velocities between the fluid and solid components. Even in the unloaded state, the diffusive coefficient $K$ has values on the order of $10^{15}$ N · s/m$^4$, which helps explain why the inertia terms are omitted in Eqs. (2) (Mow et al., 1980). Under slow flow conditions, the diffusive coefficient is related to the permeability k of the tissue by the inverse relation (Lai and Mow, 1980):

$$k = \frac{1}{K(1 + \alpha)^2}. \tag{3}$$

In our (Kuei, Lai and Mow or "KLM") version of the biphasic model for articular cartilage, the solid phase is assumed to be elastic and the interstitial fluid is inviscid (Mow and Lai, 1980; Mow et al., 1980). Accordingly, assuming small strains, the isotropic stress–strain relationship for the first-order theory for the solid phase is:

$$\boldsymbol{\sigma}^s = -\alpha p\mathbf{I} + \lambda_s \mathbf{e}\mathbf{I} + 2\mu_s\mathbf{e} \tag{4a}$$

and for the fluid phase it is:

$$\boldsymbol{\sigma}^f = -p\mathbf{I}, \tag{4b}$$

where $p$ is the apparent fluid pressure, $\lambda_s$ and $\mu_s$ are the elastic moduli of the solid matrix in the mixture and $\mathbf{e}$ is the infinitesimal strain tensor describing the deformation of the solid matrix. It is also assumed that the tissue is spatially homogeneous, so $\lambda_s$ and $\mu_s$ are constants.

Because of the generality of the formulation of our biphasic model, other terms can be included in the linearized constitutive laws, Eqs. (4), which can incorporate, for example, a viscoelastic solid matrix, diffusive couples and capillary forces. Also, the isotropic case is presented here, but formulas for the more general case of biphasic anisotropic stress–strain laws are available elsewhere (Mow et al., 1980). The significant anisotropic structure of cartilage, as manifested, for example, in split-line patterns, or anisotropic tensile properties (Woo et al., 1976; Kempson, 1979; Roth and Mow, 1980), have not been pursued in deference toward the simpler isotropic biphasic theory, which is aimed at the historical need for elucidating the role of fluid motion in the observed viscoelastic creep and stress–relaxation behavior of cartilage during compression (Bär, 1926; Coletti et al., 1972; Elmore et al., 1963; Göcke, 1927; Hirsch, 1944;

Sokoloff, 1963, 1966; Linn and Sokoloff, 1965; Hayes and Mockros, 1971; Kempson et al., 1971; Parsons and Black, 1977, 1979). Other generalizations, such as finite deformation of the solid matrix, can also be undertaken using the existing general biphasic theory. However, we find that even with the restrictive assumptions embodied in Eqs. (4), our resulting biphasic model of articular cartilage (Mow and Lai, 1980) adequately describes the observed creep and stress–relaxation behavior in compression under isothermal and constant electrolytic conditions. For convenience, we refer to this as the linear KLM model for cartilage (Mow and Lai, 1980).

It should be emphasized, however, that the biphasic assumptions of the linear KLM model are only approximately correct. For example, Hayes and Bodine (1978) and Mow and co-workers (1983) found that, in shear, the tissue is slightly viscoelastic, with a small phase angle $\delta$ bounded by $0.10 < \tan \delta < 0.35$, so a more accurate model of articular cartilage should include terms to describe the intrinsic viscoelastic behavior of the solid matrix. However, we believe that in compression the predominant mechanism giving rise to the observed viscoelastic behavior of the cartilage can be attributed to the diffusive drag caused by the interstitial fluid flowing through the solid matrix, and not to the viscoelastic properties of the solid matrix itself. In any case, with these assumptions, the task remains to determine the diffusive coefficient $K$ and elastic constants $\lambda_s$, $\mu_s$ of the KLM model for articular cartilage, to test the accuracy and general applicability of the model, and to see how the constants are affected by changes in the structural integrity and composition of the tissue.*

## Permeation Experiment

The movement of interstitial fluid through cartilage plays a fundamental role in controlling the mechanical response of the tissue, the lubrication between the two articulating surfaces and the transport of nutrients and biological viability of the tissue itself (Honner and Thompson, 1971; Ogata et al., 1978; Salter et al., 1980). Consequently, the permeability of the tissue, as it is a macroscopic measure of the ease with which fluid flows through the 10Å to 60 Å interstices of the matrix, has received considerable attention in the cartilage literature (Edwards, 1967; Maroudas et al., 1968; Maroudas, 1970, 1975, 1979; Mansour and Mow, 1976; Lai and Mow, 1980; Torzilli et al., 1982). The approach in each of these studies is basically the same: taking, say, a cylindrical disc of cartilage that is removed from the bone and forcing fluid to flow through the specimen by applying a direct fluid pressure $P_A$ across the tissue. For one-

---

* Henceforth, the superscripts and the subscript s will be dropped for convenience.

dimensional flows through a sample of thickness $h$, the apparent permeability $k_a$ that is measured in these experiments is determined using Darcy's law, which states that:

$$k_a = \frac{Qh}{AP_A},$$ (5)

where $Q$ is the volume flux of permeated fluid through a surface area $A$ of the cartilage. The difficulty in determining the permeability for soft biological tissues with this procedure is that the permeation process could give rise to a drag force (that force exerted by the fluid on the solid as it flows through the tissue) of significant magnitude to compact the soft, permeable solid matrix in a nonuniform manner (see Fig. 4.1). This compaction would decrease the permeability within the tissue, and the decrease would vary with the distance from the surface, making the measured value of $k_a$ an average, lumped-parameter value. This effect is particularly important for soft tissues such as articular cartilage where substantial compaction of the matrix can easily occur. Experimentally, this is manifested by the dependence of $k_a$ on the driving pressure $P_A$ that was first observed for articular cartilage by Mansour and Mow (1976).

To separate the effects of direct compression, i.e., the clamping strain of magnitude $\varepsilon_c$, used to hold the specimen discs in the permeation experiment, and applied pressure $P_A$, Mow and co-workers (1980) obtained a detailed family of permeability curves $k_a(\varepsilon_c; P_A)$ with $P_A$ as the parameter. In doing this, it was empirically demonstrated that there is an exponential decrease of the permeability function with $\varepsilon_c$. Permeability decreases as a function of $\varepsilon_c$ for various parametric values of the constant pressure gradient $P_A$ used to maintain steady permeation. The empirical exponential law used to curve-fit these data is:

$$k_a = A(P_A) \exp[-\alpha(P_A)\varepsilon_c].$$ (6a)

To eliminate the dependence of the permeability on $P_A$, Lai and Mow (1980) introduced the concept of intrinsic permeability $k$ defined as:

$$k = \lim_{P_A \to 0} k_a(\varepsilon_c, P_A) = k_0 \exp(M\varepsilon),$$ (6b)

where $k_0 = A(0)$, $M = \alpha(0)$ and $\varepsilon = -\varepsilon_c$ is the dilatation field. The coefficient $M$ has been defined as the nonlinear flow-limiting parameter for soft tissues such as cartilage (Lai et al., 1981). It is important to note that this function is defined only in the theoretical limit $P_A \to 0$ and may be obtained parametrically from Fig. 4.2A by extrapolating to the limit. To verify the intrinsic permeability concept, one must be able to predict the explicit function for Eq. (6a) from Eq. (6b) from a model for the steady permeation experiment or from another totally different experiment utilizing the concept of intrinsic permeability. In this chapter, we wish to utilize the dependence of compressional viscoelastic behavior of articular cartilage on the flow of interstitial fluid (in particular, the compressive stress–relaxation phenomenon) to assess $k_0$ and $M$ and to compare them with those obtained from a model of the steady permeation experiment.

## Nonlinear Theory for Steady Permeation

With the empirical determination of the functional dependence of the permeability on the strain, we now consider how well the resulting nonlinear KLM biphasic model compares with the steady experimental results for permeation of cartilage. At the same time the values for the permeability constants $k_0$ and $M$ will be obtained.

Let us consider a typical one-dimensional filtration experiment, in the $z$-direction, where a cylindrical plug of tissue, ~200 $\mu$m in thickness and 6.35 mm in diameter, is tested. The constitutive equations, Eqs. (4.4), for the stress in the cartilage in this case reduce to:

$$\sigma_{zz} = -\alpha p + H_A \frac{du}{dz} \tag{7a}$$

and

$$\sigma_{zz}^f = -p, \tag{7b}$$

where $u$ denotes the $z$-component of the displacement of the solid matrix and the aggregate equilibrium compressive modulus, $H_A = \lambda_s + 2\mu_s$. For the steady permeation experiments, where a constant pressure drop $P_A$ is applied across the specimen, the fluid velocity $V$ is constant. With this and Eqs. (7), the equations of motion, Eqs. (2), for the biphasic mixture become:

$$H_A \frac{d^2u}{dz^2} = -\frac{V}{k_0(1 + \alpha)} \exp\left(-M \frac{du}{dz}\right), \tag{8a}$$

and

$$\frac{dp}{dz} = -\frac{V}{k_0(1 + \alpha)^2} \exp\left(-M \frac{du}{dz}\right). \tag{8b}$$

Integrating these nonlinear ordinary differential equations, the pressure distribution in the cartilage is:

$$p(z) = \frac{H_A}{M(1 + \alpha)} \ln\left[1 - \frac{VM(z - h)}{k_0(1 + \alpha)H_A} \exp\left(\frac{MP_A}{H_A}\right)\right]. \tag{8c}$$

Assuming $P(0) = P_A/(1 + \alpha)$ and $\varepsilon_c = u(0)/h$ (Lai and Mow, 1980), we have from Eq. (5) the predicted apparent permeability function,

$k_a(\varepsilon_c, P_A)$
$$= k_0 \exp[-M(P_T - P_A)/H_A][1 - \exp(-MP_A/H_A)]/(MP_A/H_A), \tag{9a}$$

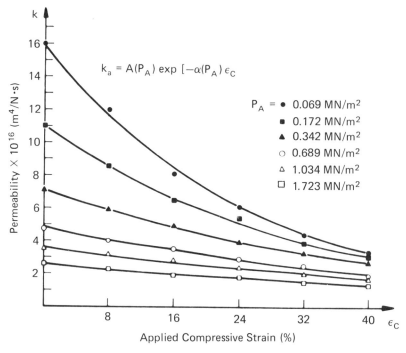

**Figure 4.2. A:** Variation of the apparent permeability $k_a$ with compressive clamping strain $\varepsilon_c$ and parameter $P_A$. (From Mow et al., 1980.)

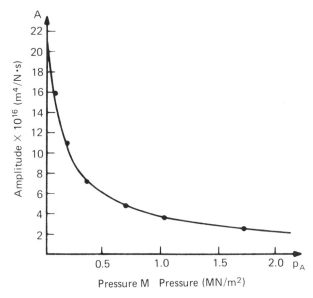

**Figure 4.2. B:** Variation of the amplitude function A as a function of $P_A$. (From Mow et al., 1980.)

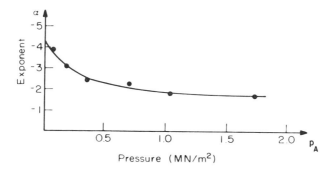

**Figure 4.2. C:** Variation of the decay exponential $\alpha$ with applied pressure $P_A$. Shut-off of permeability is greatest at low pressures and strains. (From Mow et al., 1980.)

where

$$P_T = H_A \left\{ \varepsilon_c + (P_A/H_A)/[1 - \exp(-MP_A/H_A)] - \frac{1}{M} \right\}. \qquad (9b)$$

Here $P_T$ is the total stress borne by the solid matrix at the downstream side supporting filter ($z = h$). The first term in Eq. (9b) is the pressure that results from the clamping strain $\varepsilon_c$, whereas the second and third terms together give that which results from the intrinsic permeability function, Eq. (6b). For the special case where $\varepsilon_c = 0$, from Eqs. (9), the predicted relationship between $k_a$ and $P_A$ is:

$$k_a = \frac{k_0}{(MP_A/H_A)} [1 - \exp(-MP_A/H_A)]. \qquad (9c)$$

Table 4.1 shows the comparison, for the parametric values $k_0 = 1.71 \times 10^{-15}$ m$^4$/N $\cdot$ s and $M = 4.3$, of the predicted values of $k_a$ from Eq. (9c) and the extrapolation of experimental values from Fig. 4.2. This table

**Table 4.1.** A comparison of experimentally obtained apparent permeability and the predicted apparent permeability from our nonlinear permeation theory with $k_0 = 1.7 \times 10^{-15}$m$^4$/N $\cdot$ s and $M$ = 4.3, for various values of applied pressure $P_A$

| $P_A$ | 0.172 | 0.345 | 0.670 | 1.033 | MPa[a] |
|---|---|---|---|---|---|
| $k_a$ (theoretical)[b] | 11.0 | 7.63 | 4.50 | 2.98 | $\times 10^{-16}$m$^4$/N $\cdot$ s |
| $k_a$ (experimental)[c] | 11.0 | 7.20 | 4.70 | 3.60 | $\times 10^{-16}$m$^4$/N $\cdot$ s |

[a] MPa = $10^6$ Pascals.
[b] One-dimensional analysis.
[c] Axisymmetric experiment.

shows that under reasonably small compressive strains, articular cartilage may be regarded as a nonlinearly diffusive biphasic material (Mow and Lai, 1980). Of course, the values of $k_0$ and $M$ were chosen to best-fit the experimental results. Therefore, a totally different, and independent, experimental procedure and theoretical prediction must be developed to ascertain the general validity of our nonlinear intrinsic permeability concept.

## Nonlinear Biphasic Stress Relaxation Theory

The nonlinear permeability of the cartilage has profound effects on the transient viscoelastic behavior of the tissue in compression because of the flow-limiting effects caused by the interaction of the interstitial fluid and solid matrix. One phenomenon that we have used to study these effects, as well as to develop an independent method to determine the permeability constants $k_0$ and $M$, is the observed stress–relaxation response. In these experiments we take cylindrical osteochondral plugs and compress them against a free-draining, rigid porous filter at the articular surface. This allows the fluid to exude freely ($p = 0$ at the surface). From the one-dimensional form of the constitutive equation, Eq. (7a), the compressive stress on the surface is directly related to $\partial u/\partial z$ under these conditions. This fact provides us with the method to control the rate of compression so that the deformation gradients remain within the small strain range, and therefore the theory is valid within the assumptions imposed during its derivation.

The one-dimensional deformation along the axis of the plug in the $z$-direction and the unidirectional flow for the present transient stress–relaxation problem is governed by the following nonlinear diffusion equation (Mow et al., 1982):

$$H_A \frac{\partial^2 u}{\partial z^2} = \frac{1}{k_0} \exp\left(-M \frac{\partial u}{\partial z}\right) \frac{\partial u}{\partial t}. \tag{10a}$$

The articular surface coincides with the $z = 0$ plane, and $z = h$ defines the thickness of the tissue (Fig. 4.3). The interface between the soft uncalcified cartilage and the stiff calcified cartilage is assumed to be rigid and impervious, and so we take

$$u(h, t) = 0. \tag{10b}$$

In our stress relaxation studies, a ramp displacement function is imposed on the articular surface given by:

$$u(0,t) = \begin{cases} V_0 t & 0 \le t \le t_0 \quad \text{(compression phase)} \\ V_0 t_0 & t_0 \le t \quad \text{(relaxation phase)}. \end{cases} \tag{10c}$$

Experimentally, we can control $V_0$, the rate of compression, to within

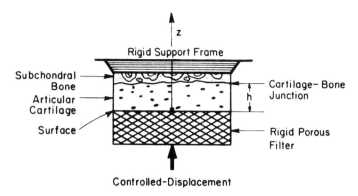

**Figure 4.3.** Model of the one-dimensional, rate-controlled, compression biphasic stress–relaxation experiment.

$0.4\mu$m accuracy per unit time (a unit time may be 20 s) for experiments ranging up to 10,000 s. Also, at the beginning of the experiment we assume

$$u(z,0) = 0. \qquad (10d)$$

That is, the tissue is allowed sufficient time ($\sim$60 min) to equilibrate fully prior to initiation of the compression stress–relaxation experiment.

The formulation of the mathematical problem for the displacement function $u(z,t)$ corresponding to our stress–relaxation experiments is now complete. However, there is no analytical solution to this nonlinear diffusion problem. Thus, it is necessary to use either numerical techniques or approximation methods to find the solution (Holmes, 1982). Before presenting the mathematical analysis of this nonlinear diffusion problem, let us recall the basic flow effects, as predicted from the linear theory, during these stress–relaxation experiments. During the compression phase of the experiment, $t \leq t_0$, fluid flow may be characterized by a massive exudation process across the surface, the highest flow rate occurring in the region of greatest compaction near the surface (Fig. 4.4). During the relaxation phase of the experiment, fluid flow is characterized by internal fluid redistribution as governed by the diffusion equation. Gel diffusion, a term often used by investigators, describes the redistribution and internal relative motion of the matrix and interstitial fluid (Tanaka and Fillmore, 1979; Grodzinsky et al., 1981).

## Asymptotic Analysis of the Nonlinear Biphasic Stress–Relaxation Phenomenon

One method we have employed to find the solution of the diffusion problem, Eqs. (10), makes use of the length of time it takes the deformation to

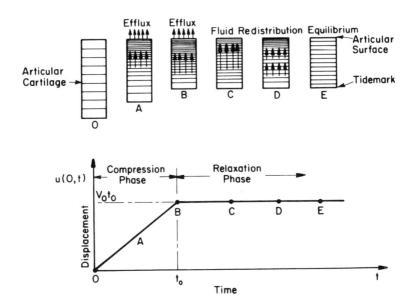

**Figure 4.4.** Schematic representation of fluid exudation and redistribution within cartilage during a rate-controlled, compression stress–relaxation experiment. The *horizontal bars* in the upper figure indicate the distribution of strain in the tissue. The lower graph shows the compression history of the plug of cartilage defined by Eq. (10c). (From Mow et al., 1980.)

diffuse through the cartilage. To assess the character of this movement, let us examine the ideal case of a constant permeability ($M = 0$) and an infinitely deep sample of this material ($h = \infty$). The solution of Eqs. (10) during the compressive stage has the following functional form (Courant and Hilbert, 1962):

$$u(z,t) = V_0 t f\left(\frac{z}{\sqrt{k_0 H_A t}}\right),\qquad(11a)$$

where the function f(s) is defined as

$$f(s) = \left(1 + \frac{1}{2}s^2\right)\text{erfc}\left(\frac{1}{2}s\right) - \frac{s}{\sqrt{\pi}}\exp\left(-\frac{1}{4}s^2\right).\qquad(11b)$$

So, for any given time $t$, $u$ decays exponentially into the linear biphasic medium. Moreover, a diffusive boundary layer exists. This means, at least for small $t$, that the boundary condition at the "tidemark," Eq. (10b), is effectively satisfied by Eqs. (11a). This solution shows that, under the imposed conditions, the largest compressive strains are occurring in the region near the surface. In fact, one can easily show that the strain $\partial u/\partial z$ at the surface, at the end of the compressive stage, is:

$$\frac{\partial u}{\partial z}(0,t_0) = -\frac{2u_0}{\sqrt{\pi k_0 H_A t_0}}, \tag{12a}$$

where $u_0 = V_0 t_0$ represents the final displacement imposed at the surface. Therefore, according to the theory of small strains, even for the linear case of a constant permeability, for fast rates of compression (so $t_0$ is relatively small), the magnitude of the surface strains could become $>100\%$! For the nonlinear permeability case, where flow-induced compaction can be significant, very high values of compression strain can occur with seemingly moderate rates of compression (Lai et al., 1981). This means that for a given $u_0$ there is a minimum time $t_0$ that can be used in these experiments and still remain within the validity of the small strain assumption used in formulating the constitutive relations, Eqs. (4). Based on the values found in the permeation experiments for this nonlinear diffusion problem (see Table 4.1), an equilibrium strain 5% should not be achieved in $<300$ s. This condition is imposed by specifying that the transient compressive strains, whose maximum is at the surface, remain $<0.25$ mm/mm—which we assume can be considered $\ll 1$.

The deformation of the solid matrix, as given by Eqs. (11), does gradually diffuse into the tissue. Since there is a finite thickness, Eqs. (11) will describe the solution only for a certain initial time interval before the diffusion front strikes the distal boundary. Thus, we can use Eqs. (11) as an approximate solution to our finite thickness problem for the case of a constant permeability, provided we specify the magnitude of error we will tolerate. For example, if we specify that the displacement at $z = h$ should be $<10\%$ of the displacement at the articular surface at the instant the compression phase ends, then the following equation must be satisfied:

$$\frac{h}{\sqrt{k_0 H_A t_0}} \geq 2.0. \tag{12b}$$

Under this condition, Eqs. (11) are reasonable approximations to the solution of Eqs. (10) in the linear case of a constant permeability if the rate of compression is such that:

$$t_0 \leq \frac{h^2}{4k_0 H_A}. \tag{12c}$$

We define a stress–relaxation experiment in which Eqs. (12) are satisfied as "fast." In this case, it is possible to take advantage of the diffusive boundary layer, as described above, to solve the nonlinear diffusion problem defined by Eqs. (10) by using an asymptotic expansion procedure. We find that the normal stress $\sigma$ at the articular surface during the compressive stage, $t \leq t_0$ (Holmes, 1982), is given by:

$$\sigma = \sigma_{zz} \sim - V_0 \sqrt{\frac{H_A}{k_0}} \left(2 \sqrt{\frac{t}{\pi}} + b_1 t + b_2 t^{3/2}\right), \qquad (13a)$$

where the constants $b_1$ and $b_2$ are given by:

$$b_1 \equiv \frac{0.386 M V_0}{\sqrt{k_0 H_A}}, \qquad (13b)$$

and

$$b_2 \equiv \frac{0.1796 M^2 V_0^2}{k_0 H_A}. \qquad (13c)$$

The restriction on the parameters for which this approximation is valid is:

$$\varepsilon_0 M \ll \frac{\sqrt{t_0 k_0 H_A}}{h}, \qquad (13d)$$

where $\varepsilon_0$ represents the magnitude of the equilibrium compressive strain imposed in the experiment. For example, based on the values obtained from the permeation experiment, Eqs. (13) describe the stress history for a 5% equilibrium compressive strain that is achieved between 400 and 800 s. This solution for the stress shows that during the initial moments of the compressive stage, the tissue deforms as if the permeability is constant. However, as $t$ increases, the nonlinear interaction between the solid and fluid, Eqs. (6), begins to play a significant role. This is due to the fact that the compaction for the fast rate is confined, principally, to the region near the articular surface and the interstitial fluid must flow past this region during the exudation process. As a consequence of this, the strains in this region are even larger in magnitude, and so is the stress, Eq. (13a), which illustrates the fundamental role of the flow-limiting effects on the deformational behavior of the nonlinearly permeable tissue.

The reverse of the inequality in Eqs. (12) represents what we define as a "slow" rate of compression. The tissue responds during the compressive stage in this case as if it were undergoing a nearly uniform compaction. From an asymptotic expansion (Holmes, 1982), we find that the stress history at the articular surface for these slow rates of compression may be described by:

$$\sigma = \sigma_{zz}(0,t) \sim - \frac{V_0 H_A}{h} (t + c_0 \exp(c_1 t)), \text{ for } \frac{h^2}{k_0 H_A} < t \leq t_0, \quad (14a)$$

where

$$c_0 = \frac{h^2}{3 k_0 H_A}, \qquad (14b)$$

and

$$c_1 = \frac{MV_0}{h}. \tag{14c}$$

Based on known typical permeation values (Lai and Mow, 1980), this expression is valid for experiments in which the compressive stage lasts longer than 1000 s.

For this slow rate it is also relatively easy to determine the solution during the relaxation phase (Holmes, 1982). We find that immediately subsequent to the start of the relaxation process,

$$\sigma = \sigma_{zz}(0,t) \sim \sigma_p - M_r \sqrt{t - t_0}, \text{ for } 0 \le t - t_0 \ll 1, \tag{15a}$$

where $M_r$ and $\sigma_p$ are defined as:

$$M_r \equiv \frac{2h\sigma_\infty}{t_0\sqrt{\pi H_A k_0 \exp(-\varepsilon_0 M)}}, \tag{15b}$$

and

$$\sigma_p \equiv -\frac{V_0 H_A}{h}(t_0 + c_0 \exp(c_1 t_0)). \tag{15c}$$

In other words, at the start of the relaxation phase, the compressive stress decreases as the square root of time from the peak compressive stress $\sigma_p$ achieved at the end of the compressive stage. Here $\sigma_\infty$ denotes the equilibrium compressive stress attained in the limit $t \to \infty$. This solution applies, roughly, to the first 100 s of the relaxation phase (see Fig. 4.7). As time increases, the compressive stress continues to decrease, and in fact it approaches exponentially its equilibrium value of $-\varepsilon_0 H_A$. We recall that stress relaxation occurs because of internal fluid redistribution, which in turn is governed by the lower permeability within the compressed tissue, $k_0 \exp(-\varepsilon_0 M)$, giving rise to a slower rate of relaxation.

## Stress–Relaxation Experiments—Results and Discussion

The two sets of asymptotic solutions, the "fast" rate given by Eqs. (13) and the "slow" rate given by Eqs. (14), provide simple analytical expressions that describe the compression phase of the stress–relaxation experiments. Note that the "fast" and "slow" rates defined here are mathematical rates relative to the rate at which the diffusion front propagates into the cartilage on initiation of compression at the articular surface, Eqs. (10). These "fast" and "slow" rates are defined for material property determinations only and are not used to describe fast and slow physiological rates of loading. We have utilized the slow rate stress history, Eqs. (14) and Eqs. (15), to describe the compressive stress–relaxation experiment. By using a nonlinear regression analysis with either Eqs. (14) for the compression phase or Eqs. (15) for the relaxation phase (as the object function), we obtain the material parameters $k_0$ and $M$. The aggregate modulus $H_A$ is obtained from the equilibrium measurement on complete stress relaxation.

Experimentally, circular osteochondral plugs, 6.35 mm in diameter (Fig. 4.5A), were removed from the medial facet of open-physis, bovine patellofemoral joints according to the method described by Armstrong and Mow (1982b). Care was taken to harvest only specimens with a glistening surface, generally exhibiting no India ink staining uptake. The plug was removed from that portion of the femoral groove where, by experience, we know that a relatively uniform layer of tissue exists and that the surface is perpendicular to the axis of the osteochondral plug. The thickness $h$ was measured by taking the average six measurements obtained around the circumference of the fully equilibrated tissue. The measuring technique used was to move the stage of a dissecting microscope so that the cross-hair in the field of view was translated from the articular surface to the cartilage–bone interface. The translation, measured by a digital micrometer, is equal to the thickness of the cartilage at that point on the circumference. Equilibration was achieved by soaking the plug in Ringer's solution at room temperature for ~30 min. The fully equilibrated plugs were tested in a bath of Ringer's solution with phenylmethylsulfonyl fluoride in our environmental chamber maintained at 20°C.

The stress–relaxation test was performed on our Rheometrics† mechanical spectrometer used in the compressional mode (Fig. 4.5A and B). The DC servo-controlled motor was interfaced with a Dynatech§ function generator with a precision ramp function signal (Fig. 4.5B). The upper head of the mechanical spectrometer can be prescribed to move vertically to within 0.4 $\mu$m accuracy through a stroke distance of 0.4 mm over a time interval ranging from $30 \times 10^{-3}$ to $10^4$ s. Thus, a precise constant strain rate experiment can be performed, via the precise ramp function signal, to satisfy the mathematically specified "slow" and "fast" rates. Typically, the thickness of the plug is 1.5 mm, and a 10% compressive strain is imposed. For example, to achieve this in 3000 s, a strain rate $\dot{\varepsilon}$ of 0.00333% s$^{-1}$ is required. This means that the mechanical spectrometer must achieve 0.4 $\mu$m every 8 sec, a limit well within the capacity of the DC servo-controlled motor.

The bony osteochondral plugs were mounted into the upper head using a manufacturer-supplied precision collet (Fig. 4.5A and B). The uncalcified cartilage was exposed for testing. The articular cartilage was interfaced against a polished sintered stainless-steel filter with 60 $\mu$m pore

---

† Rheometrics, Inc., 60 Fadem Road, Springfield, NJ 07081, U.S.A.
§ Dynatech (Exact Electronics), 2000 Arrowhead Drive, Carson City, NE 89701, U.S.A.

**Figure 4.5. A:** View of experimental configuration in the test section of our Rheometrics mechanical spectrometer with a 6.35 mm plug of osteochondral specimen in place. **B:** Schematic representation of the experimental apparatus showing specimen bathed in the environmental chamber.

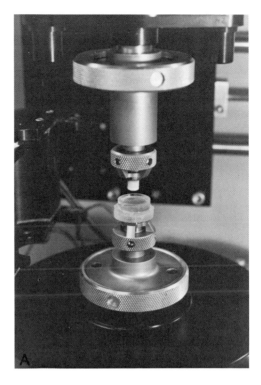

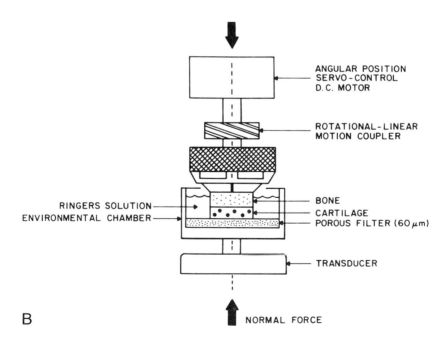

size. The stainless-steel filter was mounted into a plexiglass dish (Fig. 4.5B) containing Ringer's solution, and the cartilage specimen was completely bathed in the solution during testing. Evaporation was prevented by keeping the test specimen and the Ringer's bath in a 100% humidity environmental chamber at 20°C. This is necessary so that the electrolyte concentrations in the Ringer's solution do not increase, since mechanical properties of cartilage are very sensitive to counter-ion concentration via the Donnan osmotic effects (Maroudas, 1979; Grodzinsky et al., 1981; Lee et al., 1981). The filter-plexiglass dish was attached to a transducer with a maximum normal force range of 2000 gmf and sensitivity of ±2 gmf.

These compression experiments required that we develop a strict experimental protocol to ensure that the articular cartilage surface of the specimen made complete contact with the stainless-steel filter surface (Fig. 4.6). This is done by noting on the transducer the initial instant that a load was registered. An initial displacement adjustment of ~5 μm is usu-

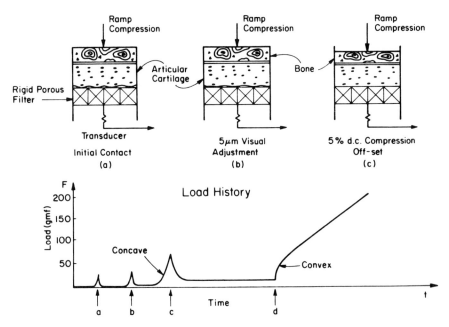

**Figure 4.6.** Schematic representation of experimental protocol to ensure that the cartilage surface is in complete contact with the rigid, porous filter. The protocol consists of: (a) initial contact of filter with sample, (b) a 5 μm displacement to achieve complete visual contact and (c) a 5% compression to interdigitate filter and articular surface completely prior to the actual stress–relaxation experiment. The *bottom curve* shows the load responses, via the transducer, during the preliminary process depicted in curves (a), (b) and (c). Controlled ramp compression begins at point (d).

ally required to achieve complete contact by visual examination. By experience, we find that another 5% DC compression offset is required to interdigitate the articular surface totally with the 60 $\mu$m porous stainless-steel filter surface. Insufficient interdigitation can cause a spurious load signal, since interdigitation brings more tissue into contact and thus more material is being compressed, producing an experimental artifact (Lai et al., 1981). Complete stress relaxation was allowed to occur (usually requiring 45–60 min) before the commencement of the actual stress–relaxation experiment. These very elaborate procedures ensured the repeatability of the sensitive measurements. We have performed numerous compression stress–relaxation studies following this protocol. All of the resultant compression stress histories follow a typical pattern (Fig. 4.7). We have also shown that repeated testing over an 8-h period does not cause overt proteoglycan leachout or significant decrease of the measured equilibrium modulus $H_A$ (Roth et al., 1981). The maximum peak load occurs at the end of the compression phase $t = t_0$, and it varies directly with strain rate $\dot{\varepsilon}$. For the "slow" rate experiment, typically, the maximum peak load was ~400 gmf and the equilibrium load was ~275 gmf. Figure 4.7 provides actual data from our experiment where $\dot{\varepsilon} = 2.08 \times 10^{-3}\% \cdot s^{-1}$ and $t_0 = 4800$ s.

For the typical slow strain rate stress history curve (Fig. 4.7), we see that immediately following the onset of the ramp compression, a parabolic load versus time curve is observed. This is described by the $t^{1/2}$ behavior in the first term of the asymptotic solution for the fast rate, Eq. (13a), which is valid in this range of time. This asymptotic behavior is essentially independent of the nonlinear permeability effect. Beyond this range, an almost linear time dependence is found (Fig. 4.7). This behavior is described by the first term of Eq. (14a). The nonlinear permeability effect does not become pronounced until $t \rightarrow t_0$. A careful examination of the data shows that, just prior to $t_0$, there is a concave curve characteristic that is predicted by the theory [the second term of Eq. (14a)] to have an exponential time dependence (Fig. 4.8). These stress-rise characteristics are governed by the kinematic rate of compression $V_0$, thickness $h$, aggregate modulus $H_A$ and intrinsic permeability parameters $k_0$ and $M$. The nonlinear flow-limiting parameter $M$ is responsible for the rise of the stress above and beyond the linear time dependence obtained with a constant permeability (Fig. 4.8).¶ For the strain rates required by the slow-rate experiment, the deviations from the linear response are relatively small during the compression phase. However, during the relaxation phase, the nonlinear intrinsic permeability function, Eq. (6b), causes a significant decrease of the rate of stress relaxation. For $\tau = (t^* - t_0)/t_0$ and $0 < \tau \ll 1$, Eqs. (15) describe the decrease of stress from the peak

---

¶ Asterisked quantities are dimensional, corresponding to those in Eqs. (13–15).

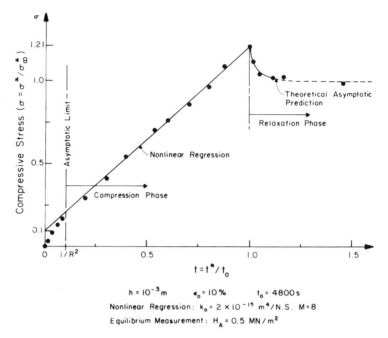

**Figure 4.7.** Typical slow strain rate stress-history curve. The asterisked quantities are dimensional, and the unasterisked quantities are dimensionless. Nonlinear regression analysis was used with Eq. (14) and the data to determine the permeability coefficients $k_0$ and $M$ for $(1/R^2) < t \leq 1$. Verification of the model and analysis is evidenced in the excellent agreement between the theoretical asymptotic prediction and the stress–relaxation data.

compressive stress $\sigma_p$. The rate of stress relaxation is proportional to $M_r$, which depends inversely on the lower constant permeability of the compressed tissue $k = k_0 \exp(-\varepsilon_0 M)$. The mechanism of stress relaxation is fluid redistribution within the tissue, and interstitial fluid flow in the compressed tissue must pass through an organic matrix with lower permeability, which slows the rate of fluid flow. These insights provide an additional method to check the validity of the nonlinear KLM theory for cartilage (Mow and Lai, 1980; Mow et al., 1980; Lai et al., 1981).

In addition to these qualitative trends, the details of the data obtained and their implications in terms of $k_0$, $M$ and $H_A$ must be verified with previous experimental data from independent tests. First, Eqs. (14) for the compression phase history permit the determination of $k_0$ and $M$ via a numerical nonlinear regression procedure, once $H_A$ has been determined by the equilibrium stress measurement. Figure 4.7 shows a typical slow rate stress history determination by this regression procedure yielding $k_0 = 2 \times 10^{-15}$ m⁴/N · s, $H_A = 0.50$ MPa and $M = 8.0$ for $h = 1.0$ mm and $t = 4800$ s. With these values, $R = [k_0 H_A t_0/h^2]^{1/2} = 2.19$, providing an a poste-

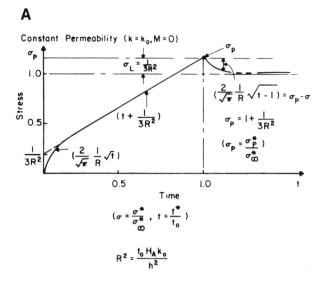

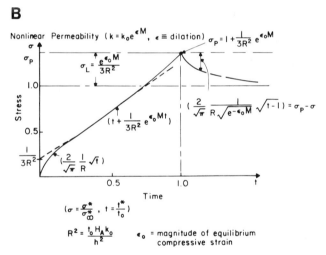

**Figure 4.8. A:** Asymptotic stress history prediction of a slow-rate compression experiment if the tissue is linearly biphasic. The stress rise in the compression phase is linear with time, and the stress intercept $(1/3R^2)$ is the same as the total stress decay during the relaxation phase. Both the initial stress rise and the initial decay are governed by the same $k_0$. **B:** Asymptotic stress history prediction of a slow-rate compression experiment if the tissue is nonlinearly biphasic (strain-dependent permeability). The stress rise in the compressive phase depends on the sum of a linear time function and an exponential time function. The stress intercept $(1/3R^2)$ is different from the total stress decay $[\exp(\varepsilon_0 M)/3R^2]$. The initial decay is at a slower rate, governed by $k_0\exp(-\varepsilon_0 M)$, than that governed by the stress rise, $k_0$. Comparison of these predictions with Figure 4.7 shows that articular cartilage must be a nonlinear biphasic material.

riori check for verifying the validity of using the asymptotic solution, Eqs. (14), to describe the stress rise for $1/R^2 < t/t_0 \leq 1$ (see Fig. 4.7). Second, these values for the intrinsic permeability coefficients $k_0$ and $M$ agree reasonably well with those measured from the direct permeability experiment using our nonlinear permeation theory (see Table 4.1). However, the present stress–relaxation experiment yields a nonlinear flow-limiting parameter $M$ consistently higher than those obtained from the direct permeability experiment. This could be due to the inherent difference in the procedure used in handling the tissue between these two experiments. For the stress–relaxation experiment, cartilage is compressed with the normal articular surface intact, and it remains on the subchondral cortex. Massive fluid exudation occurs across the densely woven collagen network of the superficial tangential zone (Edwards, 1967; Maroudas et al., 1968). For the direct permeability experiment, the superficial tangential zone is sectioned off the thin circular discs of cartilage that has been removed from the bone. Thus, the difference observed in the nonlinear flow-limiting parameter $M$ may be a reflection of these structural differences. In any case, the complete stress–relaxation experiment provides a method to check the internal consistency of the measurements and the nonlinear KLM theory for cartilage. Equations (14) were used to determine $k_0$ and $M$ during the compression phase of the experiment where the major fluid flow characteristic is exudation across the articular surface. If the nonlinear KLM theory is appropriate using these values of $k_0$ and $M$, Eqs. (15) should provide an accurate description of the stress–relaxation process where the major fluid flow is fluid redistribution within the tissue, not across the articular surface. Figure 4.7 indicates quite good agreement between the experimentally observed stress–relaxation history and the theoretically predicted stress–relaxation history.

## Summary

A new method is presented to measure the compressive strain-dependent, nonlinear, intrinsic permeability coefficients of articular cartilage. This method can be used to assess the permeability behavior of all soft, highly hydrated biological tissues, such as meniscus, nasal cartilage and intervertebral disc. For articular cartilage, the nonlinear intrinsic permeability function $k$ is assumed to have the following specific form: $k = k_0 \exp(\varepsilon M)$, where $k_0$ and $M$ are material constants and $\varepsilon$ is the dilatational field. However, the mathematical theory is equally valid for an arbitrary monotonic functional dependence, $k = k(\varepsilon)$. The method proposed depends on the biphasic nature of articular cartilage in controlling the viscoelastic stress–relaxation phenomenon in compression. With increasing compression of the solid phase of the tissue, fluid exudation from the tissue controls the measured stress rise, and, when compression stops, internal fluid redistribution causes stress relaxation. Since interstitial fluid flow is dependent on the permeability of the tissue, which is in turn dependent on the compression to which the tissue is subjected, the proposed controlled strain-rate compression stress–relaxation experiments are ideal for measuring this nonlinear tissue characteristic.

The associated experimental procedure depends on the two mathematical asymptotic solutions to the nonlinear diffusion problem derived here. These two solutions define two material testing regimes: "fast" and "slow" rates for the strain-rate controlled compression stress–relaxation experiments. Correlation between the permeability parameters determined from these transient compression stress–relaxation experiments and from steady direct-permeability experiments is good. The stress–relaxation history provides additional validation for the nonlinear permeability concept and the biphasic KLM theory for articular cartilage.

## Acknowledgments

This work is based upon research supported by grants AM 19094 and AM 26440 awarded by the National Institute of Arthritis, Diabetes, and Digestive and Kidney Diseases and grants MEA 79-19524 and MCS 81-02129 from the National Science Foundation. Any opinion, finding, conclusions or recommendations expressed in this publication are those of the authors and do not necessarily reflect the views of the National Science Foundation. We wish to thank Brendan McCormack for measuring the compression stress–relaxation parameters and Rose A. Boshoff for editorial assistance in preparing this manuscript.

## References

Armstrong CG and Mow VC (1982a). Biomechanics of normal and osteoarthrotic articular cartilage. In: *Clinical Trends in Orthopaedics* (PD Wilson Jr and LR Straub (eds.). New York: Thieme-Stratton, pp. 189–197.

Armstrong CG and Mow VC (1982b). Variations in the intrinsic mechanical properties of human articular cartilage with age, degeneration, and water content. *J Bone Joint Surg* 64A:88–94.

Armstrong CG, Mow VC, Lai WM and Rosenberg LC (1981). Biorheological properties of proteoglycan macromolecules: the viscoelastic properties of solutions of proteoglycan monomers and aggregates. *Trans Orthop Res Soc* 6:90.

Bär EW (1926). Elastizitatsprufungen der gelenkknorpel. *Arch Entwicklungsmech Organ* 108:739–760.

Bowen RM (1976). Theory of mixtures. In: *Continuum Physics, III*. AC Eringen (ed.). New York: Academic Press, pp. 1–127.

Coletti JM, Akeson WH and Woo SL-Y (1972). A comparison of the physical behavior of normal articular cartilage and the arthroplasty surface. *J Bone Joint Surg* 54A:147–160.

Courant R and Hilbert D (1962). *Methods of Mathematical Physics, II.* New York: Interscience.

Craine RE, Green AE and Naghdi PM (1970). A mixture of viscous elastic material with different constituent temperatures. *Q J Mech Appl Math* 23:171–184.

Edwards J (1967). Physical characteristics of articular cartilage. *Proc Inst Mech Eng* 181(3J):16–24.

Elmore SM, Sokoloff L, Norris G and Carmeci P (1963). Nature of 'imperfect' elasticity of articular cartilage. *J Appl Physiol* 18:393–396.

Freeman MAR and Meachim G (1979). Ageing and degeneration. In: *Adult Articular Cartilage,* 2nd ed. MAR Freeman (ed.). Kent, England: Pitman Medical, pp. 487–543.

Göcke DE (1927). Elastizitotsstudien am jungen und alten gelenkknorpel. *Verh Deutsch Orthop Gesellsch* 22:130–147.

Grodzinsky AJ, Roth V, Myers ER, Grossman W and Mow VC (1981). The significance of electromechanical and osmotic forces in the nonequilibrium swelling behavior of articular cartilage in tension. *J Biomech Eng* 103:221–231.

Hayes WC and Bodine AJ (1978). Flow-independent viscoelastic properties of articular cartilage matrix. *J Biomech* 11:407–419.

Hayes WC and Mockros LF (1971). Viscoelastic properties of human articular cartilage. *J Appl Physiol* 31:562–568.

Hirsch C (1944). The pathogenesis of chondromalacia of the patella. *Acta Chir Scand* 90 (Suppl. 83):1–106.

Holmes MH (1982). A nonlinear diffusion equation arising in the study of soft tissue. *Q J Appl Math* 61:209–220.

Honner R and Thompson RC (1971). The nutritional pathways of articular cartilage: an autoradiographic study in rabbits using 35S injected intravenously. *J Bone Joint Surg* 53A:742–748.

Kempson GE (1979). Mechanical properties of articular cartilage. In: *Adult Articular Cartilage,* 2nd ed. MAR Freeman (ed.). Kent, England: Pitman Medical, pp. 333–414.

Kempson GE, Freeman MAR and Swanson SAV (1971). The determination of a creep modulus for articular cartilage from indentation tests on the human femoral head. *J Biomech* 4:239–250.

Lai WM and Mow VC (1980). Drag-induced compression of articular cartilage during a permeation experiment. *J Biorheol* 17:111–123.

Lai WM, Mow VC and Roth V (1981). Effects of a nonlinear strain-dependent permeability and rate of compression on the stress behavior of articular cartilage. *J Biomech Eng* 103:61–66.

Lee RC, Frank EH, Grodzinsky AJ and Roylance DK (1981). Oscillatory compressional behavior of articular cartilage and its associated electromechanical properties. *J Biomech Eng* 103:280–292.

Linn FC and Sokoloff L (1965). Movement and composition of interstitial fluid of cartilage. *Arthritis Rheum* 8:481–494.

Mak AF, Mow VC, Lai WM, Hardingham TE, Muir H and Eyre DR (1982). Assessment of proteoglycan-proteoglycan interactions from solution biorheological behaviors. *Trans Orthop Res Soc* 7:169.

Mansour JM and Mow VC (1976). The permeability of articular cartilage under compressive strain and at high pressure. *J Bone Joint Surg* 58A:509–516.

Maroudas A (1970). Distribution and diffusion of solutes in articular cartilage. *Biophys J* 10:365–379.

Maroudas A (1975). Biophysical chemistry of cartilaginous tissue with special reference to solute and fluid transport. *Biorheology* 12:233–248.

Maroudas A (1979). Physicochemical properties of articular cartilage. In: *Adult Articular Cartilage,* 2nd ed. MAR Freeman (ed.). Kent, England: Pitman Medical, pp. 215–290.

Maroudas A, Bullough P, Swanson SAV and Freeman MAR (1968). The permeability of articular cartilage. *J Bone Joint Surg* 50B:166–177.

Mow VC, Kuei SC, Lai WM and Armstrong CG (1980). Biphasic creep and stress relaxation of articular cartilage in compression: theory and experiment. *J Biomech Eng* 102:73–84.

Mow VC and Lai WM (1980). Recent developments in synovial joint biomechanics. *SIAM Rev* 22:275–317.

Mow VC, Lai WM and Holmes MH (1982). Advanced theoretical and experimental techniques in cartilage research. In: *Biomechanics: Principles and Applications* R Huiskes, D Van Campen and J De Wijn (eds.). The Hague: Martinus Nijhoff, pp. 47–74.

Mow VC, Meyers ER, Roth V and Lalik P (1981). Implications for collagen-proteoglycan interactions from cartilage stress relaxation behavior in isometric tension. *Semin Arthritis Rheum* 11 (Suppl):41–43.

Mow VC, Schoonbeck JS, Koob T and Eyre DR (1983). Correlative studies on viscoelastic shear properties and chemical composition of articular cartilage. *Trans Orthop Res Soc* 8:201.

Muir H (1979). Biochemistry. In: *Adult Articular Cartilage,* 2nd ed. MAR Freeman (ed.). Kent, England: Pitman Medical, pp. 145–214.

Ogata K, Whiteside LA and Lesker PA (1978). Subchondral route for nutrition to articular cartilage in the rabbit. *J Bone Joint Surg* 60A:905–910.

Parsons JR and Black J (1977). The viscoelastic shear behavior of normal rabbit articular cartilage. *J Biomech* 10:21–27.

Parsons JR and Black J (1979). Mechanical behavior of articular cartilage: quantitative changes with ionic environment. *J Biomech* 12:765–773.

Pasternack SG, Veis A and Breen M (1974). Solvent-dependent changes in proteoglycan subunit conformation in aqueous guanidine hydrochloride solution. *J Biol Chem* 249:2206–2211.

Roth V and Mow VC (1980). The intrinsic tensile behavior of the matrix of bovine articular cartilage and its variation with age. *J Bone Joint Surg* 62A:1102–1117.

Roth V, Mow VC, Lai WM and Eyre DR (1981). Correlation of intrinsic compressive properties of bovine articular cartilage with its uronic acid and water content. *Trans Orthop Res Soc* 6:49.

Salter RB, Simmonds DF, Malcolm BW, Rumble EJ, Macmichael D and Clements ND (1980). The biological effect of continuous passive motion on the healing of full-thickness defects in articular cartilage: an experimental investigation in the rabbit. *J Bone Joint Surg* 62A:1232–1251.

Sokoloff L (1963). Elasticity of articular cartilage: effect of ions and viscous solutions. *Science* 141:1055–1057.

Sokoloff L (1966). Elasticity of aging cartilage. *Fed Proc* 25:1089–1095.

Sokoloff L (1969). *The Biology of Degenerate Joint Disease*. Chicago: University of Chicago Press.
Stahurski TM, Armstrong CG and Mow VC (1981). Variation of the intrinsic aggregate modulus and permeability of articular cartilage with trypsin digestion. In: *1981 Biomechanics Symposium*. New York: ASME, pp. 137–140.
Tanaka T and Fillmore DJ (1979). Kinetics of swelling of gels: *J Chem Phys* 70:1214–1218.
Torzilli PA, Rose DE and Dethemers DA (1982). Equilibrium water partition in articular cartilage. *Biorheology* 19:519–537.
Woo SL-Y, Akeson WH and Jemmott CF (1976). Measurement of nonhomogeneous, directional mechanical properties of articular cartilage in tension. *J Biomech* 9:785–791.

CHAPTER 5

# Intervertebral Disc Nutrition as Related to Spinal Movements and Fusion

Jill P.G. Urban and Sten H. Holm

## Introduction

The integrity of the intervertebral disc is vital to the functioning of the spine. The discs serve both as joints and as shock absorbers, and account for about a quarter to a third of the length of the spinal column. A human lumbar disc has two regions: the inner soft nucleus pulposus and the outer firm annulus fibrosus (Fig. 5.1). The major components of both nucleus and annulus are water, collagen and proteoglycans. It is the chemical nature and material properties of both collagen and proteoglycan components that enable the disc to function efficiently. The collagen of the disc is laid down in a network of fine fibers arranged in a highly specific weave (Fig. 5.1). The collagen fibers of the annulus anchor the disc to the bone. This collagen network provides the disc with the flexibility to act as a joint and yet enables it to withstand the high pressures induced during movement.

The proteoglycans of the disc, as in other load-bearing cartilages, maintain the hydration of the tissue. Proteoglycans imbibe water and thus inflate the collagen network; moreover, because they are present in high concentrations, they restrict the rate of fluid loss. Typically water, collagen and proteoglycan contents of adult human discs vary with intradiscal position and age (Fig. 5.2).

The proteoglycans are constantly being resynthesized by the disc chondrocytes. Although turnover is slow (about 2 years in an adult dog), without such replacement the proteoglycan content of the disc would gradually decrease and its mechanical function would be impaired. The integrity of the disc therefore depends to a great extent on the viability of these chondrocytes. Because the disc is large and avascular, the supply of nutrients to the chondrocytes is often thought to be barely adequate and it has been suggested that movement could improve disc nutrition and is necessary for its survival. In this chapter we examine the effects of mechanical stress, both short-term and long-term, on nutrition and metabolism of the disc.

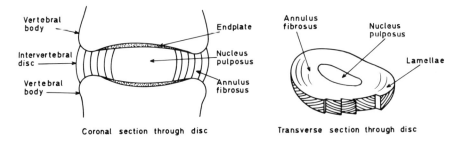

**Figure 5.1.** A schematic view of the different regions in the lumbar intervertebral disc. The intricate arrangement of the annulus lamellae with alternating directions of collagen bundles is apparent in transverse sections.

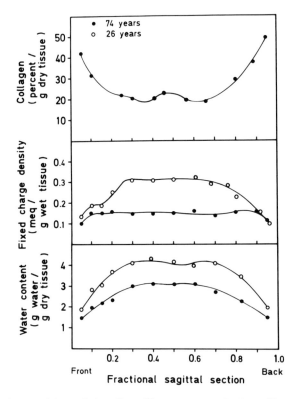

**Figure 5.2.** Composition of the disc. Shown are sagittal profiles of the glyco-saminoglycan content expressed as fixed charge density, and water content in a 26-year and a 74-year disc and collagen per dry weight in a 74-year disc. (From Urban, 1977.)

# Background

## Loads on the Lumbar Spine

In humans, the intervertebral disc is always under load. The load arises partly from body weight, and partly from muscle and ligament tension. The magnitude of this load cannot be measured directly. It has however been estimated from measurements of intradiscal pressure, myoelectric muscle activity and intraabdominal pressure (reviewed by Andersson, 1982). The load on a disc is very dependent on posture. Nachemson and Elfström (1970) found that even in a relaxed supine subject, intradiscal pressure in the L3 disc was 0.1 to 0.2 MPa, corresponding to a load of about 250 N, whereas in the same subject in unsupported sitting, the load rose to about 0.6 to 0.7 MPa, corresponding to about 700 N. Postures involving flexion and extension increase the pressure within the disc considerably. During strenuous activity, peak intradiscal pressures can rise to over 1.6 MPa.

Because of the relationship between disc pressure and posture in humans, the load on the spine tends to follow a cyclic pattern; it is at its lowest during sleep at night, and then increases during the day's activities. Little is known about the patterns of loading of animal spines, but they are also likely to follow the same cyclic pattern, being lowest during sleep, when muscular activity is lowest.

## Disc Height, Load, and Hydration

Alterations in load on the spine, which result from changes of posture and from movement, significantly affect the height of the disc since the disc deforms as the load on it is increased. Initially the deformation arises mainly from a rearrangement of the collagen network (Hickey and Hukins, 1980). However, if the increased load is maintained, the disc creeps and its volume changes slowly as fluid is squeezed out. Deformation of the disc under sustained loads depends on lumber location and degeneration state (Fig. 5.3).

Because creep results mainly from loss of fluid from the disc, its extent is governed largely by the proteoglycan content of the tissue, since proteoglycan content controls both disc hydration and the rate of fluid flow from the tissue (Urban and Maroudas, 1980). At equilibrium (condition 1) when there is no net fluid loss or gain from the disc, its swelling pressure $P_s$, exactly balances the applied pressure $P_{al}$:

$$P_{s1} = P_{al} \tag{1}$$

The swelling pressure $P_s$ results from the osmotic pressure exerted by proteoglycans which imbibe fluid and swell the disc, and from the resulting tension in the disc's own collagen network which tends to restrain the

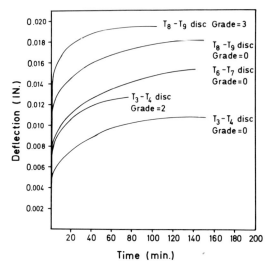

**Figure 5.3.** Constant load creep curves for discs without degeneration (grade 0) compared to discs graded as degenerated (T3–T4, T6–T7 and T8–T9 are intervertebral discs in the thoracic region of the spine). The creep rate is greater and the equilibration time shorter for degenerated discs, compared to "normal" discs. (From Kazarian, 1975.)

swelling tendencies of the proteoglycans (Maroudas and Bannon, 1981). If the applied load is increased (condition 2) so that $P_{a2} > P_{a1}$, the disc is no longer at equilibrium. Since $P_{a2} > P_{s1}$, fluid is squeezed out of the disc. As fluid is lost, the concentration of the proteoglycans increases and consequently their osmotic pressure rises. Also as the volume of the disc decreases through loss of fluid, the collagen network tension decreases and thus the force opposing the swelling tendency of the tissue is reduced. These changes tend to increase the disc's swelling pressure $P_s$. Fluid flow continues until the net pressure applied to disc equals the increased swelling pressure. Equilibrium hydration of the disc depends on applied external pressures, and hence on disc swelling pressures (Fig. 5.4). Since fluid equilibrium within the disc is reached only after many hours, physiologically it is the rate of fluid loss that is more relevant.

From results such as those in Figure 5.3, it is not possible to determine what fraction of creep results from fluid loss. However, Adams and Hutton (1982), directly measured fluid loss in vitro by comparing the fluid content of a disc loaded externally for 4 h with that of its unloaded neighbor. They found an average fluid loss of about 12%. Because of the high variability of human disc material, the standard deviations were very large. The other approach to estimating rate of fluid loss from the disc depends on modelling fluid flow in the tissue. Several models describe flow in connective tissues (McCutcheon, 1962; Kenyon, 1979; Lai and Mow, 1980). A model that describes fluid flow in the disc adequately is based on the equation derived by Fatt and Goldstick (1965) for estimating fluid flow in the cornea. They applied Darcy's law for fluid flow in a

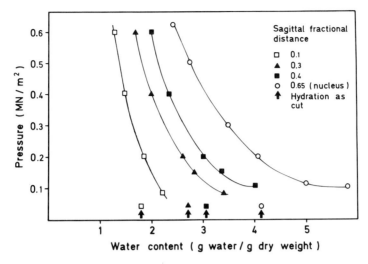

**Figure 5.4.** Swelling pressure versus hydration for different regions of the annulus and nucleus from a 54-year-old subject. (From Urban and Maroudas, 1980.)

porous material under a pressure gradient to a swelling tissue by using dry tissue thickness as the basic dimension:

$$\frac{\partial H}{\partial t} = \frac{\partial}{\partial z}\left[D(H)\,\frac{dH}{dz}\right], \tag{2}$$

where $H$ is hydration, $t$ is time, $z$ is the distance based on dry tissue volume and $D(H)$ is the water transport coefficient, analogous to a concentration-dependent diffusion coefficient, since it is a function of water content (assuming flow in $z$ direction only) and is defined by

$$D(H) = k\,\frac{\varepsilon^2}{(\varepsilon + H)}\,\frac{dP}{dH}, \tag{3}$$

where $k$ is the hydraulic permeability coefficient, $\varepsilon$ is the specific volume of the disc material and $dP$ is the pressure gradient causing flow, which by Starling's hypothesis depends on both hydrostatic and osmotic pressure differences between intradiscal fluid and fluid within the surrounding un-stressed tissue. The hydraulic permeability coefficient of fluid depends strongly on $H$ and hence on proteoglycan content (Fig. 5.5). Thus, $D(H)$ is a function of tissue composition and changes if the fluid content of the tissue changes.

## Disc Nutrition

The physiological load-bearing function of the disc depends on the integrity of the disc's matrix. Since the matrix is maintained by the cells of the

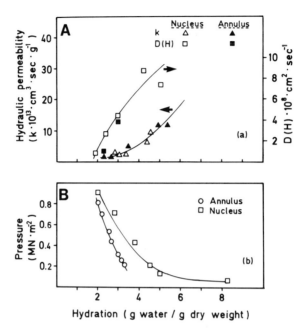

**Figure 5.5.** Variations with hydration (**A**) transport coefficient, $D(H)$ (*left curve, right ordinate*) and hydraulic permeability, $k$ (*right curve, left ordinate*) and (**B**) swelling pressure in a nucleus and inner annulus slice from a 23-year-old subject. (From Urban and Maroudas, 1980.)

disc, it is obvious that the health of the disc depends to a large extent on the viability of these cells. They are described as chondrocyte-like cells and produce proteoglycans and perhaps collagen in the adult human disc (Herbert et al., 1975; Oegema et al., 1979). These cells are not evenly distributed throughout the tissue and their concentration is highest at the periphery of the annulus. In the center of the disc their concentration is very low (about 5000 cells per mm³), being only about 1% to 4% of the volume of the tissue (Maroudas et al., 1975; Holm et al., 1981).

Since adult human disc is avascular (Schmorl and Junghanns, 1971), nutrients are supplied to these cells only by transport of necessary solutes through the disc matrix from surrounding blood vessels. Two routes into the disc have been described (Fig. 5.6), from the blood vessels surrounding the annulus, and from blood vessels in the vertebral bodies through the endplate above and below the nucleus (Urban et al., 1978). Solutes move through the disc matrix under diffusion gradients set up between the vascular supply and the disc's chondrocyte-like cells. The distances for diffusion are large. In adult human discs, some cells are as much as 6 to 8 mm from the blood supply, since a human lumbar disc is typically about

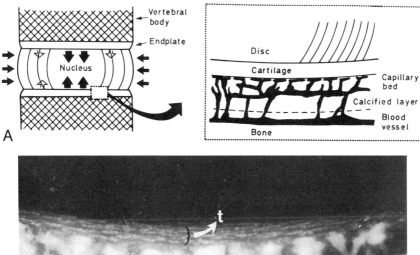

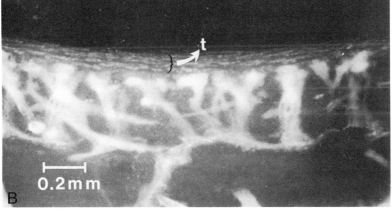

**Figure 5.6. A:** Schematic diagram of the nutritional routes into the intervertebral disc and an enlarged view of the area underneath the hyaline cartilage. **B:** Photograph of the bone–disc interface in the region of nucleus pulposus. Tetracycline was injected intravenously and the disc was excised. After histological preparation, the disc slice was viewed in a fluorescence microscope. The thickness of the cartilage is indicated by *t* in the picture. (From Holm et al., 1981.)

10 to 15 mm thick and 30 mm across its shortest diameter. Solute transport may also be aided by fluid flow, as solutes are entrained in the fluid that is pumped in and out of the disc under changing loads. Because the hydraulic permeability of disc tissue is low (Fig. 5.5), calculations imply that diffusion accounts for most of the transport of small solutes (Urban, 1977). We measured the concentrations and consumption rates of metabolites (glucose, oxygen, glycogen and lactic acid) in the tissue (Holm et al., 1981) and found steep concentration gradients of these solutes, in particular of oxygen and lactic acid (Fig. 5.7). The gradients were compatible with those expected for transport by diffusion. However, fluid flow may play a part in the transport of large solutes with low rates of diffusion, as is the case in other connective tissues.

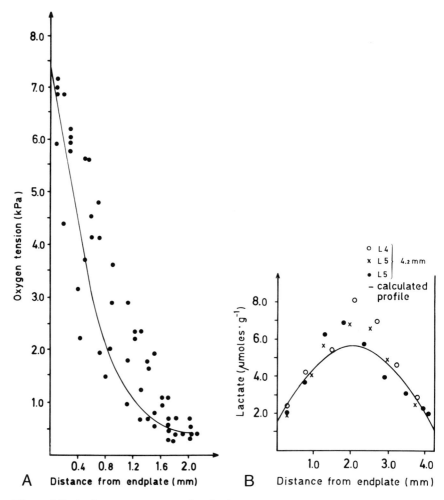

**Figure 5.7. A:** Oxygen concentration in the nucleus pulposus of a dog as a function of distance from the vertebral endplate. The solid curve was calculated theoretically. **B:** Lactate concentration in the canine nucleus pulposus as a function of distance from the vertebral endplate. The experimental points correspond to three discs of the same height obtained from three different animals. (From Holm et al., 1981.)

## Effects of Mechanical Stress on Disc Matrix

Mechanical stress may influence the structure of disc matrix directly. Mechanical overload may rupture the annulus (Adams and Hutton, 1982). Mechanical stress may also fracture the endplate of the disc (Rolander and Blair, 1975), and hence provide a path to degeneration. However, this paper will rather examine the possible effect of mechanical stress on cells of the disc. Their response to stress may influence the secretion of matrix components, and hence influence the composition and structure of the disc, or alternatively, may cause the cells to secrete enzymes that may destroy the matrix.

There is evidence that connective tissue cells may respond to changes in mechanical stress (Gillard et al., 1979; Jones et al., 1982). This may be a direct response to changes in pressure or shape that the cells experience. Alternatively, because applied mechanical stress changes the fluid content of connective tissue, it also alters the chemical environment of the cells. For instance, as fluid is lost from the tissue, the proteoglycan concentration increases. The rate of production of proteoglycans by chondrocytes is also influenced by the surrounding proteoglycan concentration (Wiebkin and Muir, 1975; Handley and Lowther, 1977). This influence could be exerted directly by the proteoglycans through receptors on the cell surface or by a response to changes in concentration of some solute present in the matrix. Because of the polyelectrolyte nature of the proteoglycans, the concentration of fixed negative charges in the tissue rises as the proteoglycan content increases. The concentration of ionic solutes is strongly related to charge density through the Gibbs-Donnan equilibrium effect (Maroudas, 1968). Thus with a decrease in hydration, the concentration of counter-cations such as $Ca^{2+}$ and $Na^+$ will rise steeply, whereas that of counter-anions such as phosphate or sulfate will fall. Proteoglycan concentration also affects the concentration of uncharged solutes in the tissue through steric effects (Maroudas, 1980). This effect is more marked with increasing solute size.

Mechanical stress may also alter the chemical environment of the cell by affecting the disc's nutrition. Fluid flow itself does not significantly affect the rate of small solute transport (Urban et al., 1982). However, fluid flow may influence the transport of some larger molecules necessary for cellular control, or it may facilitate proteoglycans transport through the matrix. Also, as fluid is expressed from the tissue, the disc loses volume. With the consequent decrease in distance for diffusion, the rate of nutrient transport into the disc will rise (Holm et al., 1981). Although changes in hydration will also affect solute diffusivity, this effect is secondary, since rate of diffusion is proportional to (disc thickness)$^2$ but only to the square root of the diffusion coefficient (Crank, 1975). Thus, small changes in dimensions may significantly affect oxygen concentration, since oxygen gradients in the tissue are very steep (Fig. 5.7). For example, proteoglycan synthesis rates depend on oxygen concentration (Lane et al., 1977).

The degree of vascularization of the vertebral bodies and other ligaments surrounding the disc may also be affected by mechanical stress. Since levels of oxygen, glucose and other substrates for disc nutrition are influenced by blood vessel contacts with the disc (Holm et al., 1981), changes in vascularization may also influence chondrocyte metabolism. Finally, exercise itself alters the concentration of blood solutes such as glucose, pH and lactic acid. These alterations of solute concentration may eventually reach the disc cells and influence them.

## Recent Studies

In this section we will discuss the results of some recent work conducted on dogs in vivo that examine the effect of applied loads on the disc.

### Does "Pumping" Increase Solute Transport through the Disc Matrix?

It has been suggested that convective movements of fluid in and out of the disc following changes of load aids nutrition of the disc by enhancing the rate of transport of solutes to and from cells. To evaluate possible effects of fluid flow on disc nutrition, the following series of tests (Urban et al., 1982) were carried out. Two groups of Labrador dogs were injected with an equivalent dose of [$^{35}$S]sulfate. One group was anesthetized for the period between injection and death. During the same period the other group ran continuously. The influence of fluid flow would be different in the two cases.

Anesthetized dogs relax loads on their spine so their discs tend to imbibe water, whereas moving dogs tend to pump water in and out of their discs. Both groups of dogs were killed at times between 1 and 6 h after injection. Their spines were removed within 10 min of death and frozen to halt diffusion. The discs were then sliced and profiles of [$^{35}$S]sulfate through the lumbar discs were measured in both sagittal and cranial-caudal directions. The measured curves were compared to those calculated on the basis that all transport into the disc was by diffusion alone.

For dogs, where the blood decay curve was log-linear with decay constant $\lambda$, the tracer concentration normalized with respect to that in serum at time $t = 0$ is predicted at any point $x$ and time $t$, employing Laplace transforms and the convolution integral (Urban, 1977):

$$u(z,T) = \frac{2K_L}{\sqrt{\pi}} \sum_{n=0}^{\infty} (-1)^n \exp(-kt)\exp(-T) \sum_{h=1}^{2} \int_0^{\infty} \frac{A(h)^2 - y^2}{A(h) \cdot B^{4y^2}} \, dy, \quad (4)$$

where

$U$ = tracer concentration
$L$ = disc radius

$z = \dfrac{x}{L}$

$T = \lambda t$
$K_L$ = partition coefficient at the disc periphery
$k$ = tracer incorporation rate
$A(1) = (2_{n+1} - z)(\lambda L^2/D)^{1/2}$
$A(2) = (2_{n+1} + z)(\lambda L^2/D)^{1/2}$
$B = \frac{1}{2}\sqrt{T}$
$y$ = fractional sagittal distance from the anterior of the disc
$D$ = diffusion coefficient of tracer in the tissue.

If fluid flow had significantly affected transport rate, the measured experimental profiles should have diverged from the calculated curves. However, there was no significant difference between measured and calculated curves for the moving and anesthetized dogs (Fig. 5.8), and thus most solute movement resulted from diffusion.

The conclusion that diffusion is the major mechanism for transport of

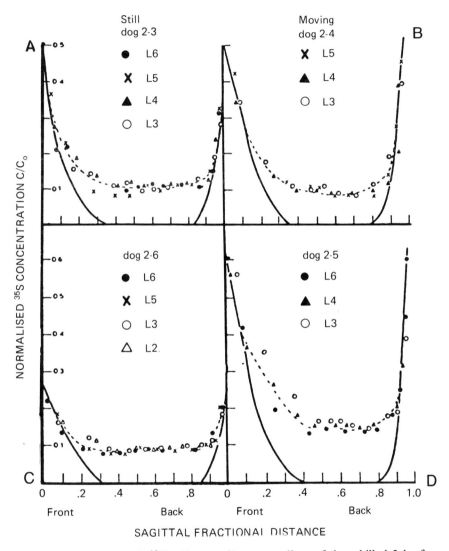

**Figure 5.8.** Normalized [$^{35}$S]sulfate profile across discs of dogs killed 2 h after tracer injection: sagittal section (——). Calculated curve for diffusion from annulus periphery (– – –). The curve was drawn through experimental points. **A, C:** Anesthetized dogs. **B, D:** Moving dogs. (L2–L6 represent intervertebral discs in lumbar region of the spine). (From Urban et al., 1982.)

solutes similar in size to sulfate in the disc is not surprising, as the fluid permeability of the tissue is very low (see Fig. 5.5). Diffusion of these small solutes through the disc is far faster than fluid flow. Moreover, since the overall direction of fluid flow is out of the disc for about 16 out of 24 hours a day in humans, it is difficult to envisage how disc cells could rely on convective transport to supply their nutritional requirements. It is possible, however, that fluid flow could aid the transport of larger solutes through the matrix.

## Long-Term Effects of Mechanical Stress on the Disc

In these experiments, the effects of long-term mechanical stress on disc metabolism were investigated. First, the effect of spinal fusion was examined (Holm and Nachemson, 1982). Fusion immobilized the involved segments and altered the mechanical stresses on both the fused and adjacent discs (Frymoyer et al., 1979). Second, the effect of an intensive exercise regimen was investigated (Holm and Nachemson, 1983). Exercise alters the mechanical stresses on the spine both during the exercise period and also afterwards as a result of muscle training. Moreover, during exercise itself, changes in blood concentration of glucose and lactic acid also affect the disc.

### Spinal Fusion

A posterior fusion (Fig. 5.9) covering three discs and their adjacent vertebral bodies was performed on adult dogs (Holm and Nachemson, 1982). Postoperatively, the dogs were allowed to move freely and later were exercised gently for 2 h a day. Dogs were killed at 3, 5 and 8 months after fusion and their discs were examined. Before the dogs were killed, they were anesthetized and their discs exposed by laparotomy. Concentration profiles of oxygen and the rates of oxygen uptake by cells were measured in vivo by inserting oxygen electrodes into the exposed discs. The rate of transport of solutes into the discs was measured by injecting [$^{35}$S]sulfate into the blood, and examining [$^{35}$S]sulfate profiles in the disc (Urban et al., 1978). The dogs were killed 3 h after [$^{35}$S]sulfate injection. Only a portion of the spine was frozen for examination of tracer and metabolite concentrations; the rest was incubated at 37°C for measurement of rates of glucose and oxygen consumption and lactic acid production. Proteoglycan and water contents of the discs were also measured to monitor changes in composition (see Holm and Nachemson, 1982, for details). Oxygen consumption rates (Fig. 5.10) and fixed charge density (Fig. 5.11), a measure of proteoglycan concentration, fell in the fused discs with time. These two parameters increased in discs adjacent to the fused segments.

### Exercise (Training)

Each of three groups of dogs was taken through a different exercise regimen daily for 3 months. One group jogged over flat ground, a second

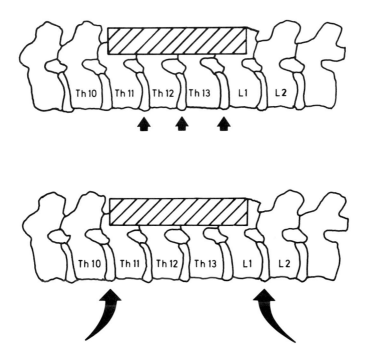

**Figure 5.9.** Schematic representation of a posterior spinal fusion, incorporating three intervertebral discs situated in the lower thoracic (Th) and upper lumbar (L) regions. *Arrows* indicate the fused discs (*above*) and the adjacent discs (*below*). (From Holm and Nachemson, 1982.)

group ran rapidly over obstacles and up-and-down steep slopes, and the third group ran a course involving many obstacles that were crawled under or jumped over. This third group of exercised dogs experienced considerable bending of the spine (Holm and Nachemson, 1983). After 3 months of training, the dogs were killed and discs in the lumbar and thoracic spines were analyzed using procedures similar to those outlined above (Holm and Nachemson, 1982) except water content and fixed charge density were not measured.

**Results**

Fusion and exercise have very different effects on the disc (Table 5.1; Figs. 5.10–5.12). In fused discs, incorporation rates of metabolites fell. Consistent with a fall in oxygen consumption rate, oxygen tension in the disc rose. These results suggest that metabolic activity per volume of disc decreased and that perhaps a proportion of the cells had died. The rate of $^{35}$S incorporation (a measure of the rate of proteoglycan synthesis) also fell. This fall is expected if some cells were less active (or dead) or if oxygen tension increased in the disc. Whatever the cause, the decreased rate of proteoglycan production causes a gradual fall in the concentration

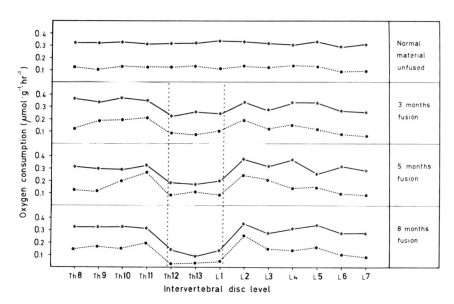

**Figure 5.10.** Oxygen consumption rates in normal, unfused and fused intervertebral discs. Discs adjacent to the fusion as well as the incorporated discs were affected already after 3 months fusion. These changes progressively increased with fusion time. After 5 months fusion the differences were significant ($p < 0.05$), both for annulus and nucleus. Results represent means for more than eight determinations. Nucleus pulposus is indicated by *filled circles*, whereas the results of annulus fibrosus periphery are marked with *stars*. Th, Thoracic discs; L, lumbar discs. (From Holm and Nachemson, 1982.)

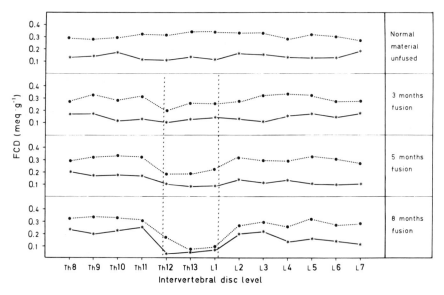

**Figure 5.11.** Fixed charge density (FCD) for normal, unfused and fused discs. Significantly decreased FCD ($p < 0.05$) in the nucleus occurred after 5 and 8 months fusion, after 8 months for the annulus fibrosus. See legend to Figure 5.10 for symbols. (From Holm and Nachemson, 1982.)

**Table 5.1.** Properties of fused and exercised discs

| Parameter | Fused discs | Exercised discs |
|---|---|---|
| $H_2O$ content | − | |
| $H_2O$ imbibition | − | |
| Fixed charge density | − | |
| Tracer concentration | + | + |
| $^{35}S$ uptake rate | − | + |
| Metabolite uptake rate | − | + |
| Lactate production rate | − | − |
| $O_2$ concentration | + | − |
| Lactate concentration | + | − |

The symbol + implies an increase relative to control discs; the symbol − implies a decrease relative to control discs. Control discs were discs from the same spinal level of nonexercised dogs or adjacent discs from the same spine in the case of fused discs.
From Holm and Nachemson, 1982, 1983.

of proteoglycans and hence of fixed charge in the matrix. Disc hydration and water imbibition decrease as fixed charge density falls (Urban and Maroudas, 1980). Loss of fixed charge also causes gain of anions, and hence tracer anion concentration (e.g., [$^{35}S$]sulfate) is higher within the disc.

The significant increase in lactic acid concentration with fusion is somewhat anomalous. Since oxygen concentration is higher than normal, the disc's metabolism may be less anaerobic (Holm et al., 1981) which is consistent with the measured fall in lactic acid production. It is therefore surprising to find that lactic acid concentration increased. A possible mechanism for this increase could be a decreased rate of transport of lactic acid from the disc. As previously discussed, a small molecule such as lactic acid moves through the disc mainly by diffusion. Although decreased water content lowers the diffusion coefficient of lactic acid in the tissue (Urban, 1977), the magnitude of the changes are not consistent with a lower rate of diffusion from the tissue. One possible explanation is that fusion gradually reduces blood supply to the disc endplate, thus partially closing one "route" for movement of solutes out of the tissue, and allowing the concentration of metabolic products to build up. In fact, all our results are consistent with a decreased nutritional supply to nucleus leading to changes in cell behavior. However, since neither blood vessel contacts nor cells were examined directly (for obvious reasons), we cannot ascertain that this is the mechanism by which fusion influenced the disc matrix.

The changes in the discs of all three groups of dogs that were rigorously exercised for 3 months were in a direction opposite to those found in fused discs. Increased transport of both charged and uncharged tracers into the discs of these trained dogs may indicate that the number of blood–disc contacts increased. Metabolites such as oxygen thus reach the

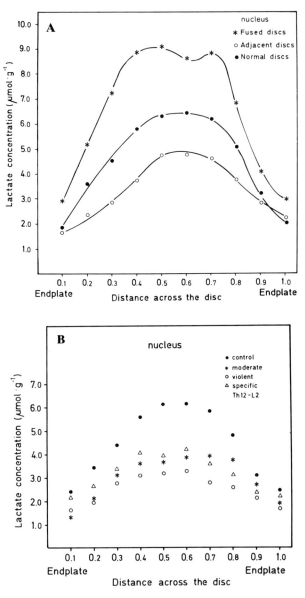

**Figure 5.12. A:** Lactate concentration profiles across the nucleus (endplate to endplate section) 8 months after fusion. In the central nucleus of the fused discs, lactate concentrations were significantly higher than normal discs and adjacent discs ($p < 0.05$). **B:** Lactate concentration profiles across the nucleus. Both discs from the control group as well as from the exercising groups (daily exercise for one-half hour) are included in the diagram. Mean values are given and each point represents more than 20 discs. (Typical values for control discs were in the central part of the nucleus $6.2 \pm 0.5$ $\mu$mol $\cdot$ g$^{-1}$ (mean $\pm$ SD) and for moderately exercised discs $3.7 \pm 0.7$ $\mu$mol $\cdot$ g$^{-1}$ (mean $\pm$ SD). In the center of the nucleus a significant reduction was found for all three exercising groups ($p < 0.05$). (From Holm and Nachemson, 1983.)

**Table 5.2.** Utilization of substrates and concentrations of metabolites in moderately exercised intervertebral discs

| | Utilization of substrates[a] | | | | | |
|---|---|---|---|---|---|---|
| | Outer annulus fibrosus | | | Central nucleus pulposus | | |
| Disc | Glucose | Oxygen | Glycogen | Glucose | Oxygen | Glycogen |
| T12-L2 | +8.6% | +13.0% | +6.1% | +11.1% | +10.7% | +7.9% |
| L3-L6 | +8.0% | +7.7% | +4.8% | +6.4% | +9.5% | +7.5% |
| L7 | +1.3% | +4.7% | +2.2% | +5.0% | +1.9% | +3.9% |

| | Concentration of metabolites[b] | | | | | |
|---|---|---|---|---|---|---|
| | Outer annulus fibrosus | | | Central nucleus pulposus | | |
| Disc | Glucose | Lactate | Oxygen | Glucose | Lactate | Oxygen |
| T12-L2 | −13.5% | −34.0%[d] | −21.1%[c] | −8.6% | −40.3%[d] | −24.7%[c] |
| L3-L6 | −12.2% | −26.8%[d] | −18.4%[c] | −11.1% | −29.7%[d] | −20.5%[c] |
| L7 | −12.9% | −19.9%[c] | −11.4% | −7.2% | −17.0%[c] | −10.6% |

[a] Utilization of glucose, oxygen and glycogen in the outer annulus and in the central nucleus of intervertebral discs from moderately exercised spines (daily exercise for half an hour). Results represent deviations (percent) from results of the nonexercised control group.
[b] Concentrations of glucose, lactate and oxygen in thoracic (T) and lumbar (L) discs. Oxygen concentration was measured as oxygen tension. Negative signs indicate reduced concentrations in comparison to discs of the nonexercised control group. Results represent deviations (percent) from the control group. Levels of significance: [c] $p < 0.05$; [d] $p < 0.01$.
From Holm and Nachemson, 1982, 1983.

disc more easily. At higher oxygen concentrations, disc metabolism is less anaerobic (Holm et al., 1981), consistent with the lowered rate of lactate production and increased oxygen consumption (Tables 5.1 and 5.2). A great degree of aerobic glycolysis would also lead to lower lactate concentration. It should be noted that in the fused spines, discs just adjacent to the fused segments behaved more like those from the exercised dogs than those farther away from the fusion (see Figs. 5.10 and 5.11).

# Summary

Altered mechanical stress affects the disc in two ways. First, under mechanical stress, the stress experienced by components of the matrix and by the cells changes, and the disc deforms. Secondly, as the load is maintained, the disc creeps, in part by expressing fluid from the tissue. Fluid loss alters the concentration of matrix constituents and affects both the environment of the cells and the physicochemical properties of the matrix. Fluid flow does not aid the transport of essential nutrients significantly (over shorter periods of time), but may influence the transport of macromolecules through the tissue. The metabolic activity of disc cells responds to long-term alterations in the mechanical stress applied to the tissue. Since the cells are responsible for renewing the matrix, altered cellular activity slowly changes the composition of the matrix.

In experimental tests, greater mechanical stress applied to the disc increased metabolic activity and small solute transport into discs. Opposite effects occurred in discs of the fused section of dog spines, where mechanical stress and movements were reduced. We suggest that these changes result from altered contact area between disc and blood supply (e.g., exercise increases this contact and thus improves nutrition). On the other hand, fusion diminishes blood contacts and nutrient supply in fused discs, leading to cellular inactivity or death.

Mechanical stress, through changes in hydration, may also alter the chemical environment of the cells. It may also affect the cells directly by deforming them through pressure gradients. These alterations in cellular behavior may therefore result from changes in cellular environment as well as (or instead of) changes in nutrition. Further tests are necessary to distinguish between these effects.

## References

Andersson GBJ (1982). Measurement of loads on the lumbar spine. In: *Idiopathic Low Back Pain,* AA White and SL Gordon (eds.). St. Louis: CV Mosby, pp. 220–251.

Adams MA and Hutton WC (1982). The mechanics of the prolapsed intervertebral disc. A hyperflexion injury. *Spine* 7:184–191.

Crank J (1975). *The Mathematics of Diffusion,* 2nd ed. Oxford: Clarendon Press, pp. 44–88.

Fatt I and Goldstick TK (1965). The dynamics of water transport in swelling membranes. *J Colloid Sci* 20:962–989.

Frymoyer JW, Hanley EN, Howe J, Kuhlmann D and Matteri RE (1979). A comparison of radiographic findings in fusion and nonfusion patients ten or more years following lumbar disc surgery. *Spine* 4:435–451.

Gillard GC, Reilly HC, Bell-Both PG and Flint MH (1979). The influence of mechanical forces on the glycosaminoglycan content of the rabbit flexor digitorum profundus tendon. *Connect Tissue Res* 7:37–46.

Handley CJ and Lowther DA (1977). Extracellular matrix metabolism by chondrocytes. III Modulation of proteoglycan synthesis by extracellular levels of proteoglycan in cartilage cells in culture. *Biochim Biophys Acta* 500:132–139.

Herbert CM, Lindberg KA, Jayson MIV and Bailey AJ (1975). Changes in the collagen of human intervertebral disc during ageing and degenerative disc disease. *J Mol Med* 1:79–91.

Hickey DS and Hukins DWL (1980). The relationship between the structure of the annulus fibrosus and the function and failure of the intervertebral disc. *Spine* 5:106–116.

Holm S, Maroudas A, Urban JPG, Selstam G and Nachemson A (1981). Nutrition of the intervertebral disc. *Connect Tissue Res* 8:101–119.

Holm S and Nachemson A (1982). Nutritional changes in the canine intervertebral disc after spinal fusion. *Clin Orthop Rel Res* 169:243–258.

Holm S and Nachemson A (1983). Variations in the nutrition of the canine intervertebral disc induced by motion. *Spine* 8:866–874.

Jones IL, Klämfeldt A and Sandström T (1982). The effect of continuous mechanical pressure upon the turnover of articular cartilage proteoglycans in vitro. *Clin Orthop Rel Res* 165:283–289.

Kazarian LE (1975). Creep characteristics of the human spinal column. *Orthop Clin North Am* 6:3–18.

Kenyon DE (1979). Mathematical model of water flux through aortic tissue. *Bull Math Biol* 41:79–90.

Lai WM and Mow VC (1980). Drag induced compression of articular cartilage during a permeation experiment. *Biorheology* 17:111–123.

Lane JM, Brighton CT and Menkowitz BJ (1977). Anaerobic and aerobic metabolism in articular cartilage. *J Rheumatol* 4:334–342.

Maroudas A (1968). Physico-chemical properties of cartilage in the light of ion-exchange theory. *Biophys J* 10:365–378.

Maroudas A (1980). Physical chemistry of articular cartilage. In: *The Joints and Synovial Fluid*, L Sokoloff (ed.). New York: Academic Press, pp. 120–149.

Maroudas A and Bannon C (1981). Measurement of swelling pressure in cartilage. *Biorheology* 18:619–632.

Maroudas A, Nachemson A, Stockwell R and Urban JPG (1975). Factors involved in the nutrition of the intervertebral disc. *J Anat* 120:113–121.

McCutcheon CW (1962). The frictional properties of animal joints. *Wear* 5:1–20.

Nachemson A and Elfström G (1970). Intravital dynamic pressure measurement in lumbar discs. *Scand J Rehab Med* Vols. 1 and 2, (Suppl. 2): 5–40.

Nachemson A, Lewin T, Maroudas A and Freeman MAR (1970). In vitro diffusion of dye through the end-plates and the annulus fibrosus of human lumbar intervertebral discs. *Acta Orthop Scand* 41:589–607.

Oegema TR, Bradford DS and Cooper KM (1979). Aggregated proteoglycan synthesis in organ cultures of human nucleus pulposus. *J Biol Chem* 254:10579–10581.

Rolander SD and Blair WE (1975). Deformation and fracture of the lumbar vertebral end-plate. *Orthop Clin North Am* 6:75–81.

Schmorl G and Junghanns H (1971). *The Human Spine in Health and Disease*. New York: Grune & Statton, pp. 29–48.

Urban JPG (1977). *Fluid and Solute Transport in the Intervertebral Disc*. Ph D. thesis. London University, London.

Urban JPG, Holm S and Maroudas A (1978). Diffusion of small solutes into the intervertebral disc. *Biorheology* 15:203–223.

Urban JPG, Holm S, Maroudas A and Nachemson A (1982). Nutrition of the intervertebral disc—effect of fluid flow on solute transport. *Clin Orthop Rel Res* 170:296–302.

Urban JPG and Maroudas A (1980). Measurement of swelling pressure and fluid flow in the intervertebral disc with reference to creep. In: *Engineering Aspects of the Spine*, Institute Mechanical Engineers Conference Publications, pp. 63–69.

Wiebkin OW and Muir H (1975). Influence on the cells on the pericellular environment. The effect of hyaluronic acid on proteoglycan synthesis and secretion by chondrocytes of adult articular cartilage. *Philos Trans R Soc Lond* 271:283–291.

CHAPTER 6

# Growth Induction of Bone and Cartilage Cells by Physical Forces

Itzhak Binderman, Dalia Somjen, and
Zvi Shimshoni

## Introduction

The adult skeleton has two major functions: (1) to provide mechanical support and protection for the organism and (2) to regulate concentrations of key blood electrolytes which include $Ca^{2+}$, $Mg^{2+}$, $H^+$ and $HPO_4^{2-}$. Bones of animals and humans undergo continuous change and remodelling. It is clear that the remodelling of the skeleton is controlled in a very complex fashion, that growth and remodelling take place in response to physical strain and that various hormones alter these processes.

Application of mechanical forces has been the classic therapeutic approach to the treatment of orthopedic and orthodontic problems. Pathological manifestations of this biological property are the loss of bone caused by immobilization and weightlessness (Uthoff and Jaworski, 1978). It is almost impossible to define the minute stresses set up in the skeletal tissue, as the physical conditions are so greatly complicated by the presence of muscles, nerves and blood supply.

Glücksmann (1938, 1942) demonstrated that the effects of mechanical stresses on skeletal tissue under the simplified conditions of culture (in vitro) were essentially the same as those found in vivo, where the situation is complicated by extraneous structures and blood flow. He found that pressure and tension, exerted on cartilage in vitro, reoriented cartilage cells, disintegrated hyaline ground substance and replaced the ground substance with fibrillar matrix. On the other hand, tensile stresses promoted bone formation and determined the pattern of osseous architecture. These classic studies suggested that mechanical forces in the living body serve as extracellular information that is transmitted to the cells, where mechanical force modulates the expression of the genetic program for growth and differentiation. Long bones of the skeleton grow in length by endochondral bone formation (Fig. 6.1) and in circumference by appositional bone formation on the periosteal surface (Fig. 6.2). Endochondral bone consists of chondroblasts and chondrocytes surrounded by proteoglycan matrix which greatly differs from the fibrous collagenous matrix

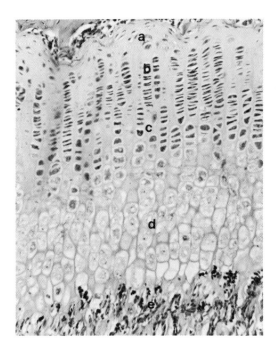

**Figure 6.1.** Sequence of endochondral bone formation: (a) mesenchymal cells (progenitors); (b) proliferating columnar chondroblasts; (c) chondrocytes, mineralized matrix; (d) hypertrophic chondrocytes; (e) newly formed bone.

around the osteoblasts in the periosteal bone. It is known today that cartilage and bone cells are chemically linked to matrix by a specific glycoprotein compound (fibronectin) that may provide the pathway of mechanical force induction at the matrix–cell interface.

The translation of the mechanical force into biochemical reactions in the cell may be explained by one of two major hypotheses. One hypothe-

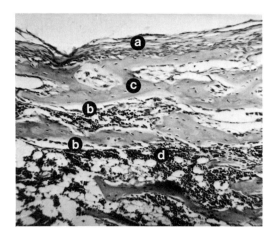

**Figure 6.2.** Lamellar bone formation. Apposition of bone cells from (a) periosteum; (b) osteoblasts; (c) osteocytes surrounded by calcified matrix; (d) bone marrow.

sis assumes that mechanical force transmitted through muscles and ligaments into the matrix causes conformational changes of macromolecules
in the cell membrane, activating enzymes for growth. The second hypothesis suggests that mechanical force generates electrical signals that produce an uneven distribution of ions across the cell membrane, and as a
result increases ion flow and causes a chain of intracellular reactions (Fig.
6.3). Our aim was to investigate the cellular biochemical reactions carried
out in bone cells in response to mechanical force and to determine
whether these reactions are similar for cartilage and bone cells.

## Background

During the early 1950s Yasuda and Fusuda (Yasuda, 1953; Fusuda and
Yasuda, 1957) found that mechanically stressed bone generated an electrical potential (piezoelectric effect). It was shown that electric currents
mimic the effects of mechanical forces on growth and remodelling of bone
(Bassett et al., 1964; Friedenberg et al., 1970).

Recently, the biochemical effects of continuous and intermittent physiological forces and mild electric perturbations on bone and cartilage rudi-
ments and on cells isolated from these tissues were examined (see review
of Rodan, 1981). Rodan and his collaborators found that continuous com-
pressive force of low magnitude ($\approx 60 \text{ g} \cdot \text{cm}^{-2}$) applied axially to a 16-day-
old chick tibia rudiment (simulating weight-bearing load) reduced glucose
consumption to about 50% compared to controls. This phenomenon was
reversible. They were the first to suggest that cyclic AMP, which is synthesized by a membrane-bound enzyme, is the chemical messenger for the
pressure effect (Rodan et al., 1975). Pressure caused a significant reduction in the rate of cyclic AMP accumulation in the epiphyseal cartilage.
Davidovitch and his associates (1976) found experimental support for this
hypothesis in a cat jaw orthodontic model in vivo. Cells isolated from
epiphyses by enzymatic digestion were exposed to hydrostatic pressure
equivalent to the effective axial compressive force ($60 \text{ g} \cdot \text{cm}^{-2}$). A signifi-

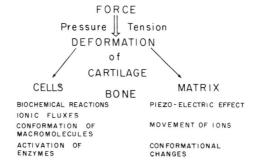

**Figure 6.3.** Diagrammatic chart
flow: transduction of mechanical
force into biochemical changes in
bone cells.

cant reduction in cyclic AMP accumulation was demonstrated only in cells isolated from the proliferative zone of the epiphysis. Investigation of a matrix-deficient chick mutant, characterized by an inability to synthesize cartilage proteoglycans, revealed a similar cyclic AMP effect (Rodan, 1981), indicating a possible direct effect of pressure on these cells.

In contrast to effects produced by continuous compressive forces, intermittent forces of the same magnitude produced a significant increase in cyclic AMP in tibia explants from normal and matrix-deficient chicks, as well as in cells isolated from these tissues (Rodan, 1981). Both studies suggest that the presence of matrix was not an absolute requirement for the pressure effect. In many cells, changes in cyclic AMP and ionic fluxes are recorded after membrane perturbation, and the two may affect each other. In the above-described studies, compressive forces induced cellular uptake of calcium irrespective of changes in cyclic AMP (Rodan, 1981). Changes in cyclic nucleotides and ionic fluxes control cell proliferation. Rodan (1981) has shown that continuous pressure is conducive to cell proliferation, whereas intermittent forces are inhibitory. Proliferative activity is inversely related to cyclic AMP levels.

## Effects of Mechanical Forces on Bone Cells

We investigated the stimulus-receptor mechanism for mechanical forces in bone cells isolated from embryonic rat periosteum and calvaria tissue by the aid of trypsin-EDTA digestion solution (Binderman et al., 1974). Normally, these cells are surrounded by fibrous collagen matrix, in comparison to cartilage cells which are embedded in a proteoglycan type of matrix. It is possible that such environmental differences in the chemical and physical properties of matrix have a profound influence on the transduction mode of the mechanical force trigger. We were able to separate several populations of osteoprogenitor cells, which under the conditions of culture, grow and differentiate, exhibit normal response to bone-seeking hormones such as parathyroid, calcitonin and prostaglandin $E_2$ ($PGE_2$) (Binderman et al., 1982). The cells adhere to the surface of the culture dishes for 24 h after inoculation and proliferate. The cells reach confluency 4 to 5 days after plating. The seeding concentration is in the range of $5 \times 10^5$ cells per 60-mm cell-culture Falcon dish. Like other normal fibroblast-like cells, the bone cells attach to the surface of the dish by pseudopodia-like extensions and contact neighbor cells via processes and extensions (Fig. 6.4).

The cells use fibronectin present in the fetal calf serum, which is included in the growth medium to facilitate their attachment to the dish surface. Later, the cells produce and secrete more of this surface glycoprotein to create a cell-to-cell and a cell-to-collagen attachment (Kleinman et al., 1978). It is possible to maintain bone cell cultures as long as 6

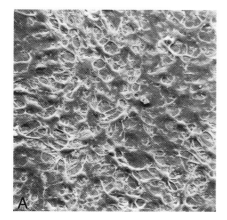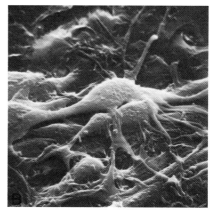

**Figure 6.4.** Bone cells in culture. SEM photomicrographs showing cell processes and cell communications of bone cells in culture. Magnifications are ×144 (A) and ×1360 (B).

weeks. During this period, the cells lay down collagen matrix which is oriented in a similar fashion as in vivo (Boyde et al., 1976).

The mechanical perturbation of these cells was achieved by irreversible deformation of the culture dish. The idea was based on the fact that the cells are tightly attached to the surface of the dish by pseudopodia-like protrusions, and by changing the geometry of the dish the distances between the attachment areas in the same cell and between cells were altered. Also, we may deform the attachment area as well. The device used here consisted of two pieces of acrylic (self-curing methyl methacrylate) connected by an orthodontic expansion screw (Fig. 6.5). This device was glued to the bottom of the dish externally with fast-curing epoxy glue (Somjen et al., 1980). By activation of the orthodontic screw (turning the key lock), the two pieces of acrylic were pulled apart, creating a tensile force on the plastic dish and producing geometric deformation of the plastic dish. Activation of the screw was discontinued when resistance to the force was maximal, before the dish broke.

Geometrical alteration of the dish triggered biochemical changes in the cell membrane. As early as 2 min after activation, a decrease in the level of $PGE_2$ in the cells was measured. $PGE_2$ in the medium increased, which suggested that $PGE_2$ was released from the cells. Subsequently, a rapid cellular synthesis of $PGE_2$ occurred, reaching a fivefold increase at 20 min, followed by a gradual decline (Somjen et al., 1980). At the same time, cellular production of cyclic AMP increased by four- to fivefold after 15 min, followed by a decline. We have found that prostaglandin synthesis determined the cyclic AMP changes. The mechanical force or $PGE_2$ induced adenyl cyclase and phosphodiesterase activities in a way

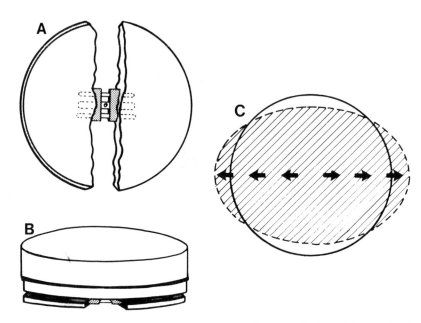

**Figure 6.5.** Diagrammatic illustration of the device. The device **(A)** was glued to the external surface of culture dish **(B)**. Activation of the orthodontic expansion screw created tensile forces on the plastic dish **(C)**.

that the net result of accumulation of cyclic AMP was achieved. We found that mechanical perturbation of bone cells in culture induced a transient accumulation of calcium in the cells (Harell et al., 1977). We also found that thymidine incorporation into DNA was significantly increased in response to mechanical forces and was inhibited by indomethacin, a prostaglandin synthesis inhibitor. These data suggest that the transduction of mechanical forces into biochemical reactions in the cell membrane is mediated by de novo synthesis of $PGE_2$. The synthesis of $PGE_2$ stimulates adenyl cyclase activity, phosphodiesterase activity and ornithine decarboxylase enzyme activity, and finally, leads to the synthesis of DNA (Fig. 6.6A).

These results indicate that compressive hydrostatic forces applied on epiphyseal cells (Rodan, 1981) induce DNA synthesis through a mechanism different from that described by us. We are aware of the fact that our cell culture system consists of several osteoprogenitor cell populations and we tested the possibility that the population responsive to perturbation is specific. Usually, primary cultures consist of cell types responsive to parathyroid (PTH), calcitonin (CT) and $PGE_2$ hormones. $PGE_2$ stimulates an eightfold increase of cellular cyclic AMP; PTH increases cyclic AMP levels by fourfold and CT by twofold (Binderman et al., 1982). An additive increase in cyclic AMP was obtained with combined hormone treatment, suggesting the presence of separate receptors for these hor-

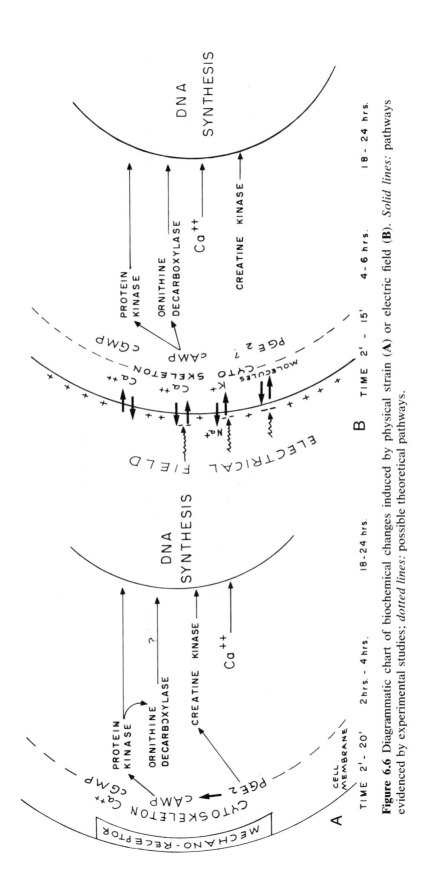

**Figure 6.6** Diagrammatic chart of biochemical changes induced by physical strain (**A**) or electric field (**B**). *Solid lines:* pathways evidenced by experimental studies; *dotted lines:* possible theoretical pathways.

mones (PGE$_2$, PTH and CT), either on the same cell type or on different cell types, or both. If the amount of cyclic AMP response represents the amount of different responsive cell types, then the PGE$_2$-responsive cell dominates the culture, and less of PTH-responsive cells and much less of CT-responsive cells exist. Other studies (Luben et al., 1976) identified the PTH-responsive cells as osteoblasts and the CT-responsive cells as osteoclasts. PGE$_2$ is known to induce many different cell types, including fibroblasts, osteoblasts and blood cells. In spite of the greater membrane response of these cultures to PGE$_2$ than to PTH (cyclic AMP effect), their effect on DNA synthesis was different. PTH stimulated DNA synthesis much more (threefold increase) than PGE$_2$ (twofold increase). Moreover, when both hormones were added to the medium, DNA synthesis increased not more than threefold, and when cells were pretreated with indomethacin, only a slight reduction in PTH stimulation of DNA synthesis occurred. However, it still remained significantly above control levels (Binderman et al., 1982). These results strongly support the premise that a cell population, which is stimulated by PGE$_2$ to synthesize DNA, is probably also PTH-responsive. Furthermore, the cell population that responds specifically to mechanical perturbation probably consists of osteoblast-like cells.

Another possibility exists whereby the cells, which are activated by mechanical perturbation and produce PGE$_2$, are not responsive to PGE$_2$ (DNA effect) and the secretion of PGE$_2$ activates neighbor cells to produce DNA. Recently, we tested this hypothesis and found that when primary cultures are subcultured, the PTH and mechanical perturbation receptor systems are not detectable. However, when the cells are cultured in medium with very low calcium concentration (0.125 mM), the PTH-responsive cells survive in two to three subcultures and their response to mechanical forces is maintained. These data support the hypothesis that osteoblast-like cells, responsive to PTH, are specifically responsive to mechanical perturbation through de novo synthesis of PGE$_2$.

Recently, we tested the stimulus–receptor mechanism present in progenitor cells of the condyle. The condylar process of the mandible consists of progenitor cells that are sensitive to mechanical stress (Meikle, 1973; Stutzman and Petrovic, 1974). Under normal conditions, mechanical stimulation is required for proliferation and differentiation of progenitor cells into chondroblasts, whereas lack of mechanical stimuli induced their differentiation into osteoblasts. Recently, we also investigated whether translation of mechanical forces in condyle cells is through the same molecular pathway found for bone cells. We isolated the condyle cells by collagenase digestion and cultured them under the same conditions normally used for bone cells (Shimshoni et al., 1984). Mechanical stimulation was performed using the same device as previously described (Fig. 6.5). Interestingly, PTH stimulated intracellular accumulation of cyclic AMP by twofold, whereas CT had no effect on these cultures. Mechanical deformation of the dish induced cellular production of cyclic AMP by 2.5-fold, and DNA synthesis by 40% to 50%. However, indomethacin failed to inhibit this DNA response (Shimshoni et al., 1983). These data indirectly suggest that the response of the condylar progenitor cells to mechanical stimulation is not mediated by de novo synthesis of prostaglandin.

In our recent experiments (Somjen et al., 1982), bone cell cultures and condyle cell cultures were electrically stimulated. We examined whether electrical stimuli can produce in our system effects similar to those generated by the mechanical forces (Fig. 6.6B). We found that variable electric fields induced changes in cellular cyclic AMP and DNA synthesis in the different populations of the bone cell cultures, as well as in the condyle cells. However, perturbation of the cell membrane by electric fields was not mediated by $PGE_2$ (Korenstein et al., 1984). Rodan (1982) proposed that perturbation of the cell membrane by electric fields in vivo produces cation ($Ca^{2+}$ and $K^+$) fluxes across the membrane or changes in cyclic nucleotides that eventually lead to DNA synthesis. We showed that many different cells of mesenchymal origin respond to electric fields of varying magnitude (Somjen et al., 1983) (Fig. 6.7). On the other hand, mechanical perturbation may redistribute ions on the cell membrane (electric field), or activate specifically a "mechano-receptor system" which stimulates synthesis of $PGE_2$. Most probably, the "mechano-receptor system" is specific for osteoblasts, whereas mechanical perturbation of cartilage cells is translated into changes in electric surface potentials on the cell membrane.

Recent observations suggest the existence of prostaglandin-producing and nonproducing subpopulations of osteoblastic cells (Aubin et al., 1982). Also, cells that produce $PGE_2$ do not respond to $PGE_2$ and cells that respond to $PGE_2$ do not produce $PGE_2$ (Rodan et al., 1982). We suggest that $PGE_2$, synthesized by a certain subpopulation of osteoblasts in response to mechanical force, induces proliferation of osteoprogenitor cells, and when released, $PGE_2$ activates osteoblasts to resorb bone.

The force applied to an organ is first transmitted to the matrix of the connective tissue (collagen or proteoglycan), where it is transmitted to the matrix–cell interface as a mechanical signal or as an electric perturbation. It is then translated into a biochemical chain of reactions within the cell membrane. We propose that in specific populations of osteoblast cells, mechanical stimulus activates synthesis of $PGE_2$, whereas in other bone and cartilage cells, mechanical stimulus activates ionic fluxes and alters cyclic nucleotides.

It is now commonly accepted that the mechanical properties of cells depend to a large extent on the integrated action of the plasma membrane and the cytoskeleton. Cytoskeletal proteins are associated with the inner face of the plasma membrane, and regulate the cascade of cyclic AMP

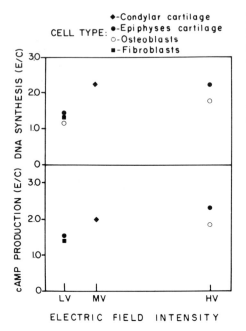

CELL TYPE:
♦-Condylar cartilage
●-Epiphyses cartilage
○-Osteoblasts
■-Fibroblasts

**Figure 6.7.** The effect of electric field perturbation on DNA synthesis (top) and cyclic AMP production (bottom). The electric field strengths used in these studies were 13 V/cm (low voltage, LV), 22 V/cm (medium voltage, MV) and 54 V/cm (high voltage, HV).

biosynthesis and action. Elevated cyclic AMP and/or ionic transmembrane fluxes and actin polymerization correlate well (for review see Geiger, 1983; Zor, 1983). Recently, Laub and Korenstein (1984) found that electric field pulses, capacitively applied to tissue cultures of embryonic bone cells, induce changes in the state of cellular actin. Figures 6.6A and 6.6B summarize cellular events at the cell membrane and the flow of mechanical or electric perturbation and its transduction into a chain of biochemical reaction starting at the cell membrane, followed by enzymatic reactions in the cytoplasm and DNA synthesis. Changes in the cell membrane ($Ca^{2+}$ transport, prostaglandin synthetase and adenyl cyclase) occur within minutes (Figs. 6.6A and 6.6B). Cytoplasmic enzyme activity (ornithine decarboxylase and creatine kinase) increases after 4 h and nuclear changes occur between 18 and 24 h (Figs. 6.6A and 6.6B). We have found that ornithine decarboxylase is induced in response to elevated levels of cellular cyclic AMP whereas creatine kinase activity is induced in response to hormones that affect growth independent of its effect on cyclic AMP. The first enzyme is important in biosynthesis of polyamines and the latter in regenerating ATP; both are involved in DNA synthesis. Creatine kinase of brain type (CK-BB) is induced 4 h after application of physical strain on cultured bone cells (Binderman et al., 1984 and unpublished results).

   The cellular reactions, in response to mechanical or electric perturbation which we described in this chapter, resemble in much detail the effects of hormones and growth factors. We feel, therefore, that it is important to study in depth the mechano-receptor system in the plasma membrane and its relationship to the cytoskeleton and to enzymes in the cell membrane. This type of information is vital for the understanding of the control of bone remodeling.

## Summary

The mammalian skeleton absorbs most of the weight-bearing load and muscular activity. The force is first transmitted to the matrix of the periosteum and bone or the perichondrium and cartilage, where it is transmitted further to the matrix–cell interface as a mechanical signal or as an electric perturbation. It is then translated into a biochemical chain of reactions within the cell membrane, including activation of adenyl cyclase, phosphodiesterase, prostaglandin synthetase and ion transport reactions which may lead to enzymatic and structural changes in the cell; changes in cytoskeleton proteins, ornithine decarboxylase and creatine kinase. These latter cellular enzyme activities propagate the synthesis of DNA and cell replication. We propose that in specific populations of osteoblasts, mechanical stimulus activates the synthesis of E series prostaglandins, whereas in other bone and cartilage cells, mechanical stimulus alters ionic fluxes and streaming potentials that signal membrane responses. We assume that electric stimulation has the capacity to circumvent the mechano-receptor system. Such changes may activate adenyl cyclase and cytoskeleton proteins and/or ionic transmembrane fluxes which induce differentiation and proliferation of different cells in the bone and cartilage environment. It is therefore possible that the electric trigger is not cell-specific, and different intensities of electric field will stimulate a variety of cell populations. Future studies should elucidate the nature of the mechano-receptor and the many intermediate pathways leading from mechanical activation to proliferation and differentiation of the activated cells.

## References

Aubin JE, Heersche JNM, Merrilees MJ and Sodek J (1982). Isolation of bone cell clones with differences in growth, hormone responses, and extracellular matrix production. *J Cell Biol* 92:452–461.

Bassett CAL, Pawluk RJ and Becker RO (1964). Effects of electric currents on bone *in vivo*. *Nature* 204:652–654.

Binderman I, Duksin D, Harell A, Sachs L and Katchalsky E (1974). Formation of bone tissue in culture from isolated bone cells. *J Cell Biol* 61:427–439.

Binderman I, Shimshoni Z and Somjen D (1984). Biochemical pathways involved in the translation of physical stimulus into biological message. *Calcif Tissue Int* 36, *Suppl* 1: S82–S85.

Binderman I, Somjen D, Shimshoni Z and Harell A (1982). The role of prostaglandins (PGE$_2$) in bone remodeling induced by physical forces. In: *Osteoporosis, Proceedings of the International Symposium on Osteoporosis.* J Menczel, M Makin, GC Robin, and R Steinberg (eds.). New York: John Wiley & Sons, pp. 195–199.

Boyde A, Jones SJ, Binderman I and Harell A (1976). Scanning electron microscopy of bone cells in culture. *Cell Tissue Res* 166:60–65.

Davidovitch Z, Montgomery PC, Eckerdal O and Gustafson GT (1976). Cellular localization of cyclic AMP in periodontal tissues during experimental tooth movement in cats. *Calcif Tissue Res* 18:316–329.

Friedenberg ZB, Andrews ET, Smolenski BI, Pearl BW and Brighton CT (1970). Bone reaction to varying amounts of direct current. *Surg Gynecol Obstet* 131:894–899.

Fusuda E and Yasuda I (1957). On the piezoelectric effect of bone. *J Physiol Soc Jpn* 12:1158–1162.

Geiger B (1983). Membrane-cytoskeleton interaction. *Biochim Biophys Acta* 737:305–341.

Glücksmann A (1938). Studies on bone mechanics in vitro; 1. Influence of pressure on orientation of structure. *Anat Rec* 72:97–113.

Glücksmann A (1942). The role of mechanical stresses in bone formation *in vitro*. *J Anat* 76:231–239.

Harell A, Dekel S and Binderman I (1977). Biochemical effect of mechanical stress on cultured bone cells. *Calcif Tissue Res Suppl* 22:202–209.

Kleinman HK, Murray JC, McGoodwin EB, Martin GR and Binderman I (1978). Attachment of bone cells to collagen. In: *Proceedings of Symposium on Mechanisms of Localized Bone Loss. Special Supplement to Calcified Tissues Abstracts.* Horton, Tarpley and David (eds.). Washington DC and London: Information Retrieval Inc. pp. 61–72.

Korenstein R, Somjen D, Fischler H and Binderman I (1984). Capacitative pulsed electric stimulation of bone cells: induction of cyclic-AMP changes and DNA synthesis. *Biochim Biophys Acta* 803:302–307.

Laub F and Korenstein R (1984). Actin polymerization induced by pulsed electric stimulation of bone cells *in vitro*. *Biochim Biophys Acta* 803:308–313.

Luben RA, Wong GL and Cohn DV (1976). Biochemical characterization with parathormone and calcitonin of isolated bone cells: provisional identification of osteoclasts and osteoblasts. *Endocrinology* 99:526–534.

Meikle MC (1973). *In vivo* transplantation of mandibular joint of the rat. An autoradiographic investigation into cellular changes at the condyle. *Arch Oral Biol* 18:1011–1020.

Rodan GA (1981). Mechanical and electrical effects on bone and cartilage cells: translation of physical signal into a biological message. In: *Orthodontics, the State of the Art.* HG Brarrer (ed.). Philadelphia: The University of Pennsylvania Press, pp. 315–322.

Rodan GA, Mensi T and Harvey A (1975). A quantitative method for the application of compressive forces to bone in tissue culture. *Calcif Tissue Res* 18:125–131.

Rodan SB, Rodan GA, Simmons HA, Walenga RW, Feinstein MB and Raisz LG (1982). Bone resorptive activity in conditioned medium from rat osteosarcoma cell line. In: *Prostaglandins and Cancer: First International Conference*. New York: Alan R. Liss, pp. 573–578.

Shimshoni Z, Binderman I, Fine N and Somjen D (1984). Mechanical and hormonal stimulation of cell cultures derived from young rat mandible condyle. *Arch Oral Biol* 29:827–831.

Somjen D, Binderman I, Berger E and Harell A (1980). Bone remodelling induced by physical stress is prostaglandin $E_2$ mediated. *Biochim Biophys Acta* 627:91–100.

Somjen D, Korenstein R, Fischler H and Binderman I (1982). Effects of electric field intensity on the response of cultured bone cells to parathyroid and prostaglandin $E_2$. In: *Current Advances in Skeletogenesis: Development, Biomineralization, Mediators and Metabolic Diseases*. M Silberman and H Slavkin (eds.). Amsterdam, Oxford and Princeton: Excerpta Medica, pp. 412–416.

Somjen D, Shimshoni Z, Levy J, Korenstein R, Fischler H and Binderman I (1983). Stimulation of cell cultures by different electric field intensities is cell specific. *Abstract, XVIIth European Symposium on Calcified Tissues, Davos, Switzerland*.

Stutzman L and Petrovic A (1974). Effets de la resection du muscle pterygoidian externe sur la croissence du cartilage condylien de jeune rat. *Bull Assoc Anat* 58:1107–1114.

Uthoff HK and Jaworski ZFC (1978). Bone response to long term immobilization. *J Bone Joint Surg* 60B:420–429.

Yasuda I (1953). Fundamental considerations for fracture treatment. *J Kyoto Med Sci* 4:395–406.

Zor U (1983). Role of cytoskeletal organization in the regulation of adenylate cyclic adenosine monophosphate by hormones. *Endocrine Rev* 4:1–21.

CHAPTER 7

# Pathophysiology of Nerve Entrapments and Nerve Compression Injuries

Lars B. Dahlin, Björn Rydevik, and
Göran Lundborg

## Introduction

Compression of peripheral nerves may induce various symptoms such as
sensory disturbances, motor weakness and pain. For example, these
symptoms are associated with trauma to limbs and nerve entrapments.
The degree and type of changes in nerve function vary with the type,
magnitude and duration of the compression trauma. However, the pathophysiology of compression-induced lesions is incompletely known. In this
chapter experimental investigations concerning the effects of compression on peripheral nerves as well as the pathophysiology of various types
of nerve compression lesions are reviewed.

## Background

The peripheral nerve trunk is a complex structure consisting of *nerve
fibers,* intraneural *connective tissue* and a rich network of *microvessels.*
Since these structures react differently to trauma, there is a broad spectrum of mechanisms which cause functional deterioration of a peripheral
nerve after trauma. Therefore, each of these structural components of
peripheral nerve will be considered separately.

### Intraneural Microanatomy

The peripheral nerve trunk (Fig. 7.1) consists of various layers of connective tissue, called the epi-, peri- and endoneurium (Sunderland, 1978). The
*epineurium* consists of rather loose connective tissue which surrounds the
so-called fascicles. The amounts of epineurial connective tissue between
different nerve trunks as well as between different levels within the same
nerve varies considerably (Sunderland, 1978). The relatively extensive
epineurium in nerve trunks where it crosses joints may bolster nerve

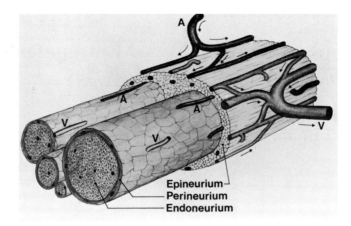

Epineurium
Perineurium
Endoneurium

**Figure 7.1.** Schematic drawing of the different connective tissue layers and segmentally approaching vessels of a peripheral nerve: arteriolar vessels (A) and venular vessels (V). The *thin arrows* indicate the direction of blood flow in the vessels. (Reproduced by permission of Dr. Claes Nordborg, Dept. of Pathology, University of Göteborg, Sweden.)

fascicles, thereby protecting the nerve mechanically from external compression (Sunderland, 1978).

Each fascicle is surrounded by a *perineurium* or perineurial sheath (Fig. 7.1), consisting of lamellated perineurial cells. These cells are joined together by tight junctions (Thomas and Jones, 1967; Shanta and Bourne, 1969). The perineurial sheath is a strong mechanical membrane and possesses properties of a diffusion barrier (Olsson and Reese, 1969, 1971; Klemm, 1970). The interstitial fluid pressure inside the fascicles, namely the endoneurial fluid pressure (EFP), is slightly greater: $+1.5 \pm 0.7$ mm Hg (Low et al., 1977; Myers et al., 1978) than that in other surrounding tissues, for example, subcutaneous tissue: $-4.7 \pm 0.8$ mm Hg (Chen et al., 1976) and muscle: $-2 \pm 2$ mm Hg (Hargens et al., 1978). EFP may increase with trauma or in certain neuropathies and this condition may affect the function of the peripheral nerve (Myers and Powell, 1981).

The *endoneurium* is the term used for the intrafascicular connective tissue elements, composed of fibroblasts and collagen fibrils (Fig. 7.1). Fibrillar content is higher in cutaneous nerves compared to deeply placed nerves, probably reflecting the extra protection required for the nerve fibers in more vulnerable superficial nerves (Sunderland, 1978).

## Intraneural Blood Flow

Both normal impulse propagation and axonal transport depend on a continuous supply of oxygen, which is provided by the rich intraneural microvascular network. The peripheral nerve receives its blood supply from vessels approaching the nerve trunk segmentally along its course (Fig. 7.1). When these vessels reach the epineurium, they divide into ascending and descending branches, which run longitudinally within the epineurium. There are frequent anastomoses between the epineurial vessels and vessels located in the perineurium as well as in the endoneurium. The endoneurial vascular bed, consisting mainly of capillaries (Fig. 7.2), communicates with extrafascicular vessels by numerous anastomoses, which often pierce the perineurial sheath obliquely (Lundborg, 1970, 1975). This anatomical arrangement may be important in neuropathies in which endoneurial pressure is elevated, since the anastomosing vessels could be partially or wholly occluded on penetration through the perineurium, thus impairing endoneurial blood flow (Lundborg, 1975).

Interference with intraneural blood flow may induce deterioration of nerve function (Eiken et al., 1964; Lundborg, 1970). However, the effects of various types of trauma on intraneural microcirculation are incompletely known. The recovery of intraneural blood flow following varying periods of tourniquet-induced ischemia in the rabbit hind limb was analyzed by Lundborg (Lundborg, 1970, 1975). Vital microscopic examination of the microcirculation in the tibial nerve revealed that intraneural

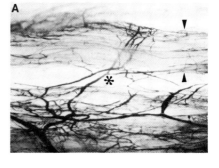

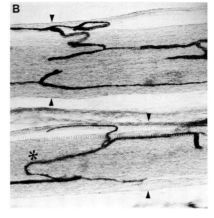

**Figure 7.2.** Microangiograms of peripheral nerves. **A:** The microvascular system of a human median nerve in the forearm—India ink perfused and clarified. The *arrows* indicate the outlines of one fascicle with a longitudinal intrafascicular capillary system. The system is supplied by segmental, extrafascicular vessels as indicated by (*). **B:** Detail of the longitudinal capillary system of two adjacent fascicles in a human ulnar nerve from the forearm. The outlines of the fascicles are indicated by *arrows* and a capillary loop is marked by (*). (Reproduced by permission of G Lundborg, *J Hand Surg* 4:34–41, 1979.)

blood flow in all layers of the nerve was rapidly restored following release of tourniquet pressure, even after ischemia periods of 8 to 10 h (Lundborg, 1970, 1975).

Surgical exposure of the whole rabbit tibial-sciatic nerve with ligation of segmental, external vessels can be performed without visible microcirculatory disturbances in the middle of the nerve (Lundborg, 1970). Transection of the tibial nerve has no apparent effect on intraneural microcirculation. Even most terminally in the cut end, normal capillary circulation is observed (Lundborg, 1970, 1975). However, if stretching is applied to the cut end of a transected nerve trunk, venular stasis is induced when the nerve is stretched to about 8% over its original length. Complete standstill of the microcirculation is induced at about 15% elongation. When the tension is relieved completely after 30 min, intraneural blood flow is restored (Lundborg and Rydevik, 1973).

The effect of pressure on the microcirculation of peripheral nerves is incompletely known. One of the few studies demonstrated that intravenously injected Evans Blue did not perfuse superficial nerve vessels during compression at 60 to 65 mm Hg (Bentley and Schlapp, 1943). However, the effects of compression on intraneural blood flow in vivo have not been investigated previously.

## Intraneural Microvascular Permeability

Under normal conditions, small amounts of serum proteins can pass through the epineurial blood vessel walls into the extravascular space. Vascular permeability to proteins in the epineurium can increase after slight trauma such as ischemia of short duration (Lundborg, 1970, 1975). This increases transcapillary fluid filtration and an epineurial edema is formed. However, such edema can not reach the endoneurial space due to the barrier function of the perineurium (Shanta and Bourne, 1969; Klemm, 1970; Olsson et al., 1971; Olsson and Reese, 1971). In contrast to the epineurial vessels, the endoneurial vascular bed is normally impermeable to proteins. Thus, the endothelium of endoneurial vessels constitutes a blood–nerve barrier which is analogous to the blood–brain barrier of the central nervous system (Olsson et al., 1971). The presence of tight junctions between the endothelial cells may provide the anatomical basis for the blood–nerve barrier in conjunction with a sparcity of pinocytotic vesicles in the endothelial cells of these vessels (Olsson and Reese, 1971). Whereas slight trauma may induce epineurial edema, more severe trauma, for example, crushed nerve (Olsson, 1966) or prolonged tourniquet ischemia (Lundborg, 1970), may induce injury to the endoneurial vessels. Endoneurial edema is a more serious condition than epineurial edema since the former affects nerve fibers more directly by various pathological mechanisms, leading to functional deterioration (Lundborg, 1970, 1975).

## The Perineurium as a Diffusion Barrier

Perineurial cells, joined together by tight junctions, provide the perineurium with its barrier properties. The barrier function of the perineurial sheath is highly resistant to various kinds of trauma such as prolonged ischemia (Lundborg et al., 1973) and dissection trauma (Rydevik et al., 1976*b*). If the perineurial barrier is broken, chronic passage of exogenous substances from surrounding tissues to endoneurial space may occur (Olsson and Kristensson, 1973; Kristensson and Olsson, 1974).

Thus, the local environment of the endoneurial space (Fig. 7.3) is normally controlled by the *blood–nerve barrier* and the *perineurial barrier* (Olsson and Kristensson, 1973; Lundborg, 1975), and injury to one or both of these barriers may have serious consequences for the nerve function (Lundborg, 1970; Rydevik et al., 1976*a*). The reaction of the barriers to acute, graded compression has not been investigated previously.

## Axonal Transport

The function of the nerve fibers is not only to conduct impulses but also to transport essential material (for example, proteins) from the nerve cell body down the axon (anterograde axonal transport) as well as in the

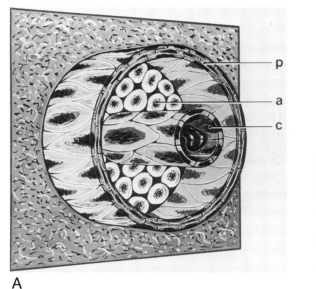
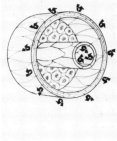

A                                                      B

**Figure 7.3.** Schematic drawings of the protective barriers of a peripheral nerve. **A:** One single fascicle with one endoneurial capillary (c) located in the center. The perineurium (p) surrounds the axons (a) and the endoneurial vessels. **B:** Barrier sites are symbolized by the curved arrows. (Reproduced by permission of G Lundborg, *J Bone Joint Surg* 57A:938–948, 1975.)

opposite direction (retrograde axonal transport). The anterograde transport consists of rapid (between 34 and 400 mm/day) components and slow (between 0.1 and 25 mm/day) components (McLean et al., 1976; Grafstcin and Forman, 1980; Brady and Lasek, 1982). The axons may have a trophic influence on the end organs, possibly via the anterograde axonal transport system (Guth, 1968). Retrograde axonal transport may provide the nerve cell body with substances from the periphery, and may affect the nerve cell body importantly (Grafstein and Forman, 1980; Varon and Adler, 1981).

Axonal transport is blocked by different toxic substances (Sjöstrand et al., 1978) or by ischemia and compression (Leone and Ochs, 1978; Hahnenberger, 1978). The reaction of the axonal transport to graded compression trauma in vivo has not been studied earlier.

## Nerve Fiber Structure and Impulse Propagation

Nerve fibers in peripheral nerves are either myelinated or unmyelinated. Myelinated nerve fibers have diameters larger than 1 to 2 $\mu$m and are surrounded by a string of longitudinally arranged Schwann cells, which form the myelin sheath. The nodes of Ranvier are regions between adjacent myelin sheaths and internodal distance (ranging between 0.2 and 2 mm) depends on the thickness and length of the nerve (Berthold, 1978; Sunderland, 1978). When several axons are submerged in longitudinally troughs along the outside of Schwann cells, these fibers are referred to as unmyelinated.

The conduction velocity of a myelinated nerve fiber is related to, among other things, the diameter of the nerve fiber (Gasser and Erlanger, 1929). In rapidly conducting myelinated nerve fibers, action potentials jump from node to node (the impulse propagation is saltatory) whereas in unmyelinated nerve fibers, impulse propagation is continuous. Large-diameter fibers are also more sensitive to compression trauma (Gasser and Erlanger, 1929), and may be subjected to greater deformation than thinner fibers at a given pressure (MacGregor et al., 1975).

Locally applied pressure on a nerve can block conduction acutely and for varying periods after pressure release (Gasser and Erlanger, 1929; Lewis et al., 1931; Bentley and Schlapp, 1943; Denny-Brown and Brenner, 1944; Causey and Palmer, 1949; Fowler et al., 1972; Sharpless, 1975). Bentley and Schlapp (1943) demonstrated that conduction block was maximal beneath the edges of a compression cuff and suggested that this was due to mechanical deformation of nerve fibers at this site. The ultrastructural appearance of the nerve fiber injury at the edges following compression at high pressure was described by Ochoa et al. (1972). They found that the nodes of Ranvier were displaced toward the uncompressed parts of the nerve, a phenomenon that occurred at proximal as well as at distal edges (Fig. 7.4). This nodal displacement was followed by segmental

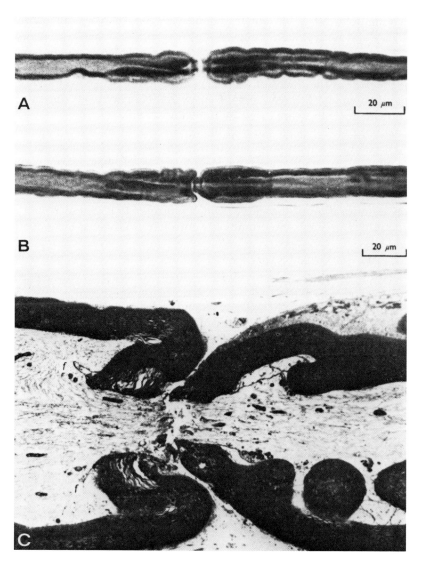

**Figure 7.4.** Injury to nerve fibers at edges of compressed segments. **A:** A light microscopic section of a normal nerve fiber with a node of Ranvier in the center. **B:** An abnormal node of Ranvier, 4 days after experimental compression with a tourniquet. The myelin sheath to the right is displaced and invaginated in the sheath to the left. **C:** Electron microscopic picture from the same area as in (*B*). There is an invagination of the paranode on the left by the one on the right, due to the pressure gradient between compressed and uncompressed part of the nerve (×4900, original magnification). (Reproduced by permission of J Ochoa et al., Anatomical changes in peripheral nerves compressed by a pneumatic tourniquet. *J Anat* 113:433–455, 1972 and by permission of Cambridge University Press.)

demyelination and a subsequent conduction block. After cuff release, recovery and remyelination occurred over a period of weeks to months. These authors claim that the basic factor responsible for conduction block after nerve compression is mechanical deformation of nerve fibers and displacement of the nodes of Ranvier. Other authors (Lewis et al., 1931; Denny-Brown and Brenner, 1944; Causey and Palmer, 1949) suggest that the conduction block is caused by ischemia.

Lundborg (1970) demonstrated that compression by a tourniquet applied around the rabbit hindlimb for 4 h may induce vascular injury and formation of an endoneurial edema of the underlying sciatic nerve, whereas the first signs of edema formation in the tibial nerve occurs after 8 h of ischemia. This endoneurial edema is followed by persistent functional deterioration of the nerve, which indicates that vascular injury in the peripheral nerve is important and contributes to the nerve conduction block.

We have performed experimental studies on intraneural blood flow (Rydevik et al., 1981), vascular permeability (Rydevik and Lundborg, 1977), axonal transport (Rydevik et al., 1980; Dahlin et al., 1982) and nerve function and structure (Rydevik and Nordborg, 1980; Dahlin et al., 1985) in association with acute, graded nerve compression. The effects of *low* (20–80 mm Hg) and *high* (200–600 mm Hg) pressure levels were investigated. The results of these studies are summarized below.


## Recent Results

### Experimental Nerve Compression Model

Rabbit tibial nerve, used in our studies of intraneural blood flow, vascular permeability and nerve fiber structure and function, was easily exposed by a medial incision between the ankle and the knee. The nerve was carefully mobilized from surrounding tissues. The rabbit vagus nerve was used for the investigations of axonal transport. This nerve was exposed on the lateral aspect of the neck along its course close to the carotid artery.

The nerve was compressed by a small compression chamber (Rydevik and Lundborg, 1977). This compression device consisted of two symmetrical halves of plexiglass onto which thin rubber membranes were glued. The two halves were placed around the nerve trunk and secured in position by four small screws. The chamber was then connected to a compressed air system, which enabled inflation of the chamber with air of varying levels of known pressure. The pressure system automatically compensated for any leakage of air and thus maintained the pressure at a constant level during the experiment. In this way the degree of nerve injury was controlled by varying the *pressure level* and *time* of application.

## Intraneural Blood Flow

The tibial nerve was exposed by incision of skin and fascia on both the medial and lateral side of the leg. In these experiments a modified transparent compression device allowed transillumination in a vital microscope (Fig. 7.5). In this way the nerve was compressed by two transparent, inflatable polyethylene cuffs connected to the previously mentioned compressed air system. This technique enabled the investigation of intraneural blood flow in epineurial/perineurial arterioles and venules as well as in endoneurial capillaries during compression. Blood flow was gradually reduced when cuff pressure was sequentially increased from zero until total ischemia of the compressed segment was induced (here we refer to ischemia as complete circulatory arrest). Ischemia was then maintained for 2 h. After pressure release, intraneural blood flow was studied

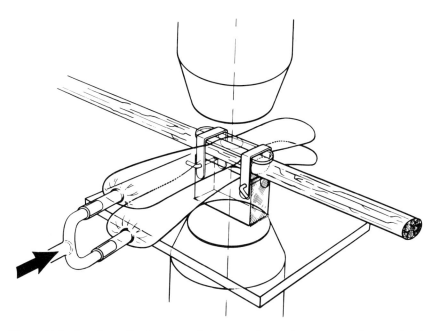

**Figure 7.5.** A schematic drawing of the experimental set up used to study the effects of compression on intraneural microcirculation. Transparent compression cuffs were placed around the nerve, and inflated with air (*arrow*) of varying pressure. (Reproduced by permission of B Rydevik et al., Effects of graded compression on intraneural blood flow. An in vivo study on rabbit tibial nerve. *J Hand Surg* 6:3–12, 1981).

for about 30 min (for details of method and results, see Rydevik et al., 1981).

Cuff application around the nerve without inflation caused no detectable impairment of intraneural blood flow. When pressure was increased to 20 to 30 mm Hg, the first signs of retarded blood flow and reduced vascular diameter were seen in epineurial venules. At this pressure level, retrograde effects on capillary circulation in the fascicles were minor or absent. Then cuff pressure was increased further; blood flow was reduced in endoneurial capillaries and feeding arterioles. At a cuff pressure of 60 mm Hg, 60% of the compressed nerves were ischemic and at 80 mm Hg, there was complete standstill of intraneural blood flow (ischemia) in the compressed segment of all nerves investigated. This cuff pressure was maintained for 2 h. Following pressure release, intraneural blood flow was rapidly restored in all layers of the nerve, except initially it was rather sluggish. However, an epineurial edema, as evidenced by decreased transparency of the nerve in the vital microscope, was observed. Nerves, compressed at 400 mm Hg for 2 h and observed 3 and 7 days after pressure release, showed no or very slow stagnant intraneural blood flow within the previously compressed segment.

## Intraneural Microvascular Permeability

Permeability properties of intraneural blood vessels, when nerves had been subjected to compression at 50, 200 and 400 mm Hg, were studied by fluorescence microscopic tracing of intravenously injected serum albumin, labelled with Evans blue (EBA) (Rydevik and Lundborg, 1977) according to a method described by Steinwall and Klatzo (1965) and Olsson (1966). The EBA solution was slowly injected into a marginal vein of the ear immediately after pressure release and the solution was allowed to circulate for 30 min. The animal was then killed and nerve specimens were fixed in 4% buffered formaldehyde for 24 h. The distribution of the EBA complex was examined in a fluorescence microscope. Using a special filter combination in the microscope, the dye complex emitted a bright red fluorescence and was easily traced. This technique thus allowed visualization of increased vascular permeability to albumin, seen as extravasation of the dye complex (for details of method and results, see Rydevik and Lundborg, 1977).

Application of the chamber around the nerve for 2 h without inflation did not cause any detectable increase in microvascular permeability of the nerve. Compression at 50 mm Hg for 2 h induced an epineurial edema. Edema was restricted to the epineurium, and was prevented from reaching the nerve fibers by the perineurial sheath. When nerves were compressed at higher pressure levels (200–400 mm Hg), macroscopical examination revealed a striking feature. There was increased blue staining at *edges* of the compressed segment, indicating vascular injury at these levels. When the central part of a compressed nerve segment was examined in the fluorescence microscope, no endoneurial edema was detected (Fig. 7.6A). However an endoneurial edema was demonstrated at the *edges* of the compressed nerve segment (Fig. 7.6B). Compression at 200 mm Hg for 2 h and 400 mm Hg for 15 min, induced edema in *some* fascicles at the edges. Edema in *all* fascicles at the edges was seen when the nerves were compressed at 400 mm Hg for 2 h. When the duration of compression at 200 mm Hg was increased to 4 and 6 h, endoneurial edema was also detected in the center of the compressed segment.

## The Perineurium as a Diffusion Barrier

After pressure release, 5 ml of EBA solution was applied around the compressed nerve segment. Two hours later, the nerve was removed and processed for fluorescence microscopic examination as described above. Compression at 400 to 600 mm Hg for 2 h or 200 mm Hg for 6 h did not cause any impairment of the perineurium barrier function to albumin (Rydevik and Lundborg, 1977).

## Axonal Transport

The fast component (~400 mm/day) of axonal transport in vagus nerves subjected to various degrees of compression was studied. Rapidly migrating proteins were labelled by microinjection of 100 $\mu$Ci of [$^3$H]leucine into the nodose ganglion of the vagus nerve. The labelled amino acids were incorporated into proteins and thereafter transported down the nerve trunk by the anterograde axonal transport system. Two hours after labelling, the nerve was subjected to compression for a period of 2 h. In some experiments, recovery from compression was allowed before proteins were labelled. In all experiments 4 h were allowed for synthesis of proteins and for axonal transport. After 4 h the whole nerve was removed and immediately cut into 2.5-mm long segments. The amount of radioactivity of each segment was measured in a Packard Tricarb liquid scintillation counter. Radioactivity in the nerve segments was plotted against the distance from the nodose ganglion, which gave a profile of the distribution of labelled proteins (for details of method and results, see Rydevik et al., 1980; Dahlin et al., 1982).

In experiments where the chamber was applied but not inflated, a profile was found that was similar to those found in untreated nerves (there was no block at the site of the cuff). Thus, cuff application itself did not block axonal transport. A similar profile was found in nerves subjected to compression at 20 mm Hg for 2 h (Fig. 7.7). However, when the nerves were compressed at 30 mm Hg for 2 h, there were various degrees of accumulation of radioactivity at the level of the compression chamber. Some of the nerves showed a profile with an accumulation at the site of

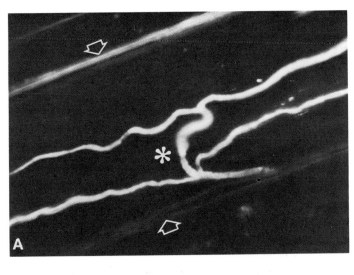

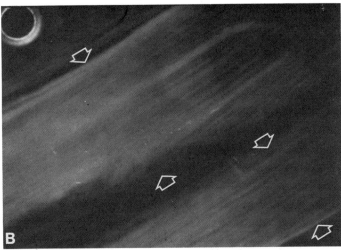

**Figure 7.6.** Fluorescence microscopic examination of rabbit tibial nerve following compression at 400 mm Hg for 2 h. Immediately after the compression, the animal was injected intravenously with Evans Blue-albumin (EBA) and frozen longitudinal sections were made. **A:** In the *central part* of the compressed segment the red fluorescent EBA-complex (*white*) has perfused the endoneurial capillaries (∗) in the fascicle. *Arrows* indicate the outlines of the fascicle. The dye-complex is strictly confined to the lumina of the endoneurial vessels, which contrast distinctly from the green nerve tissue (grayish-black), and thus, the blood–nerve barrier was unaffected. **B:** At the *edge zone* the compression induced increased permeability of the endoneurial vessels, leading to formation of an endoneurial edema. This is indicated by the diffuse orange-red fluorescence (*white*) in the endoneurial space. (Reproduced by permission of B Rydevik and G Lundborg, *Scand J Plast Reconstr Surg* 11:179–187, 1977).

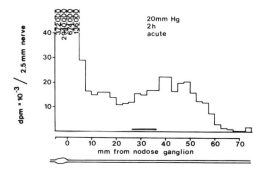 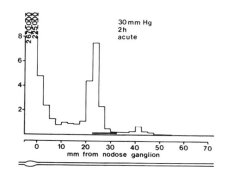

**Figure 7.7.** Demonstration of the effects of low pressure levels (20 and 30 mm Hg for 2 h) on axonal transport. The *black bar* indicates the site of compression. Units on ordinate are disintegrations per minute (dpm). Sham compression (not shown) and compression at 20 mm Hg caused no, or minimal, accumulation of axonally transported proteins, in contrast to compression at 30 mm Hg, which caused varying degrees of block (complete block shown). (Reproduced by permission of J Sjöstrand et al., in *Axoplasmic Transport in Physiology and Pathology.* Weiss and Gorio (eds.). New York: Springer-Verlag, pp. 140–145, 1982).

the cuff and a wavefront distal to this level (the block was partial), whereas in other nerves the block was more complete (Fig. 7.7). A block of axonal transport induced by 50 mm Hg was reversible within 24 h. Reversal of transport blockage occurred in most cases within 3 days after compression at 200 mm Hg for 2 h and within 7 days after compression at 400 mm Hg for 2 h.

## Nerve Fiber Structure and Impulse Propagation

Conduction velocity over a compressed segment was studied during compression at various levels for 15 min or 2 h and during a recovery period of 2 h after pressure release. The tibial nerve was stimulated at the ankle and the compound action potential was recorded at knee level. The distance between the electrodes was kept constant throughout the experiment, and therefore, the recordings of the conduction velocity during compression and recovery could be compared in percent to the pre-compression values which were regarded as 100%. The effects of compression on conduction velocity were studied in the fastest conducting nerve fibers, those that are most sensitive to compression (Gasser and Erlanger, 1929). Some of the nerves were examined by light and electron microscopy (for details of method and results, see Rydevik and Nordborg, 1980; Dahlin et al., 1985).

Application of the compression chamber, without inflation, did not affect conduction velocity. When nerves were subjected to compression at 80 mm Hg, a level known to cause total ischemia in the compressed segment, conduction velocity decreased gradually to about 87% of pre-compression value after 2 h of compression. During the first hour of the recovery period, there was a further decrease to about 80% and the conduction velocity remained constant during the rest of the observation period (Fig. 7.8).

A more pronounced impairment of nerve function was induced by compression at 200 and 400 mm Hg as compared to low pressure. Compression at 200 mm Hg for 2 h induced, on an average, a decrease in conduction velocity to about 30% of pre-compression value, followed by a slight recovery to about 45% 2 h after pressure release (Fig. 7.9). A higher pressure (400 mm Hg for 2 h) induced a complete block in all nerves after approximately 45 min with no recovery of nerve function during 2 h after release of pressure. However, if a nerve was compressed at 400 mm Hg for only 15 min, there was a decrease to only about 70% with a slight recovery following pressure release (Fig. 7.9). Morphological analysis showed the same type of nodal displacement toward the uncompressed parts of the nerve as extensively described by Ochoa and co-workers (1972) and presented in Fig. 7.4.

## Discussion

The results presented in this chapter demonstrate that acute compression of peripheral nerve can affect intraneural microcirculation, vascular permeability, axonal transport, nerve function and nerve fiber structure. These findings are discussed below and related to corresponding clinical situations.

### Effects of Low Pressure Levels (20–80 mm Hg)

The first sign of impairment of the microcirculation during compression was reduced blood flow in epineurial venules and this occurs when the nerve was compressed at 20 to 30 mm Hg cuff pressure. No retrograde effects on the capillary circulation were seen, but the applied pressure was maintained for only a short period. Impaired blood flow in the venules of a peripheral nerve during a prolonged period is considered important in the pathophysiology of the carpal tunnel syndrome (Sunderland, 1976). Disturbances in the microcirculation of venules may produce retrograde effects on the circulation of the capillaries, which in turn may reduce the supply of oxygen to the endothelial cells lining the vessel walls. An anoxic injury to these cells may increase vascular permeability with subsequent leakage of fluid and proteins into the endoneurial space, causing endoneurial edema. In other tissues, for example, subcutaneous tissue, elevated venous pressure leads to increased lymph flow, and this may prevent edema formation by protein washout (Fadnes, 1976). There are no lymphatic vessels in the endoneurial space and resorption of edema

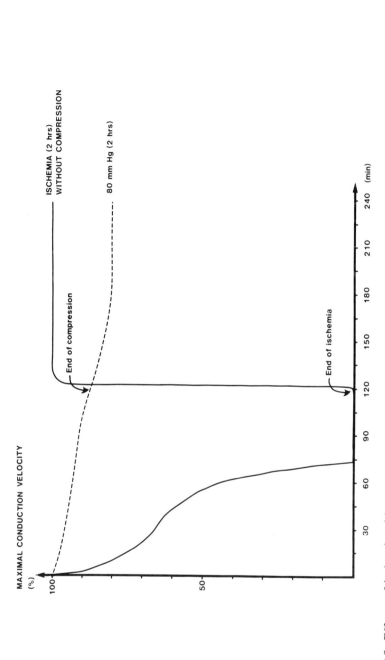

**Figure 7.8.** Effects of ischemia without compression (Lundborg, 1970) are compared with those of local compression at 80 mm Hg (Dahlin et al., 1985) on maximal conduction velocity. Local compression at 80 mm Hg is known to cause ischemia of the compressed segment.

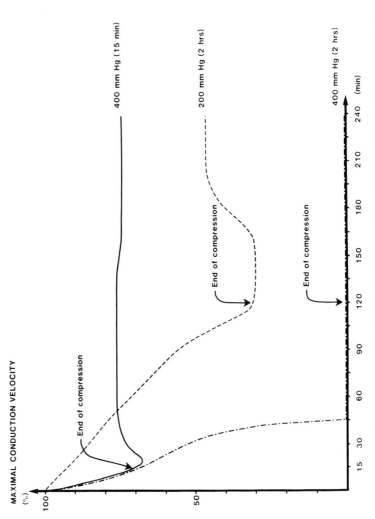

**Figure 7.9.** Effects of local compression at 400 mm Hg for 15 min, 400 mm Hg and 200 mm Hg for 2 h on maximal conduction velocity.

fluid into endoneurial blood vessels may be hindered as the blood flow in these vessels can be compromised by the edema. Due to these factors, endoneurial edema may seriously affect the various functions of the nerve fibers. Draining of endoneurial edema in an injured segment of the nerve depends on proximo-distal diffusion of fluid within the endoneurial space (Weiss et al., 1945; Olsson and Kristensson, 1973). Endoneurial edema may increase pressure within the fascicles (endoneurial fluid pressure, EFP), due to the unyielding properties of the perineurium. An increase in EFP may impair the microcirculation in the fascicles with a subsequent decrease in the delivery of oxygen and other nutrients to the nerve fibers. Elevated EFP (Myers and Powell, 1981) is found in various conditions such as toxic (hexachlorophene and lead) and metabolic (galactose) neuropathies as well as in association with nerve trauma (nerve crush with Wallerian degeneration). Although increased EFP in such neuropathies will probably not cause total collapse of the endoneurial capillaries (Low et al., 1980, 1982), EFP may be sufficiently high to reduce blood flow in the peripheral nerve (Myers et al., 1982).

Our findings agree with those reported by Bentley and Schlapp (1943), who investigated the perfusion of intravenously injected Evans Blue in a compressed peripheral nerve. They found that compression at 60 to 65 mm Hg stopped the circulation in at least the superficial vessels of the compressed nerve segment. In other tissues (for example, rabbit trachea) complete standstill occurs during compression at about 35 mm Hg pressure (Stenqvist and Bagge, 1979). Several factors might contribute to these differences in "critical pressure" for inducing ischemia. Intraneural connective tissue layers probably protect the peripheral nerve against compression. First, the fascicles are embedded in epineurial connective tissue which may protect the nerve fascicles (Sunderland, 1978). Furthermore, each fascicle is surrounded by a strong perineurial sheath and pressure inside the fascicles is positive. This arrangement contributes to the mechanical "stiffness" that protects the nerve fibers as well as the intrafascicular vessels from trauma (Rydevik et al., 1981).

Some characteristics of the intraneural microvascular anatomy should also be considered. Along the nerve trunk a few large epineurial arterioles branch rather abruptly into the endoneurial capillary system and complete impairment of endoneurial capillary circulation does not occur until these large arterioles are occluded (Rydevik et al., 1981). Thus, a high vascular perfusion pressure in a compressed nerve segment is maintained by such large arterioles even at cuff pressures that cause complete ischemia in other tissues without such arterioles (Stenqvist and Bagge, 1979; Rydevik et al., 1981). After 2 h of compression-induced ischemia, blood flow in intraneural vessels recovers within the first minutes. However, an epineurial edema is induced.

Studies on the vascular permeability in the peripheral nerve after compression at 50 mm Hg reveal edema that is restricted to the epineurium and prevented from reaching the nerve fibers due to the perineurium (Rydevik and Lundborg, 1977). Endoneurial vessels are unaffected in this situation, indicating that epineurial vessels are more susceptible to compression trauma than endoneurial vessels. This different susceptibility is also found in association with ischemia without compression (Lundborg, 1970) and dissection trauma (Rydevik et al., 1976$b$). However, compression at low pressure levels (30 and 80 mm Hg) for several hours may increase EFP due to edema which may persist for at least 24 h (Lundborg et al., 1983). Endoneurial edema may not only affect intraneural blood flow but can also alter the ionic balance around the nerve fibers which may disturb propagation of impulses as well as axonal transport. A long-standing edema may induce fibroblast invasion and conversion to intraneural fibrosis, an irreversible state.

As mentioned previously, compression at 30 mm Hg reduced intraneural blood flow (Rydevik et al., 1981) and increases vascular permeability (Lundborg et al., 1983). This pressure level corresponds well to the lowest pressure (30 mm Hg) which blocks rapid axonal transport in motor and sensory fibers of rabbit vagus nerves (Hahnenberger, 1978; Dahlin et al., 1982). Microcirculatory disturbances in the compressed nerve segment probably play an important role in blocking axonal transport at low pressure levels (Rydevik et al., 1980), but some degree of nerve fiber deformation may also contribute to these disturbances (Hahnenberger, 1978).

It is well known that normal axonal transport is dependent not only on a continuous supply of energy (Ochs, 1974), but also on an isotonic environment (Edström, 1975) and a proper concentration of $Ca^{2+}$ (Ochs and Worth, 1978). Endoneurial edema may affect the axonal transport by disturbing the local ionic balance which may contribute to the block of axonal transport. Nerves that are compressed at 50 mm Hg for 2 h show a rapid recovery and a normal profile of axonal transport occurs as early as 24 h after the compression trauma. This rapid recovery also supports the concept that disturbances in microcirculation play an important role in blocking axonal transport.

Compression at 80 mm Hg induces deterioration of nerve function (Dahlin et al., 1985). Although this pressure level induces complete ischemia of the compressed nerve segment (Rydevik et al., 1981), the decrease in conduction velocity in this situation was not as rapid as in the tibial nerve during tourniquet-induced ischemia of the extremity (Lundborg, 1970). Distal to a tourniquet, there is complete absence of nerve function after about 70 min; whereas local compression at 80 mm Hg leads to a 13% reduction of conduction velocity after 2 h (Fig. 7.8). This difference may be explained by the fact that oxygen and different ions diffuse into the compressed segment beneath the compression chamber (Rydevik and Nordborg, 1980; Dahlin et al., 1985). Furthermore, the temperature in these experiments was kept constant at body temperature around the compression chamber, whereas in the tourniquet experiments, the temperature in the ischemic limb gradually approached room temperature.

Following release of the tourniquet, nerve function was restored within a few minutes, but there was no restitution at all of nerve function during a 2-h recovery period following local compression at 80 mm Hg for 2 h (Fig. 7.8). This might be explained by an effect of compression per se on the nerve fibers as well as on the intraneural vascular system (Dahlin et al., 1985). As previously mentioned, compression at 80 mm Hg for 2 h and more induces an increase in the endoneurial fluid pressure due to formation of an edema in the fascicles (Lundborg et al., 1983), and this may also contribute to the noncomplete restitution of the nerve function.

### Clinical Implications

Our findings on the effects of compression at low pressure levels (30–80 mm Hg) on intraneural microcirculation, vascular permeability, axonal transport and nerve function are interesting in view of recent data concerning pressures acting on the median nerve in the carpal tunnel syndrome (Gelberman et al., 1981). Patients with carpal tunnel syndrome have a mean pressure of 32 mm Hg in the carpal tunnel, whereas that in an asymptomatic control group is only 2.5 mm Hg. Thus, there are reasons to believe that at these relatively low pressure levels, there may be considerable impairment of axonal transport and intraneural microcirculation. Intraneural edema may also be induced in nerve entrapment syndromes.

Peripheral nerves may also be subjected to compression in this pressure range in association with closed compartment syndromes of skeletal muscle (Mubarak and Hargens, 1981). A pressure of 30 mm Hg is claimed to be a threshold level at which the viability of muscle tissue and peripheral nerves is jeopardized. This level corresponds well to the pressure level in our studies at which changes occur in vascular permeability, intraneural blood flow and axonal transport in association with peripheral nerve compression.

Neural compression syndromes are also seen as a consequence of pressure impingement of spinal nerve roots, for example, in association with herniated discs and spinal stenosis. Nerve roots may be more sensitive to external compression than peripheral nerves due to the fact that spinal nerve roots lack perineurium and that the epineurium is poorly developed (Sharpless, 1975; Sunderland, 1978).

Low-pressure nerve compression in one region may reduce axonal transport, and the parts of the axons distal to a compression may thereby be deprived of axonally transported substances. This may render distal parts of the axons more sensitive to compression trauma. This has been called the *double-crush hypothesis* (Upton and McComas, 1973). This hypothesis is based on clinical observations that 73% of a group of patients with carpal tunnel syndrome also have an associated neural lesion in the neck. However to our knowledge this hypothesis has not been substantiated by any experimental data.

## Effects of High Pressure Levels (200–600 mm Hg)

Compared to low pressure levels, compression at high pressure levels induces injury not only to epineurial vessels but also to endoneurial vessels with subsequent edema formation in the endoneurial space. When compression time is limited to 2 h edema occurs only at the edges of the compressed nerve segment. However, when compression time is extended to 4 and 6 h, edema is also induced in the center of the segment. This indicates that edema formation in the center is more related to the duration of the compression. However, development of vascular injury at the edges of the segment is related to both the magnitude of the pressure *and* the duration of the compression, as indicated by the extent of the edema formation induced by compression at 400 mm Hg for 15 min and 200 to 400 mm Hg for 2 h (Rydevik and Lundborg, 1977).

The perineurium is remarkably resistant to compression injury, as revealed by the fact that very high pressures (400–600 mm Hg) for 2 h and 200 mm Hg for 6 h do not impair the barrier function of perineurium to EBA (Rydevik and Lundborg, 1977). The barrier function of the perineurium is also resistant to other types of trauma such as internal neurolysis (Rydevik et al., 1976b), stretching (Lundborg and Rydevik, 1973) and prolonged ischemia (Lundborg et al., 1973). Preservation of perineurial barrier function is important in the pathophysiology of compression-induced lesions. An epineurial edema induced by slight trauma is prevented from reaching the nerve fibers in the endoneurial space by the perineurium which protects the nerve fibers. On the other hand, an intact barrier function of the perineurium prevents drainage of endoneurial edema since the endoneurial space lacks lymphatic vessels (Lundborg, 1975; Sunderland, 1978). The consequences of endoneurial edema have been extensively discussed previously.

Endoneurial edema formation may also explain the no-reflow phenomenon seen in the vital microscope 3 and 7 days after compression at 400 mm Hg for 2 h (Rydevik et al., 1981). Such secondary ischemia may contribute to the functional deterioration after compression, although the importance of the ischemic factor has been questioned in acute compression injuries of peripheral nerves (Williams et al., 1980).

Compression at high pressure levels causes marked deterioration of nerve function compared to effects at low pressure levels (Rydevik and Nordborg, 1980; Dahlin et al., 1985). An important cause of this incomplete recovery of nerve function, besides vascular injury and endoneurial edema, is mechanical deformation of the nerve fibers. Ultrastructural investigation (Rydevik and Nordborg, 1980) of the nerve fibers showed the same type of deformation of axons as that extensively described by Ochoa and co-workers (Ochoa et al., 1972). Paranodal myelin sheath invagination is located at the edges of the compressed segment. The mechanical basis for injury to nerve fibers and to intraneural vessels probably relates to the pressure gradient between the compressed and noncompressed parts of the nerve (Ochoa et al., 1972; Rydevik and Lundborg, 1977). The location of the lesions, namely, injury to nerve fibers and intraneural vessels at the tourniquet edges with sparing at the center of the compressed segment, can be termed the "edge effect" (Fig. 7.10).

The importance of pressure gradients at the edges is obvious if we compare experiments of Grundfest (1936) and those of other authors using different modes of compression. Grundfest found that isolated oxygenated frog nerves enclosed in a pressure chamber withstand very high pressures without impairment of conduction, whereas relatively slight pressures applied *locally* block conduction (Lewis et al., 1931; Bentley and Schlapp, 1943; Denny-Brown and Brenner, 1944; Rydevik and Nordborg, 1980). Thus the pressure as such is not harmful, but rather the mechanical tissue deformation induced by locally applied pressure. Both the magnitude of the applied pressure and the duration of the compression determine the degree of nerve injury induced by compression. A pressure of 400 mm Hg applied for 2 h induced more deterioration of nerve function than 200 mm Hg applied for the same time. Experimental data and clinical experience concerning the effects of tourniquet application on extremities

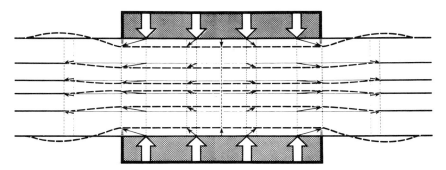

**Figure 7.10.** Schematic drawing of tissue deformations caused by compression of a peripheral nerve. The longitudinally running *thick dotted lines* show the final contour of different tissue layers during compression. The *thin black arrows* are vectors showing the displacement of different points in the nerve due to the applied pressure. The diagram is based on computations performed by Professor Richard Skalak, Columbia University, New York, NY. (Reproduced by permission of G Lundborg and B Rydevik, *Läkartidningen* (Stockholm) 79:4035–4040, 1982.)

indicate that the risk for nerve lesion increases significantly with increasing tourniquet pressure (see review by Lundborg and Rydevik, 1982).

Compression at 400 mm Hg for 2 h also induced more deterioration of nerve function as compared to compression at the same pressure level for only 15 min (Fig. 7.9). Thus, even at high pressure levels, the duration is important; 400 mm Hg applied directly to a nerve does not induce immediate injury but has to act for a certain period of time to cause functional deterioration. When analyzing nerve compression lesions it should also be noted that it is not only the *pressure level* that is critical but also the *mode of pressure application* to the nerve. Direct compression of a nerve causes more pronounced damage than indirect compression at the same pressure level in terms of vascular injury, axonal transport block, nerve fiber injury and functional deterioration.

## Summary

After review of the microanatomy of peripheral nerve, the effects of compression on peripheral nerves and the pathophysiology of various types of nerve compression lesions are discussed. Low pressure levels (20–80 mm Hg) induce changes in intraneural microcirculation, vascular permeability, axonal transport and nerve function. Venular blood flow is reduced at 20 to 30 mm Hg compression and the lowest level for impairment of axonal transport is 30 mm Hg. Total ischemia is induced when nerves are compressed at 60 to 80 mm Hg. Impairment of intraneural circulation and axonal transport is generally reversible following pressure release after 2 h of compression at pressure levels up to 80 mm Hg. Compression at higher pressure levels (200–600 mm Hg) induces injury to nerve fibers and intraneural blood vessels at the edges of the compressed segment, producing long-standing functional deterioration of the peripheral nerve. The barrier properties of perineurium are remarkably resistant to compression even at high pressures.

## Acknowledgments

This work was supported by grants from the Swedish Medical Research Council (project no. 5188), the Swedish Work Environment Fund, the Göteborg Medical Society and the University of Göteborg.

## References

Bentley FH and Schlapp W (1943). The effects of pressure on conduction in peripheral nerve. *J Physiol (Lond)* 102:72–82.
Berthold C-H (1978). Morphology of normal peripheral axons. In: *Physiology and Pathobiology of Axons*. SG Waxman (ed.). New York: Raven Press, pp. 3–63.

Brady ST and Lasek RJ (1982). The slow components of axonal transport: movements, compositions and organization. In: *Axoplasmic Transport*. DG Weiss (ed.). Berlin, Heidelberg: Springer-Verlag, pp. 206–217.

Causey G and Palmer E (1949). The effect of pressure on nerve conduction and nerve fiber size. *J Physiol (Lond)* 109:220–231.

Chen HI, Granger HJ and Taylor AE (1976). Interaction of capillary, interstitial, and lymphatic forces in the canine hindpaw. *Circ Res* 39:245–254

Dahlin LB, Danielsen N, Ehira T, Lundborg G and Rydevik B (1985). Mechanical effects of compression of peripheral nerves. *J Biomech Engineering* (in press).

Dahlin LB, Danielsen N, McLean WG, Rydevik B and Sjöstrand J (1982) Critical pressure level for impairment of fast axonal transport during experimental compression of rabbit vagus nerve. *J Physiol (Lond)* 325:84P.

Denny-Brown D and Brenner C (1944). Paralysis of nerve induced by direct pressure and by tourniquet. *Arch Neurol Psychiatry* 51:1–26.

Edström A (1975). Ionic requirements for rapid axonal transport in vitro in frog sciatic nerves. *Acta Physiol Scand* 93:104–112.

Eiken O, Nabseth DC, Mayer RF and Deterling RA Jr (1964). Limb replantation. II. The pathophysiological effects. *Arch Surg* 88:54–65.

Fadnes HO (1976). Effects of increased venous pressure on the hydrostatic and colloid osmotic pressure in subcutaneous interstitial fluid in rats: edema-preventing mechanisms. *Scand J Clin Lab Invest* 36:371–377.

Fowler TJ, Danta G and Gilliatt RW (1972). Recovery of nerve conduction after a pneumatic tourniquet: observations on the hindlimb of the baboon. *J Neurol Neurosurg Psychiatry* 35:638–647.

Gasser HS and Erlanger J (1929). The role of fibre size in the establishment of a nerve block by pressure or cocaine. *Am J Physiol* 88:581–591.

Gelberman RH, Hergenroeder PT, Hargens AR, Lundborg G and Akeson WH (1981). The carpal tunnel syndrome. A study of carpal canal pressures. *J Bone Joint Surg* 63A:380–383.

Grafstein B and Forman DS (1980). Intracellular transport in neurons. *Physiol Rev* 60:1167–1283.

Grundfest H (1936). Effects of hydrostatic pressures upon the excitability, the recovery and the potential sequence of frog nerve. *Cold Spring Harbor Symp Quant Biol* 4:179–186.

Guth L (1968). "Trophic" influences of nerve on muscle. *Physiol Rev* 48:645–687.

Hahnenberger RW (1978). Effects of pressure on fast axoplasmic flow. An in vitro study in the vagus nerve of rabbits. *Acta Physiol Scand* 104:299–308.

Hargens AR, Akeson WH, Mubarak SJ, Owen CA, Evans KL, Garetto LP, Gonsalves MR and Schmidt DA (1978). Fluid balance within the canine anterolateral compartment and its relationship to compartment syndromes. *J Bone Joint Surg* 60A:499–505.

Klemm H (1970). Das Perineurium als Diffusionsbarriere gegenuber Peroxydase bei epi- und endoneuraler Applikation. *Z Zellforsch* 108:431–445.

Kristensson K and Olsson Y (1974). Retrograde transport of horse-radish peroxidase in transected axons. 1. Time relationships between transport and induction of chromatolysis. *Brain Res* 79:101–109.

Leone J and Ochs S (1978). Anoxic block and recovery of axoplasmic transport and electrical excitability of nerve. *J Neurobiol* 9:229–245.

Lewis T, Pickering GW and Rothschild P (1931). Centripetal paralysis arising out of arrested blood flow to the limb, including notes on a form of tingling. *Heart* 16:1–32.

Low PA, Dyck PJ and Schmelzer JD (1980). Mammalian peripheral nerve sheath has unique responses to chronic elevations of endoneurial fluid pressure. *Exp Neurol* 70:300–306.

Low PA, Dyck PJ and Schmelzer JD (1982). Chronic elevation of endoneurial fluid pressure is associated with low-grade fiber pathology. *Muscle Nerve* 5:162–165.

Low PA, Marchand G, Knox F and Dyck PJ (1977). Measurement of endoneurial fluid pressure with polyethylene matrix capsules. *Brain Res* 122:373–377.

Lundborg G (1970). Ischemic nerve injury. Experimental studies on intraneural microvascular pathophysiology and nerve function in a limb subjected to temporary circulatory arrest. *Scand J Plast Reconstr Surg Suppl* 6:7–113.

Lundborg G (1975). Structure and function of the intraneural microvessels as related to trauma, edema formation and nerve function. *J Bone Joint Surg* 57A:938–948.

Lundborg G, Myers RR and Powell HC (1983). Nerve compression injury and increased endoneurial fluid pressure: a "miniature compartment syndrome." *J Neurol Neurosurg Psychiatry* 46:1119–1124.

Lundborg G, Nordborg C, Rydevik B and Olsson Y (1973). The effect of ischemia on the permeability of the perineurium to protein tracers in rabbit tibial nerve. *Acta Neurol Scand* 49:287–294.

Lundborg G and Rydevik B (1973). Effects of stretching the tibial nerve of the rabbit. A preliminary study of the intraneural circulation and the barrier function of the perineurium. *J Bone Joint Surg* 55B:390–401.

Lundborg G and Rydevik B (1982). The bloodless field in hand and arm surgery: theoretical and practical aspects. *Läkartidningen* (Stockholm) 79:4035–4040.

MacGregor RJ, Sharpless SK and Luttges MW (1975). A pressure vessel model for nerve compression. *J Neurol Sci* 24:299–304.

McLean WG, Frizell M and Sjöstrand J (1976). Slow axonal transport of labelled proteins in sensory fibers of rabbit vagus nerve. *J Neurochem* 26:1213–1216.

Mubarak SJ and Hargens AR (1981). *Compartment Syndromes and Volkmanns Contracture*. Philadelphia: W.B. Saunders, 232 pp.

Myers RR, Mizisin AP, Powell HC and Lampert PW (1982). Reduced nerve blood flow in hexachlorophene neuropathy. Relationship to elevated endoneurial fluid pressure. *J Neuropathol Exp Neurol* 41:391–399.

Myers RR and Powell HC (1981). Endoneurial fluid pressure in peripheral neuropathies. In: *Tissue Fluid Pressure and Composition*. AR Hargens (ed.). Baltimore/London: Williams & Wilkins, pp. 193–207.

Myers RR, Powell HC, Costello ML, Lampert PW, and Zweifach BW (1978). Endoneurial fluid pressure: direct measurement with micropipettes. *Brain Res* 148:510–515.

Ochoa J, Fowler TJ and Gilliatt RW (1972). Anatomical changes in peripheral nerves compressed by a pneumatic tourniquet. *J Anat* 113:433–455.

Ochs S (1974). Energy metabolism and supply of ~P to the fast axoplasmic transport mechanism in nerve. *Fed Proc* 33:1049–1058.

Ochs S and Worth RM (1978). Axoplasmic transport in normal and pathological systems. In: *Physiology and Pathobiology of Axons*. SG Waxman (ed.). New York: Raven Press, pp. 251–264.

Olsson Y (1966). Studies on vascular permeability in peripheral nerves. I. Distribution of circulating fluorescent serum albumin in normal, crushed and sectioned rat sciatic nerve. *Acta Neuropathol* 7:1–15.

Olsson Y and Kristensson K (1973). The perineurium as a diffusion barrier to protein tracers following trauma to nerves. *Acta Neuropathol (Berl)* 23:105–111.

Olsson Y, Kristensson K and Klatzo I (1971). Permeability of blood vessels and connective tissue sheaths in the peripheral nervous system to exogenous proteins. *Acta Neuropathol (Berl) (Suppl. V)*: 61–69.

Olsson Y and Reese TS (1969). Inaccessibility of the endoneurium of mouse sciatic nerve to exogenous proteins. American association of anatomists' eighty-second Annual Session. *Anat Rec* 163:318.

Olsson Y and Reese TS (1971). Permeability of vasa nervorum and perineurium in mouse sciatic nerve studied by fluorescence and electronmicroscopy. *J Neuropathol Exp Neurol* 30:105–119.

Rydevik B, Brånemark P-I, Nordborg C, McLean WG, Sjöstrand J and Fogelberg M (1976a). Effects of chymopapain on nerve tissue. An experimental study on the structure and function of peripheral nerve tissue in rabbits after local application of chymopapain. *Spine* 1:137–148.

Rydevik B and Lundborg G (1977). Permeability of intraneural microvessels and perineurium following acute, graded experimental nerve compression. *Scand J Plast Reconstr Surg* 11:179–187.

Rydevik B, Lundborg G and Bagge U (1981). Effects of graded compression on intraneural blood flow. An in vivo study on rabbit tibial nerve. *J Hand Surg* 6:3–12.

Rydevik B, Lundborg G and Nordborg C (1976b). Intraneural tissue reactions induced by internal neurolysis. *Scand J Plast Reconstr Surg* 10:3–8.

Rydevik B, McLean WG, Sjöstrand J and Lundborg G (1980). Blockage of axonal transport induced by acute, graded compression of the rabbit vagus nerve. *J Neurol Neurosurg Psychiatry* 43:690–698.

Rydevik B and Nordborg C (1980). Changes in nerve function and nerve fibre structure induced by acute, graded compression. *J Neurol Neurosurg Psychiatry* 43:1070–1082.

Shanta TR and Bourne GH (1969). The perineurial epithelium—a new concept. In: *The Structure and Function of Nervous Tissue, Vol. 1, Structure*. New York and London: Academic Press, pp. 379–459.

Sharpless SK (1975). Susceptibility of spinal roots to compression block. The research status of spinal manipulative therapy. *NIH-workshop*, Feburary 2–4. *NINCDS Monograph No. 15*. M Goldstein (ed.), pp. 155–161.

Sjöstrand J, Frizell M and Rydevik B (1978). Changes in axonal transport in various experimental neuropathies. In: *Peripheral Neuropathies, Vol. 1*. N Canal and G. Pozza (ed.). Amsterdam: Elsevier, North-Holland Biomedical Press, pp. 147–157.

Steinwall O and Klatzo I (1965). Double tracer methods in studies on blood-brain barrier dysfunction and brain edema. In: *Proceedings of the 17th Congress of Scandinavian Neurology, Gothenburg, 1964. Acta Neurol Scand* Suppl 13 41:591–595.

Stenqvist O and Bagge U (1979). Cuff pressure and microvascular occlusion in the tracheal mucosa. An intravital microscopic study in the rabbit. *Acta Otolaryngol* 88:451–454.

Sunderland S (1976). The nerve lesion in the carpal tunnel syndrome. *J Neurol Neurosurg Psychiatry* 39:615–626.

Sunderland S (1978). *Nerve and Nerve Injuries*. Edinburgh, London and New York: Churchill Livingstone.

Thomas PK and Jones DG (1967). The cellular response to nerve injury. 2. Regeneration of the perineurium after nerve section. *J Anat* 101:45–55.

Upton ARM and McComas AJ (1973). The double crush in nerve-entrapment syndromes. *Lancet* ii:359–362.

Varon S and Adler R (1981). Trophic and specifying factors directed to neuronal cells. In: *Advances in Cell Neurobiology, Vol. 2*. S Federoff, L Hertz (ed.), New York: Academic Press, pp. 115–163.

Weiss P, Wang H, Taylor AC and Edds MV Jr (1945). Proximo-distal convection in the endoneurial spaces of peripheral nerves demonstrated by colored and radioactive (isotope) tracers. *Am J Physiol* 143:521–540.

Williams IR, Jefferson D and Gilliatt RW (1980). Acute nerve compression during limb ischemia. An experimental study. *J Neurol Sci* 46:199–207.

CHAPTER 8

# Pressure Effects on Human Peripheral Nerve Function

Richard H. Gelberman, Robert M. Szabo, and Alan R. Hargens

## Introduction

The mechanism by which acute compression affects the function of peripheral nerve is not completely understood. The pathophysiology of nerve compression syndromes is related to both the magnitude and the duration of pressure. However, other factors such as nerve anatomy, systemic blood pressure and cardiovascular disease may modify the pressure-duration thresholds for nerve dysfunction. Recognition of these factors will have important implications for treatment of nerve compression lesions.

### Compression Thresholds of Peripheral Nerve

Mild compression of a nerve trunk initially affects the epineural microcirculation (Rydevik et al., 1981). These studies of vascular factors involved in the pathophysiology of acute nerve compression lesions indicate that intraneural microcirculation changed during and immediately after the application of compression. Experiments using graded controlled compression of rabbit tibial nerves defined pressure levels that interfered with the intraneural microcirculation of the epineurium, perineurium and endoneurium. Compression at 30 mm Hg impaired blood flow in the venules of all the nerves tested. Capillary and arteriolar blood flow was unaffected at this pressure level. Compression at 50 mm Hg completely occluded all epineurial venules. This pressure level also markedly reduced the flow velocity of endoneurial capillaries and decreased arteriolar flow. In 60% of the nerves, 60 mm Hg caused complete ischemia of the compressed segment, and 70 mm Hg caused ischemia in all nerves but one. Following the release of 2 h compression, the circulation was restored to normal in all layers of the nerve within 1 min.

Interneural microvessels generally respond to trauma with increased permeability. Epineurial vessels normally exchange serum proteins with the extravascular space. Lundborg (1975) showed that only slight trauma

was needed to induce epineurial edema rapidly. The edema was prevented from advancing into the endoneurial space by the perineurial
sheath barrier. In an experiment on rabbit tibial nerve, Rydevik and
Lundborg (1977) showed that 50 mm Hg compression for 2 h caused
epineurial edema. At this pressure the microvascular permeability of the
endoneurial layer seemed to be preserved. At pressure levels of 200 and
400 mm Hg, endoneurial edema was also noted, although its presence was
confined to the edges of the compression zone. The microcirculation in
the center of the compressed nerve segment was reinstated after release
of the pressure and no edema occurred. Therefore, the most significant
vascular effects in their experiments occurred beneath the edges of the
compression cuff.

Ochoa and co-workers (1972) explained the effects of pressure on peripheral nerve in another way. They described a mechanical lesion consisting of invagination of the nodes of Ranvier with local demyelination.
This lesion occluded the nodes and blocked ionic currents and nerve
conduction. A pressure difference between compressed and uncompressed nerve generated longitudinal driving forces at the edges, causing
extrusion of axoplasm. There was no pressure gradient in the center of the
compressed segment, and therefore longitudinal forces were not generated in this middle region (Fig. 8.1).

Acute compression of a peripheral nerve represents a complex lesion
including mechanical factors, ischemic factors or both. It is clear that
compression above capillary perfusion pressure compromises the neural
microcirculation. Mechanical forces, which are most pronounced at the
edges of the compressed region, induce increased vascular permeability,
which in turn raises intrafascicular pressure. Elevated intrafascicular
pressure obstructs flow in the intrafascicular vessels, thus causing nerve
fiber ischemia (Lundborg, 1970).

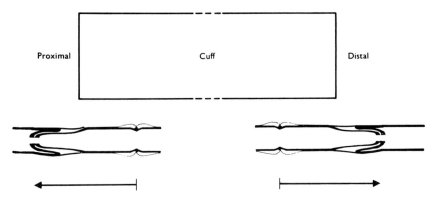

**Figure 8.1.** Diagram illustrating the direction of dislocation of the nodes of Ranvier in relation to the compressed zone. (From Ochoa et al., 1972)

When an arm tourniquet is inflated to suprasystolic levels, the nerve segment distal to the cuff becomes ischemic (Lewis et al., 1931). The segment under the cuff is not only ischemic, but is subjected to mechanical compression as well. A controversy exists as to whether the loss of distal nerve function is caused by local deformation of the nerve fiber at cuff level or by ischemia alone. This fundamental question on the effects of nerve compression has not been answered conclusively. Whatever the underlying biological mechanism, however, the threshold pressure level at which nerve fiber viability is acutely jeopardized is of great experimental and clinical significance.

## The Threshold Pressure for Nerve Compression Syndromes

The pathophysiology of acute and chronic nerve compression syndromes is an issue of considerable theoretical and clinical relevance. The clinical findings associated with chronic nerve entrapment, including the carpal tunnel syndrome, are well known (Adamson et al., 1971; Phalen, 1972; Sunderland, 1976; Hunter et al., 1978). A very interesting clinical model for acute nerve compression is the compartment syndrome. Its diagnosis, prognosis and treatment are dependent on the determination of a critical pressure threshold at which neural conduction is interrupted and nerve fiber viability is jeopardized. With the refinement of catheter techniques, intracompartmental pressure measurements are frequently relied on for diagnosing compartment syndromes and determining the need for fasciotomy (Whitesides et al., 1975a,b; Matsen et al., 1976; Hargens et al., 1977; Matsen and Krugmire, 1978; Mubarak et al., 1978).

Fundamental to determining the reversibility of acute and chronic nerve compression syndromes is the ability to distinguish clinically between the extent of ischemia and mechanical deformation. Ischemia alone may be rapidly reversible after a nerve is decompressed and intraneural microcirculation is restored. In chronic nerve compression, hypoxia of the nerve may precipitate early degenerative changes in both myelin sheaths and axons. Structural changes within the nerve, whether caused by mechanical deformation or chronic ischemia, may require a longer time to recover, and may not respond completely to operative treatment.

Most investigators agree that the microcirculation of a closed compartment is impeded when tissue pressure reaches levels equal to diastolic blood pressure. Using radioactive xenon-133, Dahn and associates (1967) found that flow stopped when external pressure equalled diastolic blood pressure. Rorabeck and collaborators (1972) demonstrated that the critical closing pressure in dogs was reached with tissue pressures in the 40 to 50 mm Hg range. In a canine compartment syndrome model, we found that nerve conduction velocity was significantly reduced at a threshold tissue fluid pressure of 30 mm Hg after 8 h of pressurization (Hargens et al., 1979). In the same model 50 mm Hg caused a complete block of nerve conduction. Lundborg and associates (1983) found that 30 mm Hg of local compression to a nerve truck for 8 h caused an increase in the endoneurial fluid pressure up to three times the original values. This pressure also impaired intraneural venular flow (Rydevik et al., 1981). We also determined that carpal canal pressure averaged 32 mm Hg in carpal tunnel syndrome patients, compared to 2.5 mm Hg in normal subjects (Gelberman et al., 1981). Compression at 30 mm Hg probably causes venous congestion and impaired oxygenation of nerve fibers, resulting in an alteration of nerve fiber conduction after prolonged periods of time. Even after prolonged periods, however, the changes occurring from this magnitude of pressure may be reversible.

Observers have noted clinically that sensibility is affected first during nerve entrapment whereas motor weakness occurs later during a more advanced stage of compression. The reasons for this are not clear. Spinner (1978) claims that peripheral axons within a compressed nerve suffer the greatest injury, whereas central fibers may be completely spared. With continued compression, heavily myelinated fibers of touch and motor function are more vulnerable than the thinly meylinated and unmyelinated pain and sympathetic fibers. The motor fibers of the median nerve, which make up 6% of the total fiber population, are located superficially on the palmar-radial aspect of the nerve (Sunderland, 1978). Therefore, they are the first to suffer from the applied pressure if local nerve topography is the critical factor. Motor fibers (A-$\alpha$) are myelinated and have a diameter of 15 to 20 $\mu$m. Myelinated sensory fibers (A-$\beta$) are 10 to 15 $\mu$m in diameter and unmyelinated pain fibers (C-fibers) are 1 to 2 $\mu$m in diameter (Dellon, 1981). If fiber size is the critical factor in determining the response to compression, the largest fibers (i.e., the motor fibers) are probably the most sensitive, and thus affected earliest in entrapment syndromes. It appears that sensory and motor fibers possess varying degrees of susceptibility to ischemia, based on factors other than anatomical location and size.

## The Clinical Assessment of Nerve Compression Syndromes

The evaluation of patients with compression syndromes depends on one's ability to measure peripheral nerve response to pressure and ischemia. There is little agreement on the reliability of sensory testing in clinical situations of peripheral nerve compression. Many authorities feel that currently used testing techniques of peripheral nerve sensibility are inconsistent and misleading (Hunter et al., 1978; Dellon, 1980, 1981). Patients with suspected nerve compression often lack abnormalities on routine testing of neuronal status. In general, sensibility testing in early compression neuropathy is less productive than provocative tests such as Phalen's wrist flexion test, Tinel's nerve percussion test or the tourniquet test. Based on a positive association in 80% of patients, Phalen (1972) states that his wrist flexion test is the most valuable sign of carpal tunnel syndrome. In a study of patients with carpal tunnel syndrome (Gelberman et al., 1981), we found that 94% had either a positive Phalen's or Tinel's test, whereas only 46% had an abnormality on standard clinical testing using the Weber two-point discrimination test.

Since 1958, the Weber two-point discrimination test has been the major clinical test of sensibility in both nerve regeneration and compression (Moberg, 1958, 1962, 1966; Werner and Omer, 1970). Although this test has provided a valid guide to functional recovery following nerve repair, it is neither consistent nor reliable in conditions of acute or chronic nerve compression. The two-point discrimination test measures the capacity of cutaneous peripheral receptors to recognize two points that are simultaneously applied to the skin. The basis for two-point discrimination depends on a complex overlapping of direct sensory units and the density of receptors in the periphery. In addition, it depends on a great deal of cortical integration of the available afferent impulses.

Although the underlying neurophysiology of sensation is not yet fully understood, several pieces of the puzzle have been provided by Mountcastle (1980). He noted that sensory receptors possess thresholds. Receptor excitation depends both on the quality and the magnitude of the stimulus. The spatial area within which a stimulus of sufficient magnitude and proper quality will evoke a discharge of impulses in a single primary afferent nerve fiber–receptor complex is called a peripheral receptive field. Peripheral branches of adjacent primary afferent nerves are intertwined and overlapped. Thus, any stimulus above threshold is likely to evoke a response in more than one fiber in a field. Peripheral receptive fields vary in size and also number of innervating nerve fibers per unit area. Central nervous system representation of a sensory field correlates directly with the peripheral innervation density. Any sensory test of spatial density relies on the innervation density of a peripheral receptive field with its corresponding peaks of activity in central neural fields. A threshold test of human sensation measures the relevant response of a primary afferent nerve fiber with its receptor cell to a quantitatively sufficient stimulus, independent of size or innervation density of its peripheral receptive field. An innervation density test depends on the size of the peripheral receptive field and, in addition, reflects higher levels of cortical integration (Mountcastle, 1980).

Percutaneous recording of mechanoreceptor activity in human peripheral nerves has revealed more information about human sensation. Nerve fibers serving the sense of touch can be divided on the basis of their adaptation to a constant touch stimulus (Dellon et al., 1972). A quickly adapting fiber signals an on-off event. A slowly adapting fiber continues its pulse response throughout the duration of the stimulus. The frequency code of the slowly adapting fiber signals stimulus amplitude. As stimulus intensity is increased, so is the role of firing of the slowly adapting fiber.

The mechanoreceptor serving the slowly adapting fiber system is the Merkel cell–neurite complex. The quickly adapting fibers can be subdivided into two groups on the basis of their response to vibratory stimuli. One group is more sensitive to low frequencies (5–40 cycles per second [cps], maximal at 30 cps) and a second group is sensitive to high-frequency stimuli (60–300 cps, maximal at 250 cps). The low-frequency receptor is thought to be the Meissner corpuscle and the high-frequency receptor the Pacinian corpuscle (Mountcastle, 1980; Dellon, 1981). Thus, several factors must be considered when evaluating information obtained from a test of peripheral sensibility (Table 8.1). In summary, these are: (1) nerve fiber populations (slowly or quickly adapting); (2) peripheral receptors (Merkel cell–neurite complex, Meissner or Pacinian corpuscle) and (3) neurophysiological correlates (threshold or innervation density). Fundamental differences between nerve regeneration and nerve compression should be reflected in testing the basic neurophysiological mechanisms. A discrepancy between the two processes forms the basis of further investigation into testing sensibility of peripheral nerve compression syndromes.

## Current Investigations

Experimental studies in our laboratory were designed to determine: (1) the relative importance of ischemia versus mechanical deformation in early peripheral nerve compression (Lundborg et al., 1982); (2) the critical threshold pressure for peripheral nerve conduction (Gelberman et al., 1983b) and (3) the clinical sensibility testing system most appropriate for evaluating and following patients with acute and chronic compressive neuropathies (Gelberman et al., 1983a, Szabo et al., 1984). Each of the

**Table 8.1.** Sensibility tests in peripheral nerve compression

| Clinical test | Sensation | Fiber type, size | Fiber population | Receptor | Type of test |
|---|---|---|---|---|---|
| Weber two-point discrimination | Constant touch | A-$\beta$ 15–20 $\mu$m | Slowly adapting | Merkel cell– neurite complex | Innervation density |
| Moving two-point discrimination | Moving touch | A-$\beta$ 15–20 $\mu$m | Quickly adapting | Meissner corpuscle | Innervation density |
| Tuning fork 256 cps | Vibration of 256 cps | A-$\beta$ 15–20 $\mu$m | Quickly adapting | Pacinian corpuscle | Threshold |
| von Frey hair or Semmes-Weinstein monofilament | Constant touch | A-$\beta$ 15–20 $\mu$m | Slowly adapting | Merkel cell– neurite complex | Threshold |

From Gelberman et al. (1983a).

studies utilized a human model for median nerve compression in the carpal tunnel (Fig. 8.2). The acute carpal tunnel syndrome model is very useful for studying the effects of compression on human nerve because the median nerve is superficial in the wrist and very accessible to controlled localized pressure. Both electrical and sensory tests of the median nerve are sensitive and reliable. Our volunteers consisted of 25 healthy subjects without any history of diabetes, alcoholism, hand trauma, symptoms of carpal tunnel syndrome or peripheral neuropathy. In addition, nine hypertensive subjects were tested (Szabo et al., 1983). A sterile wick catheter was introduced into the carpal tunnel as previously described (Bauman et al., 1981; Gelberman et al., 1981). After measurement of the resting pressure in the carpal tunnel, the hand was placed within a specially designed external compression device and localized pressure was applied to the carpal tunnel using a piece of molded rubber placed on the palmar aspect of the wrist (Fig. 8.3). The wrist rested on a layer of foam, leaving several large dorsal veins free from compression. Thus, adequate venous drainage from the hand was ensured. Compression was gradually applied to the wrist, while tissue fluid pressure was continuously measured by the wick catheter. Different levels of pressure between 30 and 90 mm Hg were used. The catheter was withdrawn when the desired pressure level was reached. Motor and sensory latencies of the median nerve at the wrist were studied by a TECA electromyograph at 10-min intervals

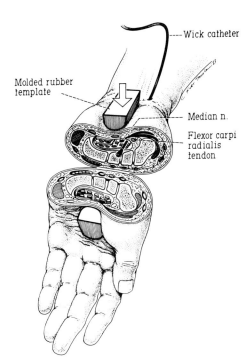

Wick catheter

Molded rubber template

Median n.

Flexor carpi radialis tendon

**Figure 8.2.** Local compression is applied over the median nerve by a molded rubber template. The wick catheter is inserted adjacent to the flexor carpi radialis tendon at level of the proximal wrist.

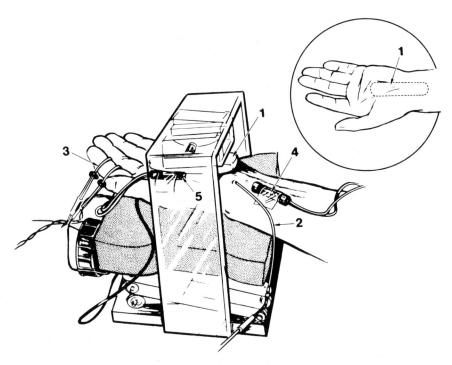

**Figure 8.3.** Controlled external compression device. Localized pressure was applied to carpal tunnel by adjusting level of lower platform toward fixed roof of compression device. (1) Molded rubber placed on the palmar aspect of the wrist. (2) Wick catheter in carpal canal just ulnar to flexor carpi radialis tendon. (3) Self-retaining spring ring digital electrode for recording and stimulating (sensory conduction tests). (4) Bar surface electrode for stimulating median nerve 3 cm proximal to wrist. (5) Bar surface electrode on thenar eminence for recording motor response. (From Gelberman et al., 1983*b*)

during compression and during the recovery phase after release of compression. A nerve stimulator delivered a rectangular pulse of 0 to 1 ms duration at the rate of 1/s to the median nerve (supramaximal intensity). Each subject was questioned as to subjective changes such as numbness, tingling or pain throughout the experiment. In the first 16 subjects, the Weber two-point discrimination test was performed on each digit using a dull-pointed eye caliper (Werner and Omer, 1970) applied in a longitudinal axis with care taken to avoid blanching the skin (Moberg, 1964; Omer, 1974, Gelberman et al., 1978). In addition, the strength of the abductor pollicis brevis was tested manually and graded on a scale from 0 to 5 (*Manual of Orthopedic Surgery,* 1972). The remaining subjects were in addition tested with a 256 cps tuning fork and the moving two-point discrimination test as described by Dellon (1978, 1981) and with Semmes-

Weinstein monofilaments (von Frey pressure test) (Werner and Omer, 1970; Levin et al., 1978; Omer, 1980). Six subjects were also tested with a fixed-frequency (120 Hz) variable-amplitude vibrometer (Bio-Thesiometer, Biomedical Instrument Co., Newbury, OH) to assess vibratory threshold (Dellon, 1981). The experiment was terminated when, after the release of compression, both subjective sensation and neurophysiological tests returned to baseline. Compression was maintained for no less than 30 min and no longer than 240 min. In three cases, local compression was used in combination with proximal tourniquet inflation. Before release of the pressure, a tourniquet was inflated around the upper arm to maintain ischemia in the previously compressed nerve segment at the wrist. Localized pressure was released and the tourniquet was kept inflated for 15 min. The tourniquet was then released and the recovery of nerve function was followed. Some subjects were studied with tourniquet inflation only in the absence of local compression.

## Mechanical Compression versus Local Ischemia

The pneumatic tourniquet was inflated around the upper arm to a pressure of 250 mm Hg and nerve function was assessed subjectively and neurophysiologically. The subjects felt paresthesias usually within 30 s, and numbness and total anesthesia of the hand followed within 10 to 15 min. Subsequent anesthesia of the arm followed a centripetal course. The fingertips became numb, followed by numbness in the hand and wrist. Subsequently, in successive order, more proximal parts of the forearm and arm followed. The deterioration of sensory response showed a course similar to the 50 to 90 mm Hg compression groups. Sensory fiber amplitudes disappeared within 20 to 30 min. Motor amplitude decreased only slightly at this time. Experiments were terminated at 30 min because of pain. Investigations carried out by Lewis and co-workers (1931) on human arms subjected to tourniquet ischemia with suprasystolic pressures revealed a disappearance of function in peripheral nerves after 15 to 45 min. In our studies, a rapid decline in nerve function also occurred after 10 to 60 min with pressures of 50 to 90 mm Hg applied to the median nerve. It appears that the acute effects of compression in this study were due to ischemia and not mechanical deformation. This concept is supported by findings in subjects who had local compression of 60 mm Hg applied at the wrist level until sensory response disappeared. The tourniquet was then inflated to maintain ischemia to the previously compressed segment of the nerve. Sensory conduction block remained as long as the tourniquet ischemia was maintained, even after the local compression was released (Fig. 8.4). Normally, relief of local compression produced an immediate return of sensory conduction. These findings indicate that continued ischemia to the median nerve at the wrist, and not mechanical-

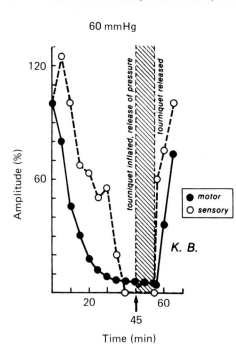

**Figure 8.4.** Representative example of subject with combined experiment to separate ischemia and mechanical-deformation compressing forces. Localized pressure was applied to median nerve at wrist, and sensory response disappeared after 40 min. At 45 min, tourniquet was inflated around upper arm to 250 mm Hg, and local pressure at wrist level was released. Sensory response remained absent and motor response continued close to zero level. When tourniquet was released at 55 min, there was rapid recovery in motor and sensory responses. (From Lundborg et al., 1982.)

structural changes in nerve fibers, was the major reason for the maintenance of the nerve conduction block.

In addition, recent studies of hypertensive subjects indicate that an increase in mean arterial pressure raises the critical threshold to nerve compression (Szabo et al., 1983). These findings confirm a direct correlation between perfusion pressure and the threshold pressure for nerve dysfunction, and furthermore favor the concept that ischemia plays the major role in the early stages of low pressure nerve compression when symptoms are still reversible.

## Critical Threshold Pressure

The pressure level at which neural tissue and muscle are acutely jeopardized in humans has not been determined conclusively. Empirical data from patients with compartment syndromes do not provide definitive information on a critical pressure limit. Estimates based on data obtained in experimental animal models (Sheridan and Matsen, 1975; Rydevik et al., 1977, 1981; Hargens et al., 1979, 1981) and a clinical study (Matsen et al., 1977) suggest a wide range of values between 30 and 60 mm Hg. At present the decision to perform a fasciotomy in compartment syndromes is guided by tissue fluid pressure measurements using one of three catheter techniques (Whitesides et al., 1975a; Matsen et al., 1976; Mubarak et al., 1978). Fascial decompression is performed in any circumstance where pressure within a compartment exceeds the tolerance limits of nerve or muscle fibers. Disagreement exists on the definition of this critical pressure. Using an infusion technique, Matsen and Krugmire (1978) measured the pressures of 29 limbs considered at risk for compartment syndrome. They found no neurovascular deficit in limbs with pressures below 50 mm Hg. Whitesides and associates (1975b) selected an absolute value of 45 mm Hg in patients with diastolic blood pressures of 70 mm Hg or the diastolic blood pressure minus 10 to 30 mm Hg as the critical pressure level. Mubarak and Hargens (1981) selected 30 mm Hg as the critical pressure level.

Which tissue, muscle or nerve is more susceptible to the effects of pressure and ischemia is a complex and not completely answered question. Some pieces of information are available from clinical observations and a few experiments but not all studies completely agree with regard to pressure–time thresholds. Although neural tissue may be more resistant than muscle to permanent injury from total ischemia, abnormalities in nerve function are demonstrated long before abnormal muscle function is detectable. Mild neurological deficits occur in dog peroneal nerve after 6 to 8 h at intracompartmental pressures of 30 mm Hg, but total conduction failure occurs at a threshold pressure of 50 mm Hg (Hargens et al., 1979). Although nerves lose their function under ischemic conditions long before muscle becomes inexcitable, continued pressure will irreversibly damage muscle more readily than nerve (Lewis, 1936). Sheridan and Matsen (1975) demonstrated that rabbit striated muscle, exposed to compartment pressures of 50 to 60 mm Hg for 24 h, exhibited necrotic changes when examined histologically. However, in a canine model, significant muscle necrosis (quantitated by pyrophosphate uptake) occurs in muscle compartments pressurized at 30 mm Hg after 8 h (Hargens et al., 1981). Although the exact effects of varying levels of pressure on muscle and nerve over different periods of time remain controversial, it is clear that following acute ischemia, nerve function is altered earlier than muscle function. Therefore, an accurate assessment of nerve function is of considerable clinical importance in evaluating compartment syndrome.

We evaluated the functional response of median nerves exposed to various levels of pressure to determine the critical pressure level for nerve viability. Compression at 90, 70, 60 and 50 mm Hg produced a consistent sequence of events. In all normotensive subjects, the sensory response disappeared 10 to 60 min after application of pressure.

The time for this response was independent of the exact pressure level as long as it was >50 mm Hg. There was a rapid decline in sensory amplitude action potentials and an increase in sensory latency. At the time of sensory loss, motor amplitude was reduced to 30 to 40% of its original value. The sensory fibers appeared resistant during the initial phases of compression. Although motor fibers were most susceptible within the first few minutes of compression, the sensory response totally disappeared first. In all cases, the sensory and motor amplitudes and latencies returned to baseline values immediately following the release of compression (Fig. 8.5). Each normotensive subject experienced either numbness or paresthesias with compression of the median nerve at or above 50 mm Hg.

When 40 mm Hg or less pressure was applied to the nerve, the findings were also consistent. No subject experienced significant changes in nerve function (defined as >50% loss) and no significant neurophysiological

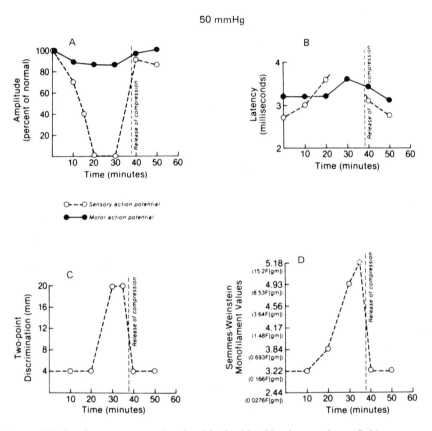

**Figure 8.5.** Sensory nerve conduction blocked by 20 min at a tissue fluid pressure of 50 mm Hg in this representative subject (**A, B**). Clinical sensibility also disappeared at this pressure level (**C, D**). **A:** Amplitudes are recorded in percentage of control baseline values. **B:** Motor (●) and sensory (○) latency in milliseconds. **C:** Two-point discrimination is recorded in millimeters. **D:** Semmes-Weinstein monofilament values are recorded in both the manufacturer's numerical markings, log 10 (force in mg), and in grams of force (in parentheses). (From Gelberman et al., 1983*b*.)

changes occurred over a period as long as 4 h (Fig. 8.6). In each case, small declines in amplitude of the sensory and motor action potentials were the earliest findings. The sensory amplitude decreased 42% (40 mm Hg compression). Sensory latencies increased by 0.2 ms. Each subject experienced mild subjective sensory abnormalities, primarily numbness in the median nerve distribution.

Two subjects were tested at both 40 and 50 mm Hg compression on separate occasions. At 40 mm Hg, the sensory amplitude of one subject remained 92% of normal at 35 min; but at 50 mm Hg, a complete sensory block had occurred by that time. Another subject maintained sensory

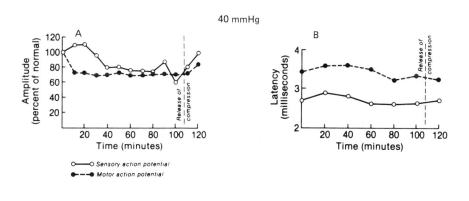

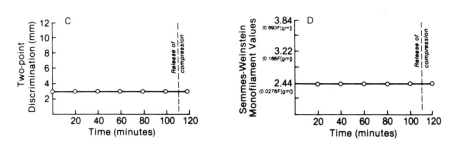

**Figure 8.6.** No significant decrease in sensory conduction or sensibility occurred at a tissue fluid pressure of 40 mm Hg in this representative subject. **A:** Amplitudes are recorded in percentage of control baseline values. **B:** Motor (●) and sensory (○) latency in milliseconds. **C:** Two-point discrimination is recorded in millimeters. **D:** Semmes-Weinstein monofilament values are recorded in both the manufacturer's numerical markings, log 10 (force in mg), and in grams of force (in parentheses). (From Gelberman et al., 1983b.)

amplitude at 87% of normal at 40 mm Hg, but had a complete sensory block after 20 min of compression at 50 mm Hg.

Subjects who were tested at 30 mm Hg compression showed a more variable response, some even demonstrating an increase in sensory and motor amplitudes. The latency times remained unchanged in this series, however. Half of the subjects tested at 30 mm Hg revealed mild symptoms of a pins-and-needles sensation toward the end of the period of compression (after 90 min). The strength of the abductor pollicis was not significantly decreased at any pressure, except in those few subjects who were compressed long enough to attain a complete motor conduction block, which was always preceded by a complete sensory block.

Human compression studies are not conducive to investigations for periods of time longer than 4 h. Our conclusions, therefore, apply to relatively short periods of time and it is possible that compression at 40 mm Hg over longer periods of time may produce greater dysfunction than is evident in these acute experiments. These results indicate that there exists a critical threshold between 40 mm Hg and 50 mm Hg at which peripheral nerve is acutely jeopardized. Compartment decompression may not be required when tissue fluid pressures are below this level.

It was interesting to note that one subject whose blood pressure was 130/90 mm Hg showed only a mild decrease in sensory and motor nerve function despite 120 min of sustained compression at 60 mm Hg. Our data were initially obtained on subjects with systemic blood pressures that ranged from 100 to 120 mm Hg systolic and 60 to 75 mm Hg diastolic. Having observed the discrepancy in the volunteer with a significantly elevated diastolic blood pressure, we actively sought out hypertensive subjects for similar studies. Our results to date in nine hypertensive subjects suggest that systemic blood pressure does affect the critical pressure at which nerve behavior is altered by compression (Szabo et al., 1983). Relationships between mean arterial blood pressure, diastolic blood pressure and the threshold pressure level for nerve dysfunction are now established (Figs. 8.7 and Fig. 8.8).

## Sensibility Testing

An unexpected finding occurred in our initial studies. In most cases, two-point discrimination remained normal even when the amplitude of the sensory fibers was reduced severely (Lundborg et al., 1982). While the subjects complained of numbness and paresthesias in the fingers, the two-point discrimination test constituted an "all-or-none function." As long as any peripheral input remained, function was integrated by the intact cortical link. This ability disappeared abruptly only when the last large sensory fibers deteriorated. Clinically, several authors have noted that two-point discrimination is most often normal in carpal tunnel syndrome

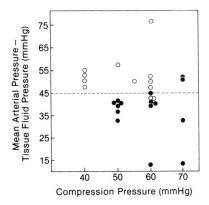

**Figure 8.7.** Relationship between mean arterial pressure minus tissue fluid pressure, and tissue fluid pressure (compression pressure). Summary of all tests performed between 40 and 70 mm Hg tissue fluid pressure (compression pressure). Pressure values are in mm Hg. *Open circles* signify no nerve conduction block. *Filled circles* signify nerve conduction block. (From Szabo et al., 1983.)

and, if abnormal, usually indicates advanced disease (Adamson et al., 1971; Hunter et al., 1978; Dellon, 1981). Utilizing the human model for median nerve compression, we evaluated four standard tests of sensibility to determine the objective sensory abnormalities of peripheral compression. It was our intention to establish the optimum test with which to monitor compression syndromes. Subjects were tested at pressures ranging from 40 to 70 mm Hg. Subjective and clinical findings were compared with neurophysiological tests, including distal sensory and motor amplitudes and latencies.

The earliest indication of impaired nerve function on electrical testing was decreased sensory action potential amplitude. This finding had previously been noted by Nielson and Kardel (1974). The pattern of sensory amplitude change was similar in all subjects tested. Each subject experienced some degree of numbness, tingling and paresthesias in the distribution of the median nerve at the time subjective sensations were first noted. Median sensory amplitude was 87% of the baseline value (Fig. 8.9).

Abnormalities in Semmes-Weinstein monofilament testing (the von

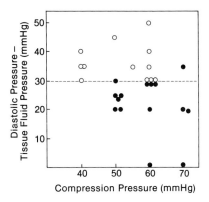

**Figure 8.8.** Relationship between diastolic blood pressure minus tissue fluid pressure, and tissue fluid pressure (compression pressure). Summary of all tests performed between 40 and 70 mm Hg tissue fluid pressure (compression pressure). Pressure values are in mm Hg. *Open circles* signify no nerve conduction block. *Filled circles* signify nerve conduction block. (From Szabo et al., 1983.)

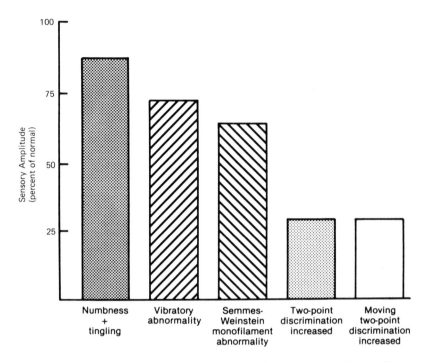

**Figure 8.9.** Subjective complaints and objective findings versus the median sensory amplitude as percent of normal baseline amplitude (summary of 12 subjects). (From Gelberman et al., 1983a.)

Frey test) were detected shortly after the first subjective sensations appeared in the median nerve distribution. The median sensory amplitude at this time was 65% of the baseline value. The monofilament range noted was between 2.83 and 3.61 units corresponding to 0.068 to 0.408 g of force (normal: 2.44 units or 0.0276 g of force). In all subjects, vibratory testing with a 256 cps tuning fork closely paralleled the Semmes-Weinstein monofilament tests (Fig. 8.10).

There was no significant difference in the findings noted with the static and moving two-point discrimination tests. Two-point discrimination remained normal at a time when sensory fiber amplitude was decreased by 70%. Two-point discrimination values increased suddenly, concomitant with a total loss of sensory fiber recording. In each subject, two-point discrimination was the last of the sensibility tests to reflect abnormalities in nerve function (Fig. 8.11).

The sensory tests we evaluated had fundamental differences with respect to the fiber populations and receptor systems under investigation. Moving two-point discrimination and vibration tests evaluate the quickly adapting fibers of touch (Dellon, 1978), which represents the greatest per-

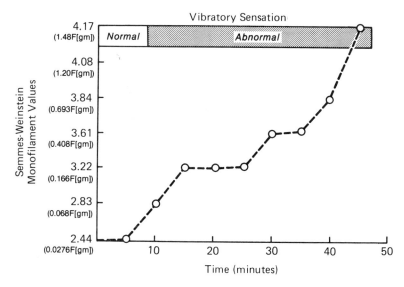

**Figure 8.10.** As compression is applied in a representative subject at 50 mm Hg, sensation gradually decreases as detected by the monofilaments. Abnormal tuning fork perception correlates well with this time interval. Semmes-Weinstein (S-W) monofilaments are recorded in both the manufacturer's numerical markings, log 10 (force in mg), and in grams of force (in parentheses). Vibration is indicated as normal or abnormal. (From Gelberman et al., 1983a.)

centage of nerve fibers. Static two-point discrimination and Semmes-Weinstein monofilaments evaluate the slowly adapting fibers (Dellon, 1981). Both static and moving two-point discriminations are innervation density tests, however. Although these tests are reliable in assessing functional nerve regeneration, neither was sensitive to the gradual decrease in nerve function created by the external compression device in our model. Fundamental differences between nerve regeneration and nerve compression form the basis for the different results obtained with sensory testing in each situation. Discrete areas of peripheral sensation correspond to specific localized points in the cerebral cortex. After a peripheral nerve laceration and subsequent regeneration, brain input is radically altered. A complete disorganization of the somatotopic regeneration within the central cortex occurs (Paul et al., 1972). In contrast, the sensory relay system to the cortex is uninterrupted in compression neuropathy and cortical organization remains intact. Static and moving two-point discrimination may remain intact if only a few fibers are conducting normally to their correct cortical endpoints.

The von Frey and vibratory tests are threshold tests that probably detect a gradual and progressive change in sensation as a greater proportion of nerve fibers are lost, while other fibers maintain their correct

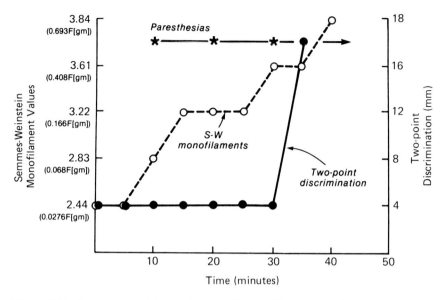

**Figure 8.11.** In a representative subject at 50 mm Hg compression, the monofilaments gradually detect median nerve dysfunction secondary to compression, whereas two-point discrimination rapidly diminishes at a later time. S-W monofilaments are recorded in both the manufacturer's numerical markings, log 10 (force in mg), and in grams of force (in parentheses). The appearance of paresthesias is indicated by an asterisk. (From Gelberman et al., 1983a.)

central connections. These tests differ in that the monofilaments measure the slowly adapting fiber system whereas vibration measures the quickly adapting fiber system. Yet both consistently reflect decreased nerve function in our model. Other investigators have contributed information to confirm clinically what we have demonstrated experimentally. Dellon (1978) noted that although only 50% of his patients with carpal tunnel syndrome had abnormal two-point discrimination, 72% had abnormal vibratory perception. Hunter and collaborators (1978) found that most patients with median nerve compression had abnormal monofilament pressure measurements but many had normal two-point discrimination. On a theoretical basis, we felt that vibration is at least as effective in detecting nerve compression as the Semmes-Weinstein monofilaments, as vibration measures a greater proportion of the fibers, i.e., the quickly adapting fiber system. There is a problem, however, with the quantitation of vibratory stimuli and response, because the results are recorded in terms of increased or decreased perception of a tuning fork. The stimulus amplitude varies with how forcefully the tuning fork is struck, and thus its amplitude is not precisely controlled. We therefore explored the use of a calibrated fixed-frequency (120 Hz) variable-amplitude vibrometer which is used for certain clinical situations (Daniel et al., 1974, 1977). All of the previously described sensory tests were performed in addition to the vibratory thresholds. The vibratory threshold values reflected the earliest clinical abnormalities and correlated well with the less quantitative tuning fork measurements (Fig. 8.12). Amplitudes of the sensory compound action potential and sensory latencies changed along with the changes in the vibrometer readings.

The information obtained both on critical pressure and sensibility testing with the human model for peripheral nerve compression leads us to adopt the following approach to acute upper extremity compartment and acute carpal tunnel syndromes. In alert, normotensive patients in whom sensory monitoring is possible, forearm intramuscular fluid pressures and

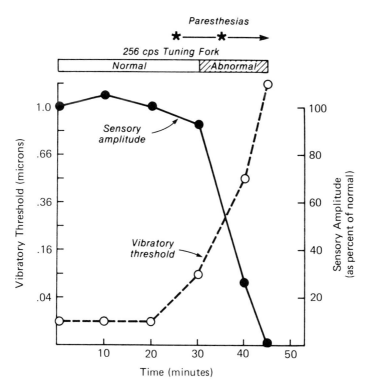

**Figure 8.12.** Representative subject with compression of median nerve at 50 mm Hg. Vibratory threshold, paresthesias and 256 cps tuning fork perception and sensory amplitude versus time. Vibratory threshold is in microns of vibratory amplitude. Paresthesias are indicated by an asterisk. Tuning fork perception is shown as normal or abnormal. Increasing vibratory threshold parallels decreasing sensory amplitude. Sensory amplitude is the most sensitive indicator of nerve dysfunction correlating closely with paresthesias. Vibratory sensibility is quantitatively detected by the vibrometer and qualitatively detected by the tuning fork. (From Szabo et al., 1984.)

carpal tunnel pressures <50 mm Hg are observed with sensory examinations using Semmes-Weinstein monofilaments, the 256 cps tuning fork and vibrometer. Repeat measurements of tissue fluid pressure are performed if any deterioration in sensory function is detected. We recognize that pressures may need to be interpreted differently in hypertensive patients or in patients in hypotensive states such as shock. The decision for fasciotomy is based on information obtained from both pressure and sensory studies. A similar approach to lower extremity compartment syndromes may be followed. However, an accurate and reproducible sensory testing scheme in the lower extremity has not yet been established. Understanding the effects of mechanical compression on peripheral nerve is not only of theoretical relevance but is also important for decision-making processes in many clinical situations.

## Summary

Previous studies in animals document the effects of acute compression on peripheral nerve. However, controversy exists with respect to the relative importance of ischemia versus mechanical factors in compression-related nerve dysfunction. Our recent investigations of median nerve function in normotensive and hypertensive subjects demonstrate significant motor and sensory dysfunction at a threshold tissue fluid pressure consistently 30 mm Hg below diastolic blood pressure. For example, sensory responses were completely blocked at threshold pressures of 40 to 50 mm Hg in normotensive subjects and 60 to 70 mm Hg in hypertensive subjects.

These studies also identify the most sensitive techniques for assessing peripheral nerve compression syndromes. Threshold tests for sensibility (vibration and Semmes-Weinstein monofilament testing) yielded gradual loss of nerve function whereas innervation density tests (two-point discrimination and moving two-point discrimination) produced essentially all-or-nothing responses. These studies also help identify tissue fluid pressure thresholds for decompression of acute compartment syndromes.

## Acknowledgment

This work is supported by the Veterans Administration and by USPHS/NIH grants AM-25501, AM-26344, and RCDA AM-00602 to A.R.H.

## References

Adamson JE, Srouji SJ, Horton CE and Mladick RA (1971). The acute carpal tunnel syndrome. *Plast Reconstr Surg* 47:332–336.
Bauman TD, Gelberman RH, Mubarak SJ and Garfin SR (1981). The acute carpal tunnel syndrome. *Clin Orthop* 156:151–156.

Dahn I, Lassen NA and Westling H (1967). Blood flow in human muscles during external pressure or venous stasis. *Clin Sci* 32:467–473.

Daniel CR, Bower JD, Pearson JE and Holbert RD (1974). Vibrometry and neuropathy. *J Miss State Med Assoc* 18:30–34.

Daniel CR, Bower JD, Pearson JE and Holbert RD (1977). Vibrometry and peripheral neuropathy. *South Med J* 70:1311–1313.

Dellon AL (1978). The moving two-point discrimination test: clinical evaluation of the quickly adapting fiber/receptor system. *J Hand Surg* 3:474–481.

Dellon AL (1980). Clinical use of vibratory stimuli to evaluate peripheral nerve injury and compression neuropathy. *Plast Reconstr Surg* 65:466–476.

Dellon AL (1981). *Evaluation of Sensibility and Re-education of Sensation in the Hand.* Baltimore: Williams & Wilkins, pp. 95–167.

Dellon AL, Curtis RM and Edgerton MT (1972). Evaluating recovery of sensation in the hand following nerve injury. *Johns Hopkins Med J* 130:235–243.

Gelberman RH, Hergenroeder PT, Hargens AR, Lundborg GN and Akeson WH (1981). The carpal tunnel syndrome. A study of carpal tunnel pressures. *J Bone Joint Surg* 63A:380–383.

Gelberman RH, Szabo RM, Williamson RV and Dimick MP (1983a). Sensibility testing in peripheral-nerve compression syndromes: an experimental study in humans. *J Bone Joint Surg* 65A:632–638.

Gelberman RH, Szabo RM, Williamson RV, Hargens AR, Yaru NC and Minteer-Convery MA (1983b). Tissue pressure threshold for peripheral nerve viability. *Clin Orthop* 178:285–291.

Gelberman RH, Urbaniak JR, Bright DS and Levin LS (1978). Digital sensibility following replantation. *J Hand Surg* 3:313–319.

Hargens AR, Mubarak SJ, Owen CA, Garetto LP and Akeson WH (1977). Interstitial fluid pressure in muscle and compartment syndromes in man. *Microvasc Res* 14:1–10.

Hargens AR, Romine JS, Sipe JC, Evans KL, Mubarak SJ and Akeson WH (1979). Peripheral nerve-conduction block by high muscle-compartment pressure. *J Bone Joint Surg* 61A:192–200.

Hargens AR, Schmidt DA, Evans KL, Gonsalves MR, Cologne JB, Garfin SR, Mubarak SJ, Hagen PL and Akeson WH (1981). Quantitation of skeletal-muscle necrosis in a model compartment syndrome. *J Bone Joint Surg* 63A:631–636.

Hunter JM, Schneider LH, Mackin EJ and Bell JA (1978). *Rehabilitation of the Hand.* St. Louis: CV Mosby, pp. 273–291.

Levin S, Pearsell G and Ruderman RJ (1978). Von Frey's method of measuring pressure sensibility in the hand: an engineering analysis of the Weinstein-Semmes pressure aesthesiometer. *J Hand Surg* 3:211–216.

Lewis T (1936). Effects of circulatory arrest. In: *Vascular Disorders of the Limbs,* 2nd ed. London: Macmillan, pp. 17–25.

Lewis T, Pickering GW and Rothschild P (1931). Centripetal paralysis arising out of arrested blood flow to a limb. Including notes on a form of tingling. *Heart* 16:1–32.

Lundborg G (1970). Ischemic nerve injury. Experimental studies on intraneural microvascular pathophysiology and have function in the limb subjected to temporary circulatory arrest. *Scand J Plast Reconstr Surg (Suppl)* 6:1–113.

Lundborg G (1975). Structure and function of the intraneural microvessels as related to trauma, edema formation and nerve function. *J Bone Joint Surg* 57A:938–949.

Lundborg G, Gelberman RH, Minteer-Convery M, Lee YF and Hargens AR (1982). Median nerve compression in the carpal tunnel—functional response to experimentally induced controlled pressure. *J Hand Surg* 7:252–259.

Lundborg G, Myers R and Powell H (1983). Nerve compression injury and increased endoneurial fluid pressure: a "miniature compartment syndrome." *J Neurol Neurosurg Psychiatry* 46:1119–1124.

*Manual of Orthopedic Surgery* (1972). Chicago: American Orthopaedic Association.

Matsen FA III and Krugmire RB Jr (1978). Compartmental syndromes. *Surg Gynecol Obstet* 147:943–949.

Matsen FA III, Mayo KA, Krugmire RB Jr, Sheriden GW and Kraft GH (1977). A model compartmental syndrome in man with particular reference to the quantification of nerve function. *J Bone Joint Surg* 59A:648–653.

Matsen FA III, Mayo KA, Sheriden GW and Krugmire RB Jr (1976). Monitoring of intramuscular pressure. *Surgery* 79:702–709.

Moberg E (1958). Objective methods for determining the functional value of sensibility in the hand. *J Bone Joint Surg* 40B:454–476.

Moberg E (1962). Criticism and study of methods for examining sensibility in the hand. *Neurology* 12:8–19.

Moberg E (1964). Evaluation and management of nerve injuries in the hand. *Surg Clin North Am* 44:1019–1029.

Moberg E (1966). Method for examining sensibility of the hand. In: *Hand Surgery*. Flynn JE (ed.). Baltimore: Williams & Wilkins, pp. 435–449.

Mountcastle VB (1980). *Medical Physiology*, 14th ed. St Louis: CV Mosby, Chapter 11.

Mubarak SJ and Hargens AR (1981). *Compartment Syndromes and Volkmann's Contracture*. Philadelphia: WB Saunders, pp. 1–232.

Mubarak SJ, Owen CA, Hargens AR, Garretto LP and Akeson WH (1978). Acute compartment syndromes: diagnosis and treatment with the aid of the wick catheter. *J Bone Joint Surg* 60A:1091–1095.

Nielson VK and Kardel T (1974). Decremental conduction in normal human nerves subjected to ischemia? *Acta Physiol Scand* 92:249–262.

Ochoa J, Fowler TJ and Gilliatt RW (1972). Anatomical changes in peripheral nerves compressed by a pneumatic tourniquet. *J Anat* 113:433–455.

Omer GE Jr (1974). Injuries to nerves of the upper extremity. *J Bone Joint Surg* 56A:1615–1624.

Omer GE Jr (1980). Sensibility testing. In: *Management of Peripheral Nerve Problems*. GE Omer Jr and M Spinner (eds.). Philadelphia: WB Saunders, pp. 3–15.

Paul RL, Goodman H and Merzenich M (1972). Alterations in mechanoreceptor input to Brodmann's areas one and three of the postcentral hand area of *Macaca mulatta* after nerve section and regeneration. *Brain Res* 39:1–19.

Phalen GS (1972). The carpal-tunnel syndrome. Clinical evaluation of 598 hands. *Clin Orthop* 83:29–40.

Rorabeck CH, Macnab I, and Waddell JP (1972). Anterior tibial compartment syndrome: a clinical and experimental review. *Can J Surg* 15:249–256.

Rydevik B and Lundborg G (1977). Permeability of intraneural microvessels and perineurium following acute, graded experimental nerve compression. *Scand J Plast Reconstr Surg* 11:179–187.

Rydevik B, Lundborg G and Bagge U (1981). Effects of graded compression on intraneural blood flow. An in vivo study on rabbit tibial nerve. *J Hand Surg* 6:3–12.

Sheridan GW and Matsen FA III (1975). An animal model of the compartmental syndrome. *Clin Orthop* 113:36–42.

Spinner M (1978). *Injuries to the Major Branches of the Forearm,* 2nd ed. Philadelphia: WB Saunders.

Sunderland S (1976). The nerve lesion in the carpal tunnel syndrome. *J Neurol Neurosurg Psychiatry* 39:615–626.

Sunderland S (1978). *Nerves and Nerve Injuries,* 2nd ed. Edinburgh: ES Livingstone.

Szabo RM, Gelberman RH, Williamson RV, Dellon AL, Yaru NC and Dimick MP (1984). Vibratory sensory testing in acute peripheral nerve compression. *J Hand Surg* 9A:104–109.

Szabo RM, Gelberman RH, Williamson RV and Hargens AR (1983). Effects of increased systemic blood pressure on the tissue fluid pressure threshold of peripheral nerve. *J Orthop Res* 1:172–178.

Werner JL and Omer GE Jr (1970). Evaluating cutaneous pressure sensation of the hand. *Am J Occup Ther* 24:347–356.

Whitesides TE Jr, Haney TC, Harada H, Holmes HE and Morimoto K (1975a). A simple method for tissue pressure determination. *Arch Surg* 110:1311–1313.

Whitesides TE Jr, Haney TC, Morimoto K and Harada H (1975b). Tissue pressure measurements as a determinant for the need of fasciotomy. *Clin Orthop* 113:43–51.

# CHAPTER 9

# Edema and the Tissue Resistance Safety Factor

Aubrey E. Taylor, James C. Parker, and Bengt Rippe

## Introduction

The formation of interstitial edema is a complex phenomenon that involves not only increased capillary filtration into the tissues, but also the changes that can occur in the tissue's ability to hold water coupled to the lymphatic drainage characteristics of the particular organ. Fifty years ago, Landis (1934) developed the concept that capillary pressure, usually controlled experimentally by altered venous pressure, must be elevated to some critical level before observable interstitial edema develops. He postulated that tissues react to increased capillary filtration by raising their tissue pressure, lowering their tissue colloid osmotic pressure (Starling, 1896) and increasing their lymphatic draining to provide the organ with a "margin of safety" in which observable edema is avoided even when capillary pressure increases by 15 to 20 mm Hg.

## Edema Safety Factors

This concept was revitalized and developed into a clear mathematical framework by Guyton and co-workers (1966, 1971, 1975), who described the ability of tissue pressure, tissue colloids and lymph flow to oppose edema in terms of "edema safety factors." These investigators defined the basic Starling equation for the capillary wall as:

$$J_V = K_{FC}[(P_c - P_t) - \sigma_d(\pi_p - \pi_t)] \tag{1}$$

where $J_V$ is volume flow across the capillary wall, $K_{FC}$ is capillary filtration coefficient, $P_c$ is microvascular pressure (referred to here as capillary hydrostatic pressure), $P_t$ is interstitial fluid pressure, $\sigma_d$ is the osmotic reflection coefficient for the proteins at the capillary wall* and $\pi_p$ and $\pi_t$

---

* The reflection coefficient describes the selectivity of a membrane to a particular solute. If $\sigma_d = 1$, the membrane is impermeable to the solute and when $\sigma_d = 0$, the membrane has no selectivity and the molecule is as permeable as water (Kedem and Katchalsky, 1958).

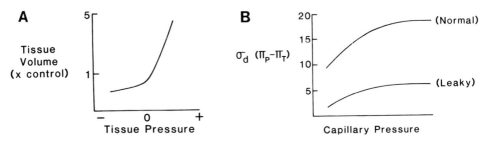

**Figure 9.1. A:** This curve illustrates how tissue fluid pressure changes as tissue volume increases (times control). Note that tissue fluid pressure changes markedly in the negative pressure range (low compliance), but when tissue fluid pressure becomes positive, tissue volume increases greatly. Ambient pressure equals zero tissue fluid pressure. **B:** These curves illustrate how the colloid osmotic tissue safety factor, $\sigma_d(\pi_p - \pi_t)$, changes as a function of capillary pressure. For leaky capillaries, $\sigma_d(\pi_p - \pi_t)$ does not change greatly; in fact, in absolute magnitude, it is considerably less than seen at normal pressures in nonleaky capillaries.

are colloid osmotic pressures of plasma and tissue fluid, respectively (Kedem and Katchalsky, 1958; Taylor et al., 1973; Granger and Taylor, 1980).

Normally, capillary filtration is equal to lymph flow. When $P_c$ is elevated, $P_t$ and $(\pi_p - \pi_t)$ will increase (Fig. 9.1). This occurs in several different capillary beds and the maximum changes of these "safety factors" following capillary pressure elevation are listed in Table 9.1 for various organs. Note that $\sigma_d (\pi_p - \pi_t)$ provides the major safety factor against edema formation in all organs with the exception of the liver and subcutaneous tissue. From these data, it is apparent that elevated interstitial fluid pressure and decreased tissue colloid osmotic pressure play ma-

**Table 9.1.** Percentage contributions of transcapillary colloid osmotic pressure gradient, interstitial fluid pressure and lymph flow to prevention of interstitial edema following elevations of venous pressure in the indicated organs

| Organ | Increased colloid osmotic pressure gradient (%) | Increased interstitial fluid pressure (%) | Increased lymph flow (%) |
|---|---|---|---|
| Colon[a] | 52 | 44 | 4 |
| Liver[b] | 0 | 58 | 42 |
| Lung[c] | 50 | 33 | 17 |
| Small intestine[d] | 45 | 35 | 20 |
| Subcutaneous tissue[e] | 14 | 62 | 24 |

Data from [a] Richardson et al. (1980); [b] Laine et al. (1979); [c] Drake and Taylor (1977); [d] Mortillaro and Taylor (1976); [e] Chen et al. (1976).

jor roles in opposing edema formation. However, the other major mechanism that provides another edema safety factor, lymph flow, is at present poorly understood (Taylor et al., 1973; Taylor, 1981).

## Lymphatic Safety Factor

When capillary pressure is elevated, lymph flow increases in all organs (Fig. 9.2). Usually lymph flow attains a plateau value (maximum lymphatic carrying capacity) that is characteristic for the particular organ under study. How is lymph flow determined by the capillary pressure operating across the capillary wall?

Classically, it was assumed that the imbalance in all forces to the right in Eq. (1): $(P_c - P_t) - \sigma(\pi_p - \pi_t)$ was responsible for lymph formation or flow (Guyton et al., 1971; Taylor et al., 1973). In general terms,

$$\text{Lymph flow} = K_{FC}\,\Delta P, \tag{2}$$

or

$$\Delta P = \text{Lymph flow}/K_{FC}. \tag{3}$$

The imbalance in Starling forces $\Delta P$ changes for different $K_{FC}$ values and different lymph flows (Fig. 9.3). Many physiologists erroneously assume that small lymph flows cannot provide any substantial safety factor. Figure 9.3 and Eq. (3) indicate the fallacy of this reasoning since small lymph flows and small $K_{FC}$ values allow large $\Delta P$ values to exist across the capillary wall–lymphatic system. $K_{FC}$ for skeletal muscle is 0.01 ml/min/mm Hg/100 g, so if lymph flow is 0.1 ml/min/100 g muscle, then $\Delta P$ would be 10 mm Hg, which is a considerable force.

## Tissue Resistance to Fluid Movement

The above approach for determining the order of magnitude of the lymphatic safety factor has been used for several years. However, several experimental findings have appeared in the literature that indicate that this approach is apparently too simplistic to explain lymph flow responses to changes in Starling forces. First, when Starling forces are measured or

**Figure 9.2.** Plot of lymph flow (times control) as a function of tissue pressure. Lymph flow increases several-fold as tissue fluid pressure approaches zero, but levels off at positive pressures.

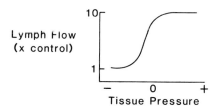

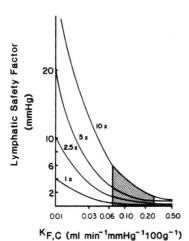

**Figure 9.3.** Representation of the lymphatic safety factor ($\Delta P$) as a function of the filtration coefficient ($K_{FC}$) for different lymph flows (1, 2.5, 5 and 10 times normal). The *dark area* indicates the range of values predicted for lung tissue when $K_{FC}$ is calculated using a balance of forces or weighed organs. The lymphatic safety factor is small even for high lymph flows if $K_{FC}$ is high. (Reprinted from Taylor and Drake, 1978 by courtesy of Marcel Dekker, Inc.)

calculated in a given organ, and divided into the corresponding lymph flow according to Eq. (2), $K_{FC}$ is sometimes 10 to 20 times that measured using other techniques in that particular organ (Erdmann et al., 1975; Taylor and Drake, 1978). Second, Gibson (1974) and Taylor and Gibson (1975) demonstrated that a decrease in $\pi_p$ of 11 mm Hg caused a greater change in lymph flow draining the dog paw than did a 50 mm Hg increase in venous outflow pressure (Fig. 9.4). Decreased $\pi_p$ should not provide a greater change in Starling forces than that imposed by the 50 mm Hg increase in venous pressure. The finding that colloids produce greater changes in lymph flow than elevated venous pressures has been confirmed in intestine, lung and other organ systems (Granger et al., 1979; Kramer et al., 1981). Third, lymph flow always increases to a greater extent when capillary pressure is elevated in capillaries that are more permeable to plasma proteins than in capillaries that are less permeable (Fig. 9.5).

Is there any common ground between these anomalies that may explain the apparent differences, relative to the lymphatic's ability to remove capillary filtrate (interstitial fluid) from tissues? How can $\Delta P$ be large when estimated by one procedure, yet orders of magnitude smaller when measured in a more direct way? If lymph flow can increase, then why doesn't it do so to provide a greater lymphatic safety factor?

Perhaps the one common factor in these experimental findings is that the lymphatic's ability to remove capillary filtrate is not described by Eq. (3) (Taylor et al., 1982). Lymph flow is not only determined by capillary filtration, but it is also a function of how easily fluid moves through the interstitium, the filling pressure of the initial lymphatics and the lymphatic's intrinsic ability to propel lymph away from the tissues (Casley-Smith, 1977; Nicoll and Taylor, 1977).

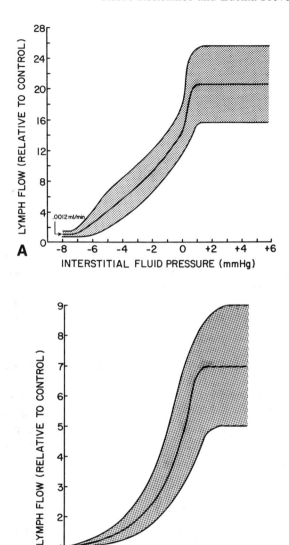

**Figure 9.4. A:** Lymph flow (times control) as a function of interstitial fluid pressure (measured using implanted capsules) for plasma proteins decreases, averaging 12 mm Hg. **B:** Plot of lymph flow as a function of interstitial fluid pressure for a 50 mm Hg increase in venous pressure. Lymph flow increased to a greater extent for the same tissue pressure when plasma colloids were decreased as compared to only increased capillary pressure. (Reproduced with permission of Gibson, 1974.)

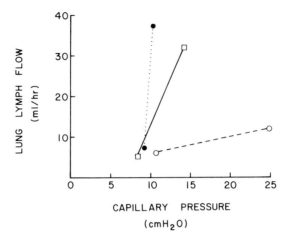

**Figure 9.5.** Plot of lung lymph flow as a function of capillary pressure for normal (○) and "leaky capillary" lungs (●, □). For the same rise in capillary pressure, lymph flows are greater when the capillaries are leaky to plasma proteins. (From Taylor and Parker, 1985. The data were modified from Brigham et al., 1974 by copyright permission of The American Society for Clinical Investigation.)

## Tissue Resistance and the Lymphatic Safety Factor

Guyton and co-workers (1966) have established that interstitial resistance is extremely high in normal tissues but decreases by orders of magnitude when the tissues begin to swell in the early phase of edema formation. Therefore, the proper $K_{FC}$ value to use in Eq. (2) is a composite of filtration coefficients of the capillary wall and tissue:

$$\Delta P = \frac{\text{Lymph flow}}{\left( K_{FC} \cdot K_{FT} \middle/ K_{FC} + K_{FT} \right),} \tag{4}$$

where $K_{FC}$ is the filtration coefficient of the capillary and $K_{FT}$ is the filtration coefficient of the tissue. Since $K_{FT}$ is a function of both the length and the radius to the fourth power of "interstitial fluid channels," then $K_{FT}$ may be quite small in dehydrated tissues and the denominator in Eq. (4) (in parentheses) will be smaller than the smallest $K_{FC}$. As the tissues swell, $K_{FT}$ increases greatly and $K_{FC}$ predominates (Taylor et al., 1982).

## Change of Tissue Resistance with Hydration

The effect of tissue resistance on lymph formation may explain how $K_{FC}$ could be large and yet lymph flow still could provide a substantial safety factor until the tissues swell and large fluid channels form. A model for lung tissue fluid regulation that incorporates tissue fluid resistance into the formation of lymph is available (Fig. 9.6). Note that a pressure gradient exists between the filtering capillaries and the more distant perivascular spaces containing the pulmonary lymphatics. If one measures lymph flow and divides by $\Delta P$ across the capillary wall in this model, a small $K_{FC}$ is calculated at normal tissue hydration. $K_{FC}$ increases as the tissues expand and $K_{FT}$ increases to values 1,000 to 10,000 times larger than control.

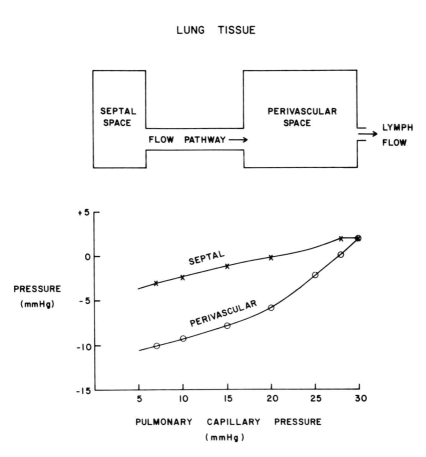

**Figure 9.6.** Replot of Guyton and co-workers' model (1976) which describes how tissue resistance can alter the lymph flow safety factor. The compartment on the left represents the filtering capillary sites. The fluid must flow through long pathways to enter the lymphatics. The major safety factor is equal to the drop in pressure between the filtering region and the more distant interstitial spaces. However, as capillary pressure increases, the pressures become equal and the capillary filtration (or lymph flow) is determined by the filtration coefficients of the capillary wall ($K_{FC}$). (From Taylor, 1981 by permission of The American Heart Association, Inc.)

## Decreased Plasma Colloid Osmotic Pressure versus Increased Capillary Pressure

Can tissue resistances explain why decreased plasma colloid osmotic pressure produces higher lymph flow than corresponding elevations of venous pressures? When venous pressure is elevated, tissue volume immediately increases, which is a function of venous capacity. This increased venous volume may rapidly change tissue fluid pressure, decrease the size of tissue channels (increase tissue resistance), alter lymphatic filling pressure by changing intralymphatic pressure to a greater degree than the surrounding pressure or somehow inhibit lymphatic drainage. These events do not occur with plasma dilution. At the present time, it is unclear which mechanism(s) is responsible for the greater effect of decreased $\pi_p$ on lymph flow as compared to increased venous pressure. However, some or all of these mechanisms may explain the results. Of course, the lymphatics' ability to pump and remove tissue fluid actively may also be affected by tissue protein content, different hormones, etc. Whatever the cause, future research should focus on these possible mechanisms, since the information will be extremely important for our understanding of basic lymphatic physiology (Wiederhielm, 1972; Granger, 1979).

## "Leaky" Capillaries and the Edema Safety Factor

Finally, the observation that lymph flow is higher in "leaky capillaries" for the same increase in capillary pressure can be explained by the following mechanism. First, when capillaries are leaky, plasma proteins rapidly move into tissues, saline follows, the tissues swell and tissue resistance decreases. When venous pressure is elevated, tissue spaces are less compressed as compared to normal tissues and tissue resistance does not change much. In addition, interstitial compliance may be altered, as some compounds that cause capillary walls to increase their permeability to plasma proteins may originate from leukocytes and their subsequent release of superoxide radicals. Superoxide radicals are known to destroy basement membranes and glycosaminoglycans (Granger et al., 1981). Therefore, tissue resistance is probably greatly decreased in different types of pulmonary edema. Since $K_{FC}$ of the capillary wall also increases under these circumstances, then Eq. (4) reduces to:

$$\cong \frac{\text{Lymph flow}}{\uparrow K_{FC}}. \tag{5}$$

If lymph flow does not increase more than $K_{FC}$, then $\Delta P$ will be smaller, even during increased lymph flow.

## Summary and Conclusions

From the foregoing discussion, it is evident that alterations in tissue fluid resistance play an important role in opposing edema formation. Everyone observes that elevation of an edemateous limb causes fluid to move away from the formerly dependent area. Yet, under normal conditions, fluid movement from one area of the tissues to another occurs only with difficulty. It is fairly easy to visualize how similar events occur in microscopic tissue spaces. Lymph flow is a complex phenomenon that is related to capillary filtration, pressure gradients that exist within the tissues, tissue fluid resistance, tissue compliance characteristics, pressure gradients for lymphatic filling, the lymphatics' intrinsic ability to contract and propel lymph and the effects of various tissue and blood-borne factors on lymphatic activity and/or capillary filtration (Taylor et al., 1973; Casley-Smith, 1977; Nicoll and Taylor, 1977).

The questions raised in this chapter provide some very formidable research problems, and future research promises to provide much new and exciting information concerning the effect of tissue resistance on lymph formation, and consequently, knowledge concerning etiologies of tissue edema.

## Acknowledgment

B. Rippe is the recipient of a Parker B. Francis Fellowship.

## References

Brigham K, Woolverton W, Blake L and Staub N (1974). Increased sheep lung vascular permeability caused by *Pseudomonas* bacteremia. *J Clin Invest* 54:792–804.

Casley-Smith JR (1977). The functioning of the lymphatic system under normal and pathological conditions: its dependence on the fine structures and permeabilities of the vessels. In: *Progress in Lymphology*. Ruttiman A. (ed.). Stuttgart: George Thieme, p. 348–359.

Chen HI, Granger HJ and Taylor AE (1976). Interactions of capillary, interstitial and lymphatic forces in the canine hindpaw. *Circ Res* 38:245–254.

Drake RE and Taylor AE (1977). Tissue and capillary force changes during the formation of intra-alveolar edema. *In Progress in Lymphology* Mayall RC and Witte MH (eds.). New York: Plenum Press, pp. 13–18.

Erdmann AJ III, Vaughan TR, Brigham KL, Woolverton WC and Staub NC (1975). Effect of increased vascular pressure on lung fluid balance in unanesthetized sheep. *Circ Res* 37:271–284.

Gibson WH (1974). *Dynamics of Lymph Flow, Tissue Pressure and Protein Ex-*

*change in Subcutaneous Connective Tissues*. Ph.D. Dissertation, University of Mississippi.

Granger DN, Parker RE, Quillen EW, Bracc RA and Taylor AE (1979). Lymph transients. In: *Lymphology*. Malick P, Bartos V, Weisslender H and Witte MH (eds.). Stuttgart: George Thieme, pp. 61–63.

Granger DN, Rutili G and McCord JM (1981). Superoxide radicals in feline intestinal ischemia. *Gastroenterology* 81:22–29.

Granger DN and Taylor AE (1980). Permeability of intestinal capillaries to endogenous macromolecules. *Am J Physiol* 238:H457–H464.

Granger HJ (1979). Role of the interstitial matrix and lymphatic pump in regulation of transcapillary fluid balance. *Microvasc Res* 18:209–216.

Guyton AC, Granger HJ and Taylor AE (1971). Interstitial fluid pressure. *Physiol Rev* 51:527–563.

Guyton AC, Scheel K and Murphree D (1966). Interstitial fluid pressure: III. Its effect on resistance to tissue fluid mobility. *Circ Res* 19:412–419.

Guyton A, Taylor A, Drake R and Parker J (1976). Dynamics of subatmospheric pressure in the pulmonary interstitial fluid. *Ciba Symp* 38:77–100.

Guyton AC, Taylor AE, Granger HJ (1975). *Circulatory Physiology, Vol II*. Philadelphia: WB Saunders, pp. 18–52.

Kedem O and Katchalsky A (1958). Thermodynamic analysis of the permeability of biological membranes to nonelectrolytes. *Biochim Biophys Acta* 27:229–246.

Kramer GC, Harms BA, Gunther RA, Renkin EM and Demling RH (1981). The effects of hypoproteinemia on blood-to-lymph fluid transport in sheep lung. *Circ Res* 49:1173–1180.

Laine GA, Hall JT, Laine S and Granger HJ (1979). Transsinusoidal fluid dynamics in canine liver during venous hypertension. *Circ Res* 45:317–323.

Landis E (1934). Capillary pressure and capillary permeability. *Physiol Rev* 14:404–481.

Mortillaro NA and Taylor AE (1976). Interaction of capillary and tissue forces in the cat small intestine. *Circ Res* 39:348–358.

Nicoll PA and Taylor AE (1977). Lymph formation and flow. *Annu Rev Physiol* 39:73–95.

Richardson PDI, Granger DN, Kvietys PR and Mailman D (1980). Permeability characteristics of colonic capillaries. *Am J Physiol* 239:G300–G305.

Starling EH (1896). On the absorption of fluid from the connective tissue spaces. *J Physiol (Lond)* 19:312–326.

Taylor AE (1981). Capillary fluid filtration: Starling forces and lymph flow. *Circ Res* 49:557–575.

Taylor AE and Drake RE (1978). Fluid and protein movement across the pulmonary microcirculation. In: *Lung Biology in Health and Disease, Vol. 7: Lung Water and Solute Exchange*. Staub N (ed.). New York: Marcel Dekker, pp. 129–182.

Taylor AE and Gibson H (1975). Concentrating ability of lymphatic vessels. *Lymphology* 8:43–49.

Taylor AE, Gibson WH, Granger HJ and Guyton AC (1973). The interaction between intracapillary and tissue forces in the overall regulation of interstitial fluid volume. *Lymphology* 6:192–208.

Taylor AE and Parker JC (1985). Pulmonary interstitial spaces and lymphatics.

In: *Handbook of Physiology, Sect. 3, The Respiratory System*. Fishman AP and Fisher AB (eds.), pp. 167–217.

Taylor AE, Parker JC, Kvietys PR and Perry MA (1982). The pulmonary interstitium in capillary exchange. *NY Acad Sci* 384:146–165.

Wiederhielm CA (1972). The interstitial space. In: *Biomechanics: Its Foundations and Objectives*. (Fung YC, Perrone N, Anliker M (eds.). Englewood Cliffs, New Jersey: Prentice-Hall, pp. 273–286.

CHAPTER 10

# Fluid Dynamics and Stress in Synovial Joints with Special Reference to the Immature Hip

David H. Gershuni and Alan R. Hargens

## Introduction

Synovial joints as a class include the majority of the important joints in the body. These articulations respond to physiological and pathological factors elsewhere in the body and may themselves influence surrounding and adjacent structures such as ligaments, bones, physes and articular cartilage. This chapter reviews the present state of knowledge of synovial fluid production and resorption, the effects of simulated effusion on the surrounding soft and hard tissues and the inflammatory response of the synovium with respect to fluid production and subsequent changes in intraarticular pressures. Particular emphasis will be placed on studies concerning the hip joint and interpretation of the effects of induced effusions with and without synovitis on the joint capsule and immature bony capital femoral epiphysis.

## Background

A synovial joint is characterized as an articulation between two bones covered by hyaline cartilage and linked by a synovial lined capsule. The synovium in some areas is arranged in folds and villi, which increase overall absorption area and provide a larger interface between the underlying blood supply and the synovial fluid (Fig. 10.1). The synovium and joint cavity, however, should not be compared to other body cavities such as those lined by peritoneum or pleura. This is because the synovial cavity develops embryologically as a cleft within the undifferentiated mesenchymal tissue of the joint interzone (Haines, 1947). The cleft appears in the human embryo at about 6 weeks of age and is dependent on movement of muscles of the limb. The lining cells of the cavity undergo some differentiation into a synovium consisting of an intimal layer with an abundant blood supply but no underlying basement membrane (Barland et al., 1962; Wyllie et al., 1966; Ghadially and Roy, 1966). This layer is

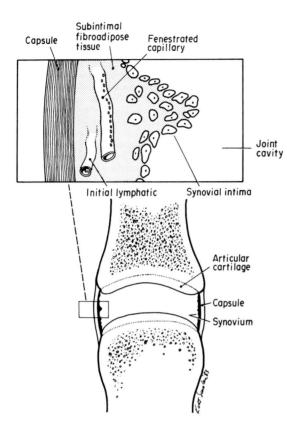

Figure 10.1. Schematized synovial joint and magnified detail of the synovium. The latter is seen raised up into a villus projecting into the joint cavity. Underlying the villus is a fibroadipose tissue with contained capillary and initial lymphatic. The fibrous capsule finally bounds the joint.

interrupted in places by gaps of varying size (Lever and Ford, 1958; Simkin, 1979). The capillaries beneath the intimal layer may control the diffusion of solute by adjusting their fenestration diameters (Fig. 10.1) which conveniently face the intimal layer (Sutter and Majno, 1964). The synovium is completed by a subintimal supportive layer of fibroadipose tissue, which is less vascular than layers nearer the capsule but contains lymphatics. Functionally synovial fluid is not actively secreted by the synovium but is an ultrafiltrate of plasma to which hyaluronic acid has been added by the synovial cells.

In summary then, the synovial cavity develops as a simple cleft lined by a layer of cells with no basement membrane (unlike epithelium or mesothelium). The synovium in a nonselective manner allows the transport of synovial fluid. The synovial cavity therefore has embryological and functional features likening it to an interstitial space. It is thus logical to discuss fluid transport across the synovial membrane in classic Starling terms.

The complex mechanism of production and resorption of a synovial effusion is critically important in understanding any possible effects of a joint tamponade, especially in the immature hip with its unique vascular microanatomy. A synovial effusion is a form of localized edema where the fluid is retained in a large interstitial space, the joint cavity (Bauer et al., 1940; Lipson et al., 1965). Thus, like other forms of edema, fluid passes across the semipermeable synovium following a disturbance of transcapillary pressures according to the Starling equilibrium (Starling, 1896). Therefore, in analyzing the pathophysiological aspects of effusions, one must consider capillary and intraarticular hydrostatic pressures and plasma and synovial fluid colloid osmotic pressure (Fig. 10.2). Following a synovitis, the synovial vascular bed dilates and hence intracapillary hydrostatic pressure increases. With an accompanying increased capillary permeability (Sharp, 1963; Lipson et al., 1965) related to production of prostaglandin $E_1$, bradykinin and histamine (Grennan et al., 1977) and slightly negative intraarticular pressure (Bauer et al., 1940; Eyring and Murray, 1964; Levick, 1979), water, readily diffusible substances and proteins cross into the synovial cavity. Thus, the colloid osmotic pressure of the synovial fluid increases. Intraarticular hydrostatic pressure also rises secondary to excess volume of fluid.

The mechanism of resorption of an effusion is somewhat more controversial. Colloid osmotic pressure of synovial fluid is consistently less than that of plasma in patients with rheumatoid and nonrheumatoid joint effusions (Lipson et al., 1965; Palmer and Myers, 1968). Jensen and Zachariae (1959) also found that effusions within osteoarthritic joints had colloid osmotic pressures below the normal range of 9 to 10 mm Hg. Although the osmotic gradient between synovial fluid and plasma therefore probably favors resorption, the gradient is not considered the principal factor in secretion or resorption (Lipson et al., 1965) because hydrostatic pressures in the synovial vascular bed or in the joint cavity are of greater magnitude.

SYNOVIAL CAPILLARY

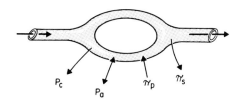

**Figure 10.2.** Capillary system in the synovium and the transcapillary pressure relationships involved. *Arrows* indicate direction of each Starling pressure parameter $P_c$, $P_a$, $\pi_p$, and $\pi_s$.

$P_c$ — Capillary blood pressure

$P_a$ — Intra-articular pressure

$\pi_p$ — Plasma oncotic pressure

$\pi_s$ — Synovial fluid oncotic pressure

Synovial fluid flow occurs passively down pressure gradients, there being no evidence for active transport as occurs, for example, in the generation of cerebrospinal fluid (Bauer et al., 1940; Levick, 1979). The synovial microcirculation is one pathway for fluid resorption; the second is through the synovium to tissues outside the synovium by way of intercellular gaps permeable to hydrophilic solutes (Lever and Ford, 1958; Ball et al., 1964; Cochrane et al., 1965; Levick, 1980a). The extrasynovial interstitial space then provides a quasi-infinite cavity to accommodate large volumes of absorbed fluid (Levick, 1980b). One must then consider transendothelial and interstitial channels as being important pathways with absorption of synovial fluid via lymphatic vessels being judged as insignificant (Levick, 1979, 1980b). Some writers however feel that lymphatic blockage may reduce resorption (Kuhns, 1933; Bauer et al., 1940; Lipson et al., 1965).

Intraarticular hydrostatic pressure is a most important determinant of transsynovial fluid movement. The sensitivity of this flow to pressure increases sixfold at a critical level around 7 mm Hg, the so-called "breaking point" (Edlund, 1949; Levick, 1979). At this point a rapid increase in synovial hydraulic conductivity occurs related to enlargement of the intercellular channels, and this allows a much more rapid flow of fluid from the joint cavity. Any joint movement that increases intraarticular pressure (Caughey and Bywaters, 1963; Eyring and Murray, 1964; Jayson and Dickson, 1970; Levick, 1979; Knight and Levick, 1982) will also stimulate efflux of an effusion from the joint.

The particular problem of production and resorption of synovial fluid in relation to a transient synovitis and Legg-Calvé-Perthes' syndrome will be discussed. Legg-Calvé-Perthes' syndrome is a process spontaneously occurring in the hips of young children (Gershuni et al., 1978), small breeds of dogs (Hulth et al., 1962; Mickelson et al., 1981) and pigs (Thomasen, 1939). The precise etiology of Legg-Calvé-Perthes' syndrome is unknown but at some point involves a vascular interruption leading to necrosis of part or all of the femoral capital epiphysis—a sine qua non of the condition (Jonsater, 1953; McKibbin and Ralis, 1974). Transient synovitis similarly has a varied etiology resulting in an inflammation of the synovial lining cells but without the presence of bony necrosis (Fox and Griffin, 1956; Spock, 1959; Valderrama, 1963).

The relationship between Legg-Calvé Perthes' syndrome and transient synovitis is well documented (Fox and Griffin, 1956; Spock, 1959; Valderrama, 1963; Kemp and Boldero, 1966; Jacobs, 1971). Both conditions affect children, most commonly between the ages of 4 and 8 years, resulting in hip pain, limp and mild to moderate limitation of motion. The early radiological sign of enlargement of the femoral head-acetabulum distance may be all that is noted in both conditions (Waldenström, 1938; Anderson and Stewart, 1970; Kemp, 1973) and usage of radioisotopes demonstrating blood flow and mineral accretion disturbances in the hip joint may be the only means to distinguish transient synovitis from Legg-Calvé-

Perthes' syndrome (Gershuni, 1980; Lamont et al., 1981; Deutsch et al., 1981). The two conditions can coexist and, more importantly, Legg-Calvé-Perthes' syndrome evolves from a preceding episode or episodes of transient synovitis with an incidence of 1.5% to 18% of cases (Spock, 1959; Valderrama, 1963; Kemp and Boldero, 1966; Jacobs, 1971).

The close relationship and consecutive occurrence of transient synovitis and Legg-Calvé-Perthes' syndromes led several investigators to hypothesize that, as in other inflammatory states, a significant outpouring of transudate occurs in transient synovitis of the hip. In the closely confined environs of the joint, such an effusion might cause an increase of intraarticular pressure which could occlude intracapsular, extraosseous blood vessels. In the 4- to 8-year age group particularly susceptible to Legg-Calvé-Perthes' syndrome, the most significant or exclusive blood supply to the immature femoral capital epiphysis is via the lateral epiphyseal vessels (Fig. 10.3) originating from ascending cervical vessels running in a subsynovial plane along the femoral neck (Trueta, 1957; Chung, 1976; Crock, 1980). The acetabular artery gives a branch that becomes the artery of the ligamentum teres. This branch, a less important provider of capital epiphyseal nutrition (Trueta, 1957; Wertheimer and Lopes, 1971; Kemp, 1973; Chung, 1976), also lies subsynovially (Fig. 10.3). Vessels cease to penetrate the femoral capital physis to supply the epiphysis from approximately the age of 18 months until the physis finally closes at maturity (Trueta, 1957; Ogden, 1974; Chung, 1976; Crock, 1980). It was therefore hypothesized that the subsynovial ascending cervical vessels are uniquely vulnerable to the effects of an effusion at a high intraarticular pressure; subsequent loss of blood flow would be expected to cause necrosis of the capital epiphysis (Kemp, 1973).

Several experimental models were designed to raise intraarticular pressure in the hip joints of animals to test the tamponade hypothesis (Woodhouse, 1964; Tachdjian and Grana, 1968; Kemp, 1973; Singleton and Jones, 1979; Borgsmiller et al., 1980; Kemp, 1981). Kemp (1973, 1981) found that isotonic saline, glucose solution and dextran-40 were unsuitable joint infusates if the tamponade pressure was to be maintained for any length of time (presumably due to reabsorption of these solutions); therefore he finally used an ethylene glycol bee's wax suspension to maintain tamponade for 12 to 18 h. Infusing the same bee's wax suspension, Singleton and Jones (1979) found that the raised intraarticular pressure so produced tended to fall gradually and further injections of the wax suspension were necessary to maintain the pressure. Tachdjian and Grana (1968) similarly found that a very high viscosity, nonabsorbable material was necessary to maintain the requisite intraarticular pressure. They injected silicone into canine hips for this purpose.

Most authors required that tamponade be maintained at approximately 150 to 200 mm Hg (Tachdjian and Grana, 1968; Borgsmiller et al., 1980), that is, arterial pressure levels, to produce total ischemia of the osseous

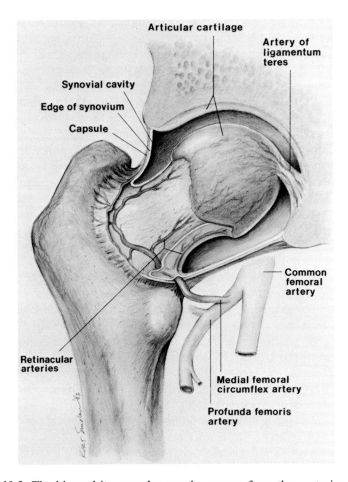

**Figure 10.3.** The hip and its vascular supply as seen from the posterior aspect. Note the vessels, running along the femoral neck to reach the head, in the subsynovial plane. The artery of the ligamentum teres is also intracapsular but extrasynovial.

femoral capital epiphysis and such pressures had to be maintained for 10 h to obtain subsequent bone necrosis (Tachdjian and Grana, 1968). Singleton and Jones (1979) used lower pressures in puppies, a maximum of 60 mm Hg for 10 h, and found some trabeculae with empty lacunae but no definite femoral head necrosis. Kemp (1973) showed that intracapsular tamponade at a pressure of 40 mm Hg inhibited the perfusion of the osseous capital femoral epiphyseal vessels as demonstrated by the Spalteholz technique (Spalteholz, 1914). Although he apparently noted some changes in bone after 6 h of tamponade he could not produce the complete picture of epiphyseal necrosis as in classic Legg-Calvé-Perthes' syndrome. Bassett et al. (1969) found that in puppies, 40 mm Hg tamponade pressure certainly did not affect femoral capital epiphyseal flow as judged by radioisotope uptake and in some animals up to 110 mm Hg intraarticular pressure did not obstruct blood flow. Launder et al. (1981) showed that elevated intracapsular pressure (44 mm Hg) in the immature dog's hip obstructed venous outflow and decreased femoral head blood flow but they agreed that the haemodynamic changes of the magnitude involved in a transient synovitis have not been shown to induce Legg-Calvé-Perthes' syndrome. Woodhouse (1964), also working with puppies, was the sole author to find that a tamponade of only 50 mm Hg prolonged for 12 h caused femoral head necrosis.

There has thus evidently been some difficulty in producing and maintaining an experimental model of hip tamponade, defining the pressure and time period required to produce a necrotic femoral capital epiphysis and explaining the relevance of the studies to clinical transient synovitis and Legg-Calvé-Perthes' syndrome as occurs in the child.

We reexamined the problem by producing a more valid tamponade model in the immature pig hip, and then followed changing pressure–volume relationships within the joint. In the light of the new data obtained, we question the hypothesis that tamponade might occur in transient synovitis and be a cause of Legg-Calvé-Perthes' syndrome (Gershuni et al., 1983).

We used 20 immature, 6-week-old pigs, weighing 8.4 to 11.4 kg, for the study. Each animal was laid on its side with the hip on which the experiment would be performed uppermost and the limbs lying in neutral position. Premedication with atropine 0.05 mg/kg and acepromazine 4 mg/kg by intramuscular injection was followed by induction of general anesthesia with ketamine 20 mg/kg intravenously and continued at a dose of 10 mg approximately every 20 min. The hip was approached by a posterior incision, splitting gluteus maximus and transecting the short external rotator muscles. A 16-gauge needle, connected via a three-way stopcock and thence to a Sage continuous infusion pump (Model 341) and a pressure transducer (Hewlett-Packard Model HP 1280) by inextensible tubing, was inserted via the cartilagenous posterior acetabular lip into the joint cavity (Fig. 10.4). Prior to insertion of the needle, the system was filled with autologous plasma colored by 1% methylene blue. Because synovial fluid is essentially a dialysate of plasma (Bauer et al., 1940; Gardner, 1950; Levick, 1979), autologous plasma was used as the infusion fluid. After allowing time for needle and intraarticular pressure to equilibrate, a basal reading of intraarticular pressure was obtained. Infusion was then commenced at the rate of 0.25 cc/min, utilizing the Sage continuous infusion pump, while graphically recording the pressure changes within the joint on a Hewlett-Packard four-channel chart recorder (Model HP 7754A). Distension of the capsule by the colored plasma and any possible leakage of infusate from around the needle was easily detected. If the latter occurred the experiment was terminated. Infusion continued until a pres-

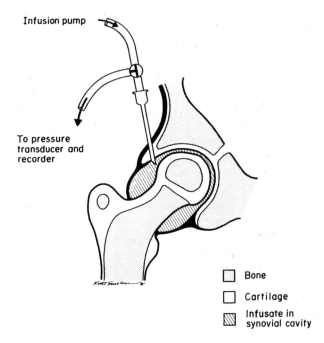

Infusion pump

To pressure
transducer and
recorder

Bone

Cartilage

Infusate in
synovial cavity

**Figure 10.4.** Method of tamponade production and monitoring of intraarticular pressure in the pig's hip. (From Gershuni et al., 1983.)

sure of 50, 100 or 200 mm Hg was attained in each of three groups of animals. Infusion was then stopped and the decrease of intraarticular pressure was monitored until it reached a pressure of 35 mm Hg (Fig. 10.5). At that point, pressure recording ceased and the remaining joint infusate was aspirated as exhaustively as possible and its volume recorded. The experiment was performed on the left normal hip of each animal and on the opposite hip, in which a synovitis was induced 2 weeks previously by the intraarticular injection of a suspension of surgical talc (magnesium tetrasilicate). This material is a physical, long-standing, non-toxic irritant to the synovium and thus induces a synovitis (Gershuni-Gordon and Axer, 1974; Parsons et al., 1983). The talc suspension was injected through the joint capsule following general anesthesia and exposure of the joint via a posterior approach as described above. Two weeks subsequent to the injection, the capsule was found to be hermetically sealed. Antero-posterior radiographs of both hips were taken 2 weeks following the talcum injection.

All of the above-described radiographs of the pigs' hips taken just before the tamponade experiment showed a significant enlargement of the radiological medial joint space of the synovitis affected side (>2 mm greater) as compared to the control side. This enlargement denoted the presence of a synovitis (Gershuni-Gordon and Axer, 1974).

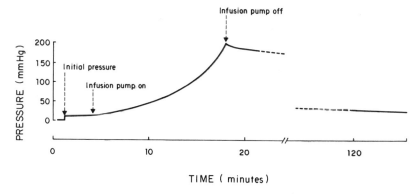

**Figure 10.5.** Initial intraarticular pressure in the hip, subsequent pressure achieved and rate of its decrease with time. (From Gershuni et al., 1983.)

The initial intraarticular pressures in the control and synovitis-affected hips were not significantly different (Table 10.1). The highest initial intraarticular pressure recorded was 10 mm Hg in one hip affected by the synovitis.

The volume of plasma infused to attain the required intraarticular pressure was, on average, greater on the synovitis-affected side but did not reach a statistically significant difference (Tables 10.2–10.4). Likewise, the time to decrease to 35 mm Hg from the prescribed pressure tended to be slower in the synovitis-affected hips and the volume of plasma aspirated at the end of pressure decrease was greater in those hips but not significantly so on statistical testing (Tables 10.2–10.4). The volume of fluid aspirated from the hips at the end of the experiment varied from 50% to 60% of the volume originally infused. The volume aspirated tended to comprise a greater percentage of the infusate in the higher as compared to the lower pressure groups (Tables 10.2–10.4).

Pressure elevation within the joint during infusion showed a slow initial rise with a subsequent steeper curve especially in the experiments conducted at 200 mm Hg (Fig. 10.5). This was reflected in joint compliance ($dV/dP$) which gradually decreased through the pressure range 25 to 200

**Table 10.1.** Initial intraarticular pressure

|  | Initial pressure (mm Hg) |
| --- | --- |
| Synovitis-affected hips (n = 17) | $1.7 \pm 1.1^{a}$ |
| Control hips (n = 20) | $1.9 \pm 0.69^{a}$ |

[a] Mean pressures are not statistically different (p > 0.50).
(From Gershuni et al., 1983.)

**Table 10.2.** Experiment conducted at 50 mm Hg pressure

|  | Infusion volume (cc) | Time period to reach 35 mm Hg (min) | Volume aspirated (cc) |
|---|---|---|---|
| Synovitis-affected hips (n = 5) | 1.8 ± 0.3 | 4.2 ± 2.3 | 1.0 ± 0.2 |
| Control hips (n = 6) | 1.6 ± 0.3 | 3.0 ± 1.0 | 0.8 ± 0.2 |
| Student *t* test | p > 0.50 | p > 0.50 | p > 0.50 |

Student *t* test comparing synovitis-affected hips with control hips.
(From Gershuni et al., 1983.)

mm Hg (Table 10.5). Although the compliance values for the synovitis-affected hips tended to be greater than those of the control side, statistical significance was noted only at the 50 mm Hg level (p < 0.05). On cessation of infusion, there was an initial rapid decrease of pressure followed by a slower phase (Fig. 10.5).

Tables 10.1 to 10.5 contain unpaired statistical analyses comparing all control with all synovitis-affected hips because not every animal had a successful study on both hips. Nevertheless, paired testing of those animals with successful studies of both hips yielded statistical results that were almost identical to those reported in Tables 10.1 to 10.5.

## Discussion

The hip can be considered as a closed compartment. The elasticity of this enclosed space or, in other terms, the compliance of its walls, can be represented as a change in volume per unit change in pressure ($dV/dP$). During initial stages of infusion into the joint in the above experiment, passive filling of the cavity was readily accomplished and compliance was high. After a threshold volume was reached, the capsule began to resist the distending force of the fluid and compliance decreased rapidly. Hip joint compliance decreased, as intraarticular pressure increased, in a simi-

**Table 10.3.** Experiment conducted at 100 mm Hg pressure

|  | Infusion volume (cc) | Time period to reach 35 mm Hg (min) | Volume aspirated (cc) |
|---|---|---|---|
| Synovitis-affected hips (n = 5) | 4.2 ± 1.0 | 43.8 ± 12.0 | 2.5 ± 0.7 |
| Control hips (n = 7) | 2.9 ± 0.3 | 34.8 ± 6.9 | 1.7 ± 0.3 |
| Student *t* test | p > 0.20 | p > 0.50 | p > 0.20 |

Student *t* test comparing synovitis-affected hips with control hips.
(From Gershuni et al., 1983.)

**Table 10.4.** Experiment conducted at 200 mm Hg pressure

|  | Infusion volume (cc) | Time period to reach 35 mm Hg (min) | Volume aspirated (cc) |
|---|---|---|---|
| Synovitis-affected hips (n = 7) | 4.5 ± 0.5 | 132 ± 26.4 | 2.7 ± 0.3 |
| Control hips (n = 7) | 4.0 ± 0.5 | 122 ± 31.6 | 2.4 ± 0.5 |
| Student *t* test | p > 0.20 | p > 0.50 | p > 0.50 |

Student *t* test comparing synovitis-affected hips with control hips.
(From Gershuni et al., 1983.)

lar fashion in both control and synovitis-affected hips. There was a tendency for the synovitis-affected side to have a more compliant capsule. However, this was statistically significant only for the group subjected to 50 mm Hg pressure. This implies that hips affected by this experimental form of synovitis were not prone to a more severe tamponade for a given volume of infusate. In fact, these hips had a capsule whose collagen fibers appeared to have become weaker, probably due to the inflammatory process initiated in the synovium. Alternatively or additionally, reabsorption from the inflamed joint occurred faster than via normal synovium at any given pressure (Soccianti, 1966).

Because the literature implies that an intraarticular pressure of 200 mm Hg is necessary for stasis of the subsynovial blood supply to the capital femoral epiphysis (Tachdjian and Grana, 1968; Borgsmiller et al., 1980), this was the highest pressure utilized in our experiment. It is, however, difficult to conceive how such a pressure could be attained by the mechanism of synovial fluid production just discussed. Continual formation of the effusion could perhaps occur in the clinical situation. However, it is rare to aspirate a volume of fluid in excess of 1 to 2 cc from a child's hip affected by transient synovitis or Legg-Calvé-Perthes' syndrome. To attain an intraarticular pressure of 200 mm Hg, an infusion volume much greater than that (4–4.5 cc) was required in this experiment using a hip similar in size to that of the young child. Moreover, the data show that even if a joint pressure of 200 mm Hg could be reached, it would decrease within approximately 2 h to capillary pressure or below. With lower initial intraarticular pressures (50–100 mm Hg) the decrease to 35 mm Hg was correspondingly much more rapid, occurring in the group subjected to 50 mm Hg pressure in only a few minutes. In a study of the human knee pressurized with normal saline to 50 mm Hg, very similar pressure curves were obtained with the pressure dropping to 35 mm Hg within 15 min and then dropping more slowly (Myers and Palmer, 1972). The decrease is mainly due to the fact that the pressure of the infusion exceeds the elastic limit of the capsule so that inelastic stretching or "viscous creep" (Levick, 1978) of the capsular fibers then occurs. To a further extent, decrease is due to fluid reabsorption because only 50% to 60% of the

**Table 10.5.** Hip compliance $dV/dP$ at constant infusion rate of 0.25 cc/min

|  | 25 mm Hg | 50 mm Hg | 100 mm Hg | 150 mm Hg | 200 mm Hg |
|---|---|---|---|---|---|
| Synovitis-affected hips ± SEM | 0.042 ± 0.0057 n = 17 | 0.035 ± 0.0042 n = 17 | 0.021 ± 0.0027 n = 12 | 0.017 ± 0.0036 n = 7 | 0.013 ± 0.0045 n = 7 |
| Control hips ± SEM | 0.031 ± 0.0022 n = 20 | 0.024 ± 0.0019 n = 20 | 0.019 ± 0.0019 n = 14 | 0.016 ± 0.0023 n = 7 | 0.011 ± 0.0019 n = 7 |
| Student $t$ test | $p > 0.05$ | $p < 0.05$ | $p > 0.20$ | $p > 0.50$ | $p > 0.50$ |

(From Gershuni et al., 1983.)

infused volume of plasma was aspirated at the end of each of the infusion experiments. Knight and Levick (1982) also found that at high induced pressures in the rabbit knee, reabsorption of an isotonic infusion was very rapid and responded with great sensitivity to small increases in intraarticular volume. Finally the "breaking point" phenomenon presumably accounted in large part for the rapid decrease.

Rosingh and James (1969) have shown that the minimum period of ischemia necessary to produce osteocyte death is 6 h, although Davis et al. (1981) found that bone marrow and cortical bone remain viable after 25 h of ischemia. In our study, using a physiological solution to simulate an effusion, a tamponade could not be maintained, in synovitis-affected or in normal hips, for a time period even approaching the minimum to cause osteocyte death.

The simulation of a transient synovitis by the per-capsular injection of magnesium tetrasilicate produces definite, moderately long-standing inflammatory changes in the synovium with enlargement of the radiological medial joint space denoting articular cartilage thickening, joint incongruency and possibly excess synovial fluid (Gershuni-Gordon and Axer, 1974; Gershuni et al., 1979, 1981). Thus the synovitis model appears to mimic the human condition closely. In the present study utilizing the synovitis model, there was no difference in the initial intraarticular pressure between control and synovitis-affected hips except in the group subjected to 50 mm Hg pressure, the range being 8 to 10 mm Hg. This suggests that clinical joint synovitis also exists without an accompanying high-pressure effusion. In placing into clinical perspective high-pressure effusions, it is significant to note that pressures as low as 15 to 30 mm Hg induced in the human hip were found to be very painful (Eyring and Murray, 1964). However, children with transient synovitis do not normally suffer from excessive pain; in fact, the symptomatology may be so mild as to be ignored (Harrison and Burwell, 1981).

An important clinical observation, which has relevance to the problem, was made by Duthie and Houghton (1981). They noted that in 60 hemophiliacs, who developed hemarthrosis of the hip, subsequent osteonecrosis of the capital epiphysis never occurred. It is inferred from this observation that even hemorrhage into the hip at arteriolar pressure could not produce or maintain tamponade sufficiently high to occlude the subsynovial circulation to the femoral capital epiphysis and to cause osteocyte death.

The general and vascular anatomy of the immature pig's hip is similar to that of the young child (Salter et al., 1969), and therefore the pig's hip is a valid experimental model to study human disease processes. From analysis of our data, it is thus considered unlikely that joint tamponade is a valid explanation for the development of the femoral capital epiphyseal osteonecrosis occurring in Legg-Calvé-Perthes' syndrome. In addition, if the unique blood supply to the femoral head by the lateral epiphyseal artery was obstructed by a joint tamponade, it is difficult to explain the pathogenesis of *partial* epiphyseal necrosis, as may occur in human Legg-Calvé-Perthes' syndrome; logically an all-or-none phenomenon would be the most likely possibility.

## Summary

Synovial joints have specific anatomical characteristics that include an articular cartilage layer encompassing the related bone ends, and these tissues are enclosed in a soft tissue capsule lined by a synovial layer of cells. In the immature hip the subsynovial blood vessels, running along the femoral neck to supply the bony capital femoral epiphysis, are potentially at risk if joint tamponade occurs.

The synovial cavity is developmentally, morphologically and functionally a unique interstitial space into which and from which an ultrafiltrate of plasma (synovial fluid) flows. This fluid flow, across the synovial semipermeable membrane, is governed by the well-known Starling forces pertaining to capillary microcirculations. Intraarticular hydrostatic pressure is the most important of these forces, especially above the "breaking point" pressure of 7 mm Hg. Inflammatory changes developing in the synovium alter the dynamics of such fluid production and resorption. In addition, a significant volume of joint fluid passes through gaps in the synovial lining cells into the periarticular interstitial space. From this interstitial space the fluid may finally return to the systemic circulation by way of the lymphatics.

It has been theorized by other authors that in the clinical condition of transient synovitis, excessive production of synovial fluid could cause hip joint tamponade severe enough to obstruct subsynovial vascular circulation to the femoral capital epiphysis. If this in fact occurred, necrosis of the osseous femoral head would result, thus explaining the pathogenesis of Legg-Calvé-Perthes' syndrome in children. However, experimental evidence from studies on the immature pig's hip, involving the production of a tamponade with and without the prior induction of a synovitis as well as other clinical knowledge, refutes such a sequence of events.

## Acknowledgments

This work was supported by the Veterans Administration and by USPHS/NIH Grants AM-25501, AM-26344 and AM-00602.

## References

Anderson J and Stewart AM (1970). The significance of the magnitude of the medial joint space. *Br J Radiol* 43:238–239.
Ball J, Chapman JA and Muirden AD (1964). The uptake of iron into rabbit

synovial tissue following intra-articular injection of iron dextrans. A light and electron microscope study. *J Cell Biol* 22:351–361.

Barland P, Novikoff AB and Hammerman D (1962). Electron microscopy of the human synovial membrane. *J Cell Biol* 14:207–220.

Bassett FH, James JW, Allen BC and Azuma H (1969). Normal vascular anatomy of the head of the femur in puppies with emphasis on the inferior retinacular vessels. *J Bone Joint Surg* 51A:1139–1153.

Bauer W, Ropes MW and Waine H (1940). The physiology of articular structures. *Physiol Rev* 20:272–312.

Borgsmiller WK, Whiteside LA, Goldsand EM and Lange DR (1980). Effect of hydrostatic pressure in the hip joint on proximal femoral epiphyseal and metaphyseal blood flow. *Trans Orthop Res Soc* 26:23.

Caughey DE and Bywaters EGL (1963). Joint fluid pressure in chronic knee effusions. *Ann Rheum Dis* 22:106–109.

Chung SMK (1976). The arterial supply of the developing proximal end of the human femur. *J Bone Joint Surg* 58A:961–970.

Cochrane W, Davies DV and Palfrey AJ (1965). Absorptive functions of the synovial membrane. *Ann Rheum Dis* 24:2–15.

Crock HV (1980). An atlas of the arterial supply of the head and neck of the femur in man. *Clin Orthop* 152:17–27.

Davis RF, Berggren A, Weiland AJ and Dorfman H (1981). The effect of prolonged ischemia time on osteocyte and osteoblast survival in composite bone grafts revascularized in microvascular anastomoses. *Trans Orthop Res Soc* 6:162.

Deutsch SD, Gandsman EJ and Sparagen SC (1981). Quantitative regional blood-flow analysis and its clinical application during routine bone-scanning. *J Bone Joint Surg* 63A:295–305.

Duthie RB and Houghton GR (1981). Constitutional aspects of the osteochondroses. *Clin Orthop* 158:19–27.

Edlund T (1949). Studies on the absorption of colloids and fluid from rabbit knee joints. *Acta Physiol Scand* 18:1–108.

Eyring EJ and Murray WR (1964). The effect of joint position on the pressure of intra-articular effusion. *J Bone Joint Surg* 46A:1235–1241.

Fox KW and Griffin LL (1956). Transient synovitis of the hip joint in children. *Texas State J Med* 52:15–20.

Gardner E (1950). Physiology of movable joints. *Physiol Rev* 30:127–176.

Gershuni DH (1980). Preliminary evaluation and prognosis in Legg-Calvé-Perthes' disease. *Clin Orthop* 150:16–22.

Gershuni DH, Amiel D, Gonsalves M and Akeson WH (1981). The biochemical response of rabbit articular cartilage matrix to an induced talcum synovitis. *Acta Orthop Scand* 52:599–603.

Gershuni-Gordon DH and Axer A (1974). Synovitis of the hip joint. An experimental model in rabbits. *J Bone Joint Surg* 56B:69–77.

Gershuni DH, Axer A and Hendel D (1978). Arthrographic findings in Legg-Calvé-Perthes' disease and transient synovitis of the hip. *J Bone Joint Surg* 60A:457–474.

Gershuni DH, Axer A and Siegal B (1979). Localized regressive articular cartilage changes in the hip joint of the rabbit following synovitis. *Acta Orthop Scand* 50:179–185.

Gershuni DH, Hargens AR, Lee Y-F, Greenberg EN, Zapf R and Akeson WH (1983). The questionable significance of hip joint tamponade in Legg-Calvé-Perthes' syndrome. *J Paed Orthop* 3:280–286.

Ghadially FN and Roy S (1966). Ultrastructure of rabbit synovial membrane. *Ann Rheum Dis* 25:318–326.

Grennan DM, Mitchell W, Miller WJ and Zeiklin JJ (1977). Effects of prostaglandin $E_1$, bradykinin and histamine on canine synovial vascular permeability. *Br J Pharmacol* 60:251–254.

Haines RW (1947). The development of joints. *J Anat* 81:33–55.

Harrison HM and Burwell RG (1981). Perthes' disease: a concept of pathogenesis. *Clin Orthop* 156:115–127.

Hulth A, Norberg I and Olsson S (1962). Coxa plana in the dog. *J Bone Joint Surg* 44A:918–930.

Jacobs BW (1971). Synovitis of the hip in children and its significance. *Pediatrics* 47:558–566.

Jayson MIV and Dixon A St J (1970). Intraarticular pressure in rheumatoid arthritis of the knee. III. Pressure changes during use. *Ann Rheum Dis* 29:401–408.

Jensen CE and Zachariae L (1959). The contributions from hyaluronic acid and from protein to the colloid osmotic pressure of human synovial fluid. *Acta Rheum Scand* 5:18–28.

Jonsater S (1953). Coxa plana. A histopathologic and arthrographic study. *Acta Orthop Scand (Suppl. XII)* 1–98.

Kemp HBS (1973). Perthes' disease, an experiment and clinical study. *Ann R Coll Surg Eng* 52:18–35.

Kemp HBS (1981). Perthes' disease—the influence of intracapsular tamponade on the circulation in the hip joint of the dog. *Clin Orthop* 156:105–114.

Kemp HBS and Boldero JL (1966). Radiological changes in Perthes' disease. *Br J Radiol* 39:744–760.

Knight AD and Levick JR (1982). Pressure-volume relationships above and below atmospheric pressure in the synovial cavity of the rabbit knee. *J Physiol (Lond)* 328:403–420.

Kuhns JG (1933). Lymphatic drainage of joints. *Arch Surg* 27:345–391.

Lamont RL, Muz J, Heilbronner D and Bouwhuis JA (1981). Quantitative assessment of femoral head involvement in Legg-Calvé-Perthes' disease. *J Bone Joint Surg* 63A:746–752.

Launder WJ, Hungerford DS and Jones LH (1981). Haemodynamics of the femoral head. *J Bone Joint Surg* 63A:442–448.

Lever JD and Ford EHR (1958). Histological, histochemical and electron microscopic observation on synovial membrane. *Anat Rec* 132:525–539.

Levick JR (1978). Fluid transport across synovial tissue *in vivo*. *J Physiol (Lond)* 275:83.

Levick JR (1979). An investigation into the validity of the subatmospheric pressure recordings from synovial fluid and their dependence on joint angle. *J Physiol. (Lond)* 289:55–57.

Levick JR (1980a). Absorption of artificial effusions from synovial joints: an experimental study in rabbits. *Clin Sci* 59:41–48.

Levick JR (1980b). Contributions of the lymphatic and microvascular systems to fluid absorption from the synovial cavity of the rabbit knee. *J Physiol (Lond)* 306:445–461.

Lipson RL, Baldes EJ, Anderson JA and Polley HF (1965). Osmotic pressure gradients and joint effusions. *Arthritis Rheum* 8:29–37.

McKibbin B and Ralis Z (1974). Pathological changes in a case of Perthes' disease. *J Bone Joint Surg* 56B:438–443.

Mickelson MR, McCurnin DM, Awbrey BJ, Maynard JA and Martin RL (1981). Legg-Calvé-Perthes' disease in dogs. A comparison to human Legg-Calvé-Perthes' disease. *Clin Orthop Rel Res* 157:287–300.

Myers DB and Palmer DG (1972). Capsular compliance and pressure volume relationships in normal and arthritic knees. *J Bone Joint Surg* 54B:710–716.

Ogden JA (1974). Changing patterns of proximal femoral vascularity. *J Bone Joint Surg* 56A:941–950.

Palmer DG and Myers DB (1968). Some observations on joint effusions. *Arthritis Rheum* 11:745–755.

Parsons JR, Byhavi S, Alexander H and Weiss AB (1983). Carbon fiber debris within the synovial joint: time-dependent mechanical and histological studies. *Trans Orthop Res Soc* 8:9.

Rosingh GE and James J (1969). Early phases of avascular necrosis of the femoral head in rabbits. *J Bone Joint Surg* 51B:165–174.

Salter RB, Kostuik J and Dallas S (1969). Avascular necrosis of the femoral head as a complication of treatment for congenital dislocation of the hip in young children: a clinical and experimental investigation. *Can J Surg* 12:44–60.

Sharp GWG (1963). Effect of certain anti-arthritic compounds on the permeability of synovial membrane in the rabbit. *Ann Rheum Dis* 22:50–54.

Simkin PA (1979). Synovial physiology. In: *Arthritis and Allied Conditions*. McCarthy DJ (ed.). Philadelphia: Lea & Febiger, pp. 167–178.

Singleton WB and Jones EL (1979). The experimental induction of subclinical Perthes' disease in the puppy following arthrotomy and intra-capsular tamponade. *J Comp Pathol* 89:57–71.

Soccianti P (1966). Radioisotopes in the study of synovial fluid dynamics. *J Nucl Biol Med* 10:95–100.

Spalteholz W (1914). *Über das Durchsichtigmachen von Menschlichen und Tierischen Präparaten und seine Theoretischen Bedingungen*, Ed. 2 Leipzig: Hirzel.

Spock A (1959). Transient synovitis of the hip in children. *Pediatrics* 24:1042–1049.

Starling EG (1896). On the absorption of fluids from the connective tissue spaces. *J Physiol (Lond)* 19:312–326.

Sutter ER and Majno G (1964). Ultrastructure of the joint capsule in the rat: presence of two kinds of capillaries. *Nature* 202:920–921.

Tachdjian MO and Grana L (1968). Response of the hip to increased intra-articular pressure. *Clin Orthop* 61:199–212.

Thomasen EA (1939). Calvé-Perthes'-like changes in the head of the humerus in swine. *Acta Orthop Scand* 10:331–337.

Trueta J (1957). The normal vascular anatomy of the human femoral head during growth. *J Bone Joint Surg* 39B:358–394.

Valderrama JAF de (1963). The observation hip syndrome and its late sequelae. *J Bone Joint Surg* 45B:462–470.

Waldenström H (1938). The first stages of coxa plana. *J Bone Joint Surg* 20:559–566.

Wertheimer LG and Lopes DSLF (1971). Arterial supply of the femoral head. *J Bone Joint Surg* 53A:545–556.

Woodhouse CF (1964). Dynamic influences of vascular occlusion affecting the development of avascular necrosis of the femoral head. *Clin Orthop* 32:119–129.

Wyllie JC, More RH and Haust MD (1966). The fine structure of normal guinea pig synovium. *Lab Invest* 15:519–529.

# CHAPTER 11

# Mechanical Stress and Viability of Skin and Subcutaneous Tissue

Narender P. Reddy

## Introduction

Mechanical stresses on skin and subcutaneous tissue are of particular interest from the standpoint of decubitus ulceration. Decubitus ulcers are localized areas of cellular necrosis caused by prolonged or excessive mechanical loads on tissue. These ulcers are considered a major problem in the comprehensive rehabilitation of the patient with a spinal cord injury. Decubitus ulcers, also known as pressure sores or bed sores, impair the mobility and quality of life for a great number of handicapped and chronically disabled persons. In the United States alone, there are over 1.4 million cases of complete or partial paralysis as a result of spinal cord injury (National Academy of Sciences, 1977). In terms of economics, the yearly costs of treating these ulcers is estimated to be in the range of 750 million (Brand and Mooney, 1977) to 2 billion dollars (Krouskop et al., 1983). The prevention of this severe complication constitutes a continuing problem within the disciplines of biomedical and rehabilitation engineering. The pathogenesis of these ulcers involves biomechanical and microcirculatory factors which include the type, magnitude and duration of stresses in the affected tissues.

During sitting or reclining for extended periods of time, normal individuals relieve stresses that are potentially damaging to their tissues by periodic shifting of position. Patients with loss of sensation, such as those with spinal cord injuries, do not sense or relieve these excessive stresses. The type and magnitude of stresses generated in the tissue depend on body build and the types of cushion used to support the body (Garfin et al., 1980; Garber and Krouskop, 1982; Garber et al., 1982; Reddy et al., 1982). Garfin and co-workers (1980) observed large areas of high pressure generated over skin surfaces of human subjects lying prone and supine on various types of beds (Fig. 11.1). In certain regions surface pressures up to 200 mm Hg were observed. In seated subjects, the pressure beneath ischial tuberosities exceeded 150 mm Hg (Kosiak et al., 1958). By impairing microcirculation, lymph circulation and interstitial transport processes, these high pressures may cause breakdown of skin and subcutaneous tissue.

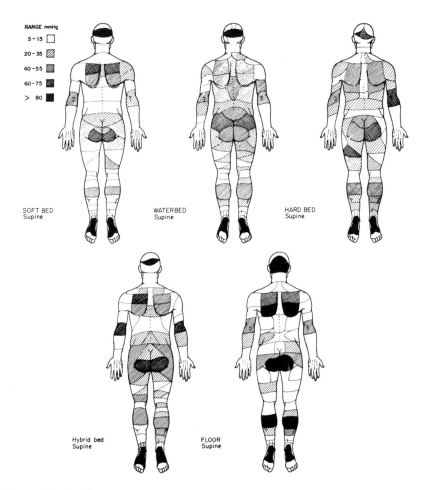

**Figure 11.1.** Surface pressure generated in supine positions while lying on various types of beds. (From SR Garfin et al., 1980. Reproduced by permission of *Arch Phys Med Rehab*.)

Although it is known that prolonged excessive stresses in tissue cause ulceration, the mechanisms of decubitus ulceration and associated damage processes are not clearly understood. The purpose of this chapter is to review possible mechanisms of stress-induced tissue necrosis.

## Background

Our understanding of the etiology of decubitus ulcer formation is fragmentary and incomplete. Although the pressure sore has perplexed physicians since antiquity, investigators developed interest in its pathophysiology only recently. Several investigators have produced pressure sores experimentally by application of excessive and prolonged loads on tissue. There is general agreement that an inverse relationship exists between the intensity and duration of load application required to produce ulceration. High external pressures require only a short duration of loading whereas lower pressures require longer application times to cause equivalent tissue damage. There is a delay of 3 to 5 days between load application and external appearance of an ulcer at the skin surface.

Groth (1942) produced pressure sores in rabbits by applying loads of various magnitudes to posterior ischii via two 15-mm diameter circular discs. He concluded that an inverse relationship exists between the load intensity and application duration required to produce ulceration. Kosiak (1959) applied external pressure of different intensities for various durations over dog's femoral trochanter and ischial tuberosities using an inverted 20-ml syringe driven by compressed air. After release of pressure, he observed edema and cellular infiltration immediately which persisted for 1 or 2 days. He sacrificed the animals 4 to 7 days after pressure application. Kosiak also found an inverse relationship between pressure intensity and the duration of application necessary to cause ulceration in dogs (Fig. 11.2A) and rats. In Kosiak's experiments (1961), ulceration generally appeared 3 or 4 days after the application of pressure. Since the intensities of applied pressure were larger than the intracapillary pressure, Kosiak advanced the hypothesis that ischemia and capillary damage were the primary factors leading to pressure-induced ulcers.

Lindan (1961) applied external pressure to rabbit ears using clips. When the clips were removed after 7 to 9 h of continuous pressure at 100 mm Hg, he noted that the underlying tissues were at first white and bloodless with hyperemia in surrounding tissues, but then blood flow returned within a few seconds. One-half hour later tissue edema was noted. After 12 to 15 h of continuous pressure and subsequent release, he observed greater damage, including edema and hemorrhage which eventually led to ulceration. Hussain (1953) found that a threshold pressure of 100 mm Hg for 2 h was required to produce first signs of tissue breakdown in rats. He also noted edema and attributed it to the effects of ischemia.

Reswick and Rogers (1976) monitored skin–cushion interface pressures on 800 normal human subjects and patients, and also found an inverse relationship between the intensity and duration of interface pressure that skin and subcutaneous tissues could tolerate. They provided a threshold curve separating acceptable and unacceptable combinations of pressure intensity and duration (Fig. 11.2B). Since then their curve has been used as a guideline for soft tissue management in various clinics across the United States.

Dinsdale (1974) observed an inverse relationship between the pressure intensity and loading duration necessary to produce ulceration in swine experimentally. In some experiments, he applied frictional force at the

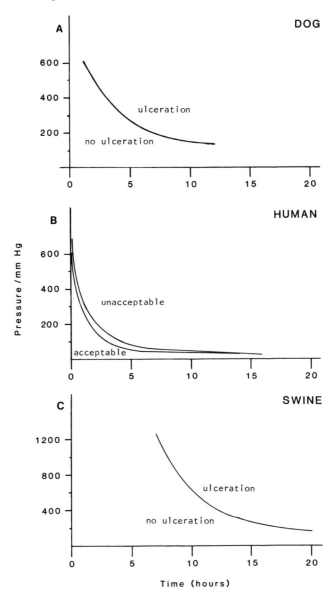

**Figure 11.2.** Threshold pressure intensity versus application duration relationship for the following conditions: **A:** Ulceration observed in experimental dogs. (From M Kosiak, 1961. Reproduced by permission of *Arch Phys Med Rehab.*) **B:** Acceptable interface pressures in human subjects. (From JB Reswick and JE Rogers, Rancho Los Amigos Hospital Technical Report, submitted to Social and Rehabilitation Service, 1976.) The two curves represent different humidity conditions at the buttock–cushion interface. **C:** Experimental production of ulcers in swine. (From RK Daniel and DD Wheatley, 1981. Reproduced by permission of *Arch Phys Med Rehab.*)

skin surface and found that friction significantly increased ulcer production. Recently, Daniel and Wheatley (1981) experimentally produced decubitus ulcers in swine using a computer-controlled electromechanical load applicator device. They also observed an inverse relationship between the critical pressure intensity and duration necessary to cause ulceration (Fig. 11.2C). Nola and Vistnes (1980) found different responses to experimental pressure sores in skin and muscle of rats. Both skin and muscle were targets for necrosis in the case of loads applied over a bony prominence.

In all of the animal experiments discussed above, there was a lag of 3 to 4 days between load application and external appearance of the irreversible tissue damage. Most investigators found that edema persisted for at least 1 day after pressure release. These observations led the investigators to believe that ischemia associated with blood vessel occlusion was the major factor in decubitus ulcer formation.

Brand (1976) applied repetitive mechanical loads to the rat's foot pad in different patterns over a period of 3 weeks. Momentary pressure applications (1100 mm Hg, 0.08 s duration) repeated 10,000 times a day caused soft tissue hypertrophy in normal rats and led to ulceration in neurectomized rats. Manley and Darby (1980) applied similar repetitive loads in neurectomized rats and observed plantar ulceration after 7 to 10 days of load application.

Studies of blood flow also illustrate the effects of external loading. Daly and co-workers (1976) and Halloway and associates (1976) measured forearm skin blood flow during external pressure loading in normal subjects using Xe-133 washout from intracutaneous injection sites. Flow decreased with increasing pressure and ceased when external pressure equalled mean arterial pressure (Fig. 11.3). Reactive hypermia occurred following pressure release of 90 mm Hg or greater, but did not occur after release at lower pressures.

External pressure creates a distribution of compressive and shear stresses that generate gradients of interstitial fluid pressure within the tissue beneath the site of load application. In the above-mentioned studies, interface loads are monitored but no attempt is made to correlate these loads with internal stress or interstitial fluid pressure. Although some investigators emphasize the importance of shear stress over compressive stress (Bennett et al., 1979; Reichel, 1958), stress distribution is not correlated with damage processes. Guyton and colleagues (1971) have proposed a theory that the total tissue pressure generated as a result of external loads is expressible as the sum of interstitial fluid pressure and solid tissue pressure. Interstitial fluid pressure in unloaded normal tissue is subatmospheric and ranges from $-2$ to $-5$ mm Hg (Scholander et al., 1968; Snashall et al., 1971; Hargens, 1981).

Early attention focused on methods for healing ulcers and few investigations were directed toward understanding the physiological mechanism

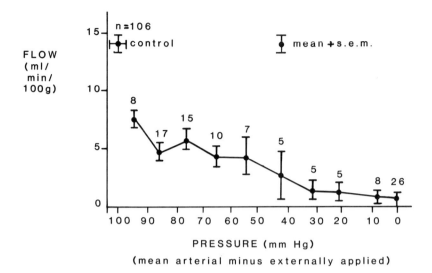

**Figure 11.3.** Forearm skin blood flow (measured by Xe-133 disappearance) during external pressure application. Flow rate is plotted against the difference between mean arterial and externally applied pressure. (From GA Halloway Jr et al., 1976. Reproduced by permission of *J Appl Physiol.*)

and damage processes underlying pressure sore formation. Of those studies that involved experimental production of pressure sores, very few attempted to study transport processes. Persistent edema and cellular infiltration indicate definite disturbances in transport mechanism.

Skin is a three-dimensional network of connective tissue fibers. Spaces between these fibers are filled with interstitial fluid and ground substance. The dermis contains blood and lymphatic vessels, nerve terminals, glands, hair, fibroblasts and other types of cells. Subcutaneous tissue is a continuation of the dermis and is composed of connective tissue and fat cells. Most investigators suggest that due to persistent edema following external pressure application, hypoxia due to blood vessel occlusion is the major factor in ulcer formation. Few workers have focused on other tissue components. In this regard the lymphatic system may play an important role in tissue breakdown (Krouskop et al., 1978).

The lymphatic system is essentially a drainage system within the body. It is a complex network of vessels and provides a major route for the transport of excess fluids and proteins from tissues. Most enzymes and many metabolic waste products are transported from the tissue of origin into the blood circulation system via the lymphatics. Lymph from most parts of the body enters the jugular vein via the thoracic duct. Whereas interstitial fluid pressure in subcutaneous tissue is usually 1 to 4 mm Hg negative with respect to the atmosphere, jugular vein pressure is usually slightly positive. Therefore, lymph in this tissue is pumped against an imposed gradient in addition to overcoming the resistance to flow offered by the vessels (Fig. 11.4). Flow in lymphatics is governed by certain extrinsic and intrinsic forces. The extrinsic forces include movements of various organs and skeletal muscle contractions which exert an external pressure. The intrinsic forces are due to active contraction of smooth muscle in the walls of the lymphatics. After a century of neglect, the intrinsic forces are now recognized as playing an important role in lymph propulsion. In addition, there are numerous valves along lymphatic vessels that allow unidirectional flow of lymph from the periphery toward the thoracic duct.

Hall and associates (1965) were the first to record intrinsic pressure pulses from lymph vessels in animal experiments. Several investigators have studied isolated lymph vessel motility in vitro: Mislin and Schipp (1967) used guinea pig mesenteric lymphatics and McHale and Roddie (1976) used bovine lymphatics. Hargens and Zweifach (1977) demonstrated active contractility in rat and guinea pig mesentery. Their studies found that elevated transmural pressures and lymphatic distention initiate contractions. These contractions are often modulated by humoral mediators such as epinephrine. Pharmacological agents, including epinephrine and caffeine, affect contractions of isolated strips of lymph vessel walls in vitro (Tirone et al., 1973; Ohhashi et al., 1978, 1980).

Our group (Reddy et al., 1975, 1977) formulated computer models of the lymphatic system using laws of mechanics and existing knowledge of lymphatic transport. This work indicated that intrinsic contractions play a dominant role in lymph propulsion and that passive or extrinsic forces play only a secondary role. Although this is true for most tissues, extrinsic forces may be important in skeletal muscle lymph flow (see Chapter 12). Recently, Hargens and co-workers (1982) measured interstitial fluid pressure up to 500 to 600 mm Hg in skeletal muscle during maximum contraction, suggesting that extrinsic forces are important in the skeletal muscle lymph flow. Distention plays an important role in coordination and smooth propagation of the contractions along the vessel walls. Intrin-

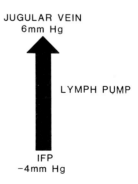

JUGULAR VEIN
6mm Hg

LYMPH PUMP

IFP
−4mm Hg

**Figure 11.4.** The lymph pump transports fluid against a pressure gradient from interstitial spaces (interstitial fluid pressure of −1 to −4 mm Hg) into the venous system (jugular venous pressure of +6 mm Hg).

sic pressure pulses in the order of 30 to 60 mm Hg have been recorded in human lymphatics (Kinmouth and Taylor, 1956; Shields, 1980). Since lymph propulsion is highly dependent on lymphatic smooth muscle activity and since smooth muscle is sensitive to ischemia, lymph flow may be impaired due to lymphatic smooth muscle damage during prolonged external loading (Krouskop et al., 1978). Thus, lymphatic damage may be a contributing factor to decubitus ulceration.

## Recent Results

### Interstitial Fluid Flow during Tissue Compression

Recently, the effects of external pressure on interstitial fluid dynamics were examined using a simple mathematical model (Reddy and Cochran, 1979; Reddy et al., 1981*a*). Our theoretical analysis of interstitial dynamics suggests that the flow of interstitial fluid and ground substance plays a role in ulcer formation. Consider a circular cylindrical slice of tissue of radius *a* with pressure applied at the top surface (Fig. 11.5). For simplicity, let the interstitial fluid pressure in this pressurized region $P_a$ be uniform over the entire volume of the cylinder. Now consider a surrounding concentric cylindrical slice of tissue of radius $R$ from the center of the pressurized region. The rate of interstitial fluid flow from the region per unit length of the cylinder is proportional to the gradient in fluid pressure from the loaded region to the surrounding region. Also, the law of conservation of mass requires that the decrease of interstitial fluid volume in the pressurized cylinder be equal to the increase of interstitial fluid volume in the surrounding unloaded tissue. From these relationships, for a given

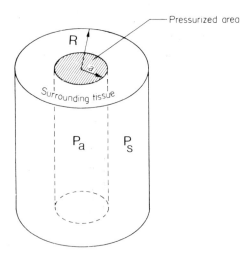

**Figure 11.5.** Tissue model for interstitial fluid flux calculations: inner cylindrical tissue slice (radius *a*) of high interstitial fluid pressure surrounded by concentric tissue ring of low interstitial fluid pressure. Interstitial fluid pressure in the inner cylindrical slice is $P_a$. The interstitial fluid pressure in the surrounding region, up to radius $R$ from the center, is $P_s$. The pressure difference $P_a - P_s$ drives fluid flow outward from the inner tissue slice into the surrounding region.

ratio of initial volume to final volume within this central pressurized region (with prescribed parameters of porosity and fluid conductivity), the product of loading duration $t$ and interstitial fluid pressure gradient between the loaded region $P_a$ and the surrounding unloaded region $P_s$ equals a constant (see Appendix at end of the chapter):

$$t(P_a - P_s) = \text{constant.} \tag{1}$$

If pressure in the surrounding region is negligible, then the product of pressure in the central region and loading duration is a constant. For example, if $P_a - P_s$ is 150 mm Hg, we calculate that the time required for interstitial volume to reach half its initial volume is approximately 1.8 h. Thus, it appears there is an inverse relationship between pressure intensity and load duration required for the interstitial fluid volume to reach a given portion of its initial volume. This relationship provides an adequate model of experimentally observed threshold pressure intensity and loading duration characteristics in decubitus ulcer formation (Fig. 11.6).

## Interstitial Fluid Pressure during Tissue Compression

The relationship between interstitial fluid pressure (measured by the wick catheter technique) and tissue stress was examined during external tissue

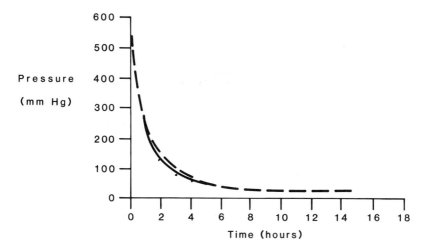

**Figure 11.6.** A comparison of theoretical (solid line) results (NP Reddy et al., 1981*a*) with experimental (dashed line) observations in humans (JB Reswick and JE Rogers, 1976). Calculations of interstitial pressure-duration relationship required for interstitial fluid volume to reach half of its initial volume are compared with a threshold pressure-application duration relationship observed in human subjects (acceptable region is below the curve and unacceptable region is above the curve). (Reproduced by permission of Pergamon Press, U.K.)

compression of the forelimbs of anesthetized Yorkshire pigs (Reddy et al., 1981*b*). We prepared wick catheters made of Dermalon fibers pulled into a polyethylene tube (PE-50, 0.58 mm internal diameter), filled with heparinized saline and connected to a pressure transducer. We calibrated the system by inserting the catheter through a rubber stopper into an intravenous tube filled with saline and connected to a pressure manometer.

Yorkshire pigs, weighing 25 kg, were anesthetized with thiopental sodium and wick catheters were placed 2 to 5 mm below the skin in subcutaneous tissue of the forelimb using a thin-walled 18-gauge needle. After equilibration, the cuff was inflated to various pressures for 10 to 15 min with simultaneous recording of interstitial fluid pressure. Sufficient time was allowed between pressure applications so as to reach steady state. In some experiments, cuff–skin interface pressures were checked with Kulite semiconductor pressure transducers.

As cuff pressure was increased, there was an initial rapid rise followed by a slow rise of interstitial fluid pressure (Fig. 11.7). Interstitial fluid pressure reached a steady state within 5 to 15 min, depending on the intensity of applied pressure. The relationship between external cuff pressure and interstitial fluid pressure is nonlinear (Fig. 11.8). In the unloaded condition, interstitial fluid pressure was $-3.9 \pm 1.4$ mm Hg. Interstitial fluid pressure reached 65% to 75% of the applied external cuff pressure. All of the points are significantly different from 100% response (dashed line). If interstitial fluid pressure were 100% of applied cuff pressure, then the data should fall on the dashed line. However, when we infused the tissue with excess fluid (0.02–0.03 ml), interstitial fluid pressure reached 100% of the cuff pressure. The cuff–skin interface pressure as measured by the semiconductor equalled cuff pressure.

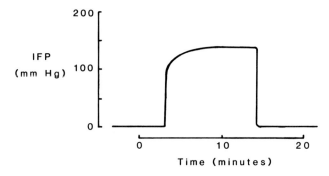

**Figure 11.7.** Subcutaneous interstitial fluid pressure-time characteristics during external pressure application. (From NP Reddy et al., 1981*b*. Reproduced by permission of *Am J Physiol*.)

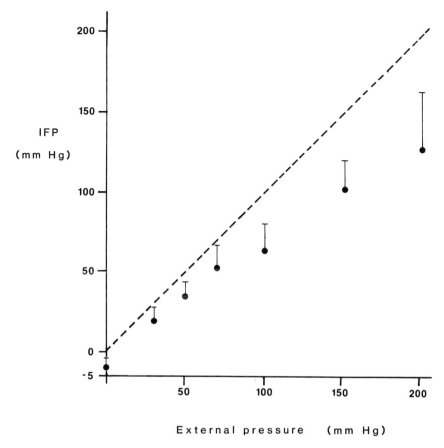

**Figure 11.8.** The relationship between external cuff pressure and subcutaneous interstitial fluid pressure (NP Reddy et al., 1981*b*). *Filled circles* represent means and *bars* indicate standard deviations. The *broken line* represents the case when interstitial fluid pressure is equal to external pressure. (Reproduced by permission of *Am J Physiol.*)

## Blood Circulation during Tissue Compression

Recently, Newson and co-workers (1981, 1982) measured skin surface $pO_2$ and blood flow during external pressure application in human subjects over the ischial tuberosity (Fig. 11.9). They used skin-mounted electrochemical transducers for $pO_2$ measurements developed by Huch and associates (1973). External pressure was applied through the oxygen transducer using a spring device such that $pO_2$ measurements could be taken at the site of load application. Load applicator ($pO_2$ sensor) was cylindrical with a blunt conical tip of 25 mm diameter. For blood flow measurements,

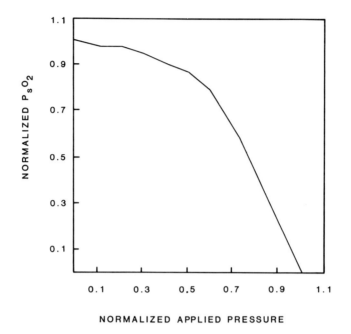

**Figure 11.9.** The relationship between mean normalized transcutaneous oxygen partial pressure ($P_sO_2$) and normalized external pressure. (TP Newson et al., 1981. Reproduced by permission of *Arch Phys Med Rehab.*)

thermal clearance and photoelectric plethysmograph methods were employed. Blood flow was completely occluded in the compressed tissue beneath the load applicator at pressures of 300 mm Hg. The time required for $pO_2$ at the surface to reach zero was of the order of a few minutes.

In normal human subjects seated on a hard surface, Bennett and collaborations (1981) measured the pressure distribution at the buttock-seat interface and correlated pressure distribution with skin blood flow distribution measured with photoplethysmography. As detected by photoplethysmography, complete cessation of flow occurred in regions where the interface pressure was of the order of 120 mm Hg (Fig. 11.10). In the case of geriatric patients, much lower pressures were required to cause flow cessation. In all of these experiments, interface pressure measurements were made and no attempt was made to correlate these pressures with internal stress states.

## Lymph Circulation

During hypoxic states, tissues release a number of humoral mediators. Although the effects of some humoral mediators on microcirculation are known, their effects on lymph propulsion are not known. Although a

**Figure 11.10.** Local skin blood flow during sitting on hard surface. (L Bennett et al. 1981. Reproduced by permission of *Arch Phys Med Rehab*.) Blood flow rate as measured by plethysmograph is plotted against local external pressure on tissue (buttock–cushion interface pressure). Although no units for blood flow were given in the paper, flow rate is believed to be in the order of 10 to 20 ml/min. **A:** Data from young and healthy (control) group. Complete flow cessation required at least 120 mm Hg. **B:** Data from geriatric patients. A pressure of 20 mm Hg was sufficient to cause flow cessation in several subjects.

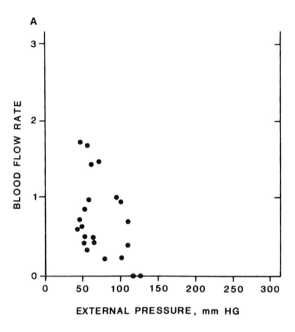

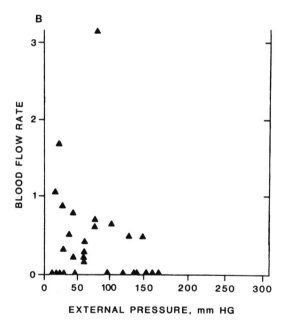

number of investigators have demonstrated that humoral mediators mod-
ulate contractility in isolated lymphatic vessel wall segments, there are
very few studies on the effect of circulating vasoactive agents. Since most
circulating vasoactive substances affect transcapillary exchange either by
changing microvascular permeability, surface area or pressure, it was
uncertain if these agents affect lymphatic motility in vivo. Recently, we
developed an experimental model to study the role of various factors on
lymph vessel motility in a living animal (Reddy and Staub, 1981). In
thoracic duct perfusion experiments on anesthetized dogs, we studied the
effects of various circulating hormones on motility of the thoracic duct. In
our perfusion experiments, inflow and outflow pressures were kept at the
same level so that there was no pressure gradient along the vessel wall.
However, transmural distending pressure was altered by changing the
inflow and outflow pressures simultaneously. In this way, only the intrinsic contractile forces were operational. Extrinsic forces, if any, were
constant throughout the experiment. We confirmed in vitro observations
that epinephrine and norepinephrine increase lymphatic motility even in
a dose that does not significantly affect systemic arterial pressure. We
observed that serotonin, histamine and Prostaglandin $E_1$ (a systemic
vasodilator) significantly inhibited lymph propulsion.

Miller and Seale (1981) injected sulfur colloid tagged with radioactive
technetium-99 m into the subcutaneous tissue in upper thighs of hindlimbs
of dogs and measured the radioactivity during external compression with
a dead weight cylindrical device. They measured radioactivity in the tissue (through an external solid state detector) at the injection site (loaded
region) and also at the regional lymph node. Technetium accumulated at
the lymph node, and therefore, they assumed that lymphatics cleared the
tracer. Lymphatics cleared the interstitial fluid until the external pressure
reached 60 to 70 mm Hg and then lymph flow was reduced to zero by any
further increase in external pressure (Fig. 11.11). It is not known how
deep the lymphatics were from the surface. Also, the precise depth of
injection site was not controlled. Nevertheless, these results suggest that
lymphatics play a role in maintaining tissue viability.

## Discussion

Cells are resistant to high hydrostatic pressures but relatively low pressure gradients may cause cellular damage by altering fluid fluxes. Cattel
(1936) investigated the effect of hydrostatic pressure on isolated tissue
enzymes and unicellular organisms, thereby avoiding pressure effects on
nutrient supply and waste product removal. Hydrostatic pressures in excess of $1.2 \times 10^9$ mm Hg were required before significant changes in
cellular function were observed, and therefore pressure sores are probably produced by pressure gradients and altered fluid fluxes, as suggested

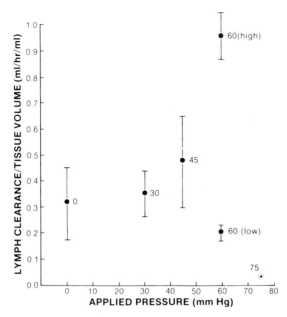

**Figure 11.11.** Tissue clearance of Tc-99m during external pressure application in experimental dogs. At 60 mm Hg, high clearance and low clearance groups were noted. (From GE Miller and J Seale, 1981. Reproduced by permission of *Lymphology*.)

by Newson and Rolfe (1982). Cellular anoxia due to blood vessel occlusion is definitely a factor in tissue necrosis. Capillaries in the skin are arranged perpendicular to the skin surface, and therefore they are more resistant to compressive stresses. Moreover, skin is extremely resistant to ischemia since epidermal cells can withstand 12 h of normothermic ischemia without necrosis (Milton, 1972).

The lymphatic system may play an important role in tissue damage produced by external compression (Fig. 11.12). A major conclusion from recent findings in lymphatic physiology is that lymph propulsion greatly depends on lymphatic smooth muscle contraction and that smooth muscle motility is highly sensitive to intravascular distention and circulating humoral mediators. In particular, motility is inhibited by serotonin, histamine and prostaglandin $E_1$, all of which are substances that are usually released during hypoxic states (Reddy and Staub, 1981). In addition, smooth muscle itself is sensitive to hypoxia.

As a result of external pressure application, hypoxia may damage lymphatic smooth muscle, causing loss of lymphatic motility and impaired lymph flow. Humoral mediators released during hypoxia may further inhibit lymphatic smooth muscle activity. Impaired lymph flow may lead to accumulation of metabolic waste products which in turn leads to the onset

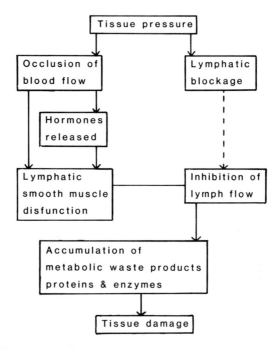

**Figure 11.12.** Hypothesis on the role of lymphatics in decubitus ulcer formation. Application of external pressure on tissue causes occlusion of blood and lymph flow. Lymphatic smooth muscle is sensitive to hypoxia. Prolonged occlusion of blood flow may cause lymphatic smooth muscle dysfunction. Due to lymphatic smooth muscle damage, lymph flow is not restored even after pressure release. In addition, humoral mediators released by the capillary and tissue during hypoxic states may further inhibit lymphatic smooth muscle contractility. With little or no lymph flow, metabolic waste products and enzymes accumulate and the tissue becomes necrotic.

of tissue necrosis. Recent results of Miller and Seale (1981) support this hypothesis. They found that lymphatics are able to remove interstitial fluid at external pressures up to 60 to 70 mm Hg and lose this ability with any further increase in external pressure.

Tissue hypoxia leads ultimately to ulceration but the quantitative relationships between stress fields in soft tissue and physiological mechanisms that produce tissue damage as a function of time are not understood. Also, the phenomenological models postulated by early investigators do not explain the observed intensity-duration effects. Halloway and associates (1976) found that skin blood flow ceases when the external pressure reaches mean arterial pressure (Fig. 11.3). If oxygen is the only factor involved, all pressure intensities in excess of the capillary closing pressure should produce ulceration and the same duration of time.

Although prolonged external loading leads to ulceration, the precise internal stress distributions (e.g., shear stress, direct stress or pressure gradients) that cause damage are not known. Our ongoing studies at Helen Hayes Hospital will correlate damage mechanisms with types of stress distributions in the tissue using in vivo indentation experiments in pigs (Cochran et al., 1980). In model experiments simulating buttock-cushion interactions, different cushion materials produced different types of stress distributions in the model buttock (Reddy et al., 1982).

There is considerable confusion in the literature regarding concepts of tissue stress and interstitial fluid pressure. Stress is defined as force per unit area and is a second-order tensor. Components of the stress tensor $\sigma_{ij}$ can be defined as the force in the $i$ direction acting on unit area normal to the $j$ direction (Fig. 11.13). The indices $i$ and $j$ can vary from one to three. The values $\sigma_{11}$, $\sigma_{22}$ and $\sigma_{33}$ are normal stresses in the three directions. $\sigma_{12}$, $\sigma_{13}$ and $\sigma_{23}$ are shear stresses. Pressure is a scalar quantity equal in all directions and measured as force exerted upon unit area.

Stress tensor $\sigma_{ij}$ can be written as the sum of an isotropic tensor $-P$ equal to the negative of the mean normal stress, and an anisotropic tensor $\sigma_{ij}$, which is a function only of deformation:

$$\sigma_{ij} = -P\delta_{ij} + \tau_{ij}, \tag{2}$$

where

$$P = -(\sigma_{11} + \sigma_{22} + \sigma_{33})/3 \tag{3}$$

and

$$\delta_{ij} = 1 \text{ if } i = j; \quad \delta_{ij} = 0 \text{ if } i \neq j. \tag{4}$$

Hydrostatic pressure $-P$ contributes to stresses in the normal direction but does not contribute to shear stresses. For compressible materials such as the subcutaneous tissues, $-P$ is identical to the hydrostatic pressure, whereas for compressible materials it includes the isotropic stress associated with changes in volume. In the case of stresses in the normal direction $\sigma_{ii}$, $\tau_{ii}$ is called the extranormal stress. In the case of a viscous fluid, $\sigma_{ii}$ is equal to $-P$ and $\tau_{ii}$ is simply zero. In the case of soft tissues, $-P$ is interstitial fluid pressure, and $\sigma_{ii}$ is total normal stress. The extranormal stress $\tau_{ii}$, depends on material properties and deformation of the solid matrix elements.

In our experiments (Reddy et al., 1981b), the relationship between interstitial fluid pressure and total normal stress was examined. Uniform compression was applied to the limb (width-to-diameter ratio of the cuff was approximately 1.4) and a wick catheter was placed close to the surface. Total normal stress equalled cuff pressure. Interstitial pressure was only 65% to 75% of the applied stress. The difference between the total normal applied stress and the interstitial fluid pressure is the extranormal stress. In our experiments, extranormal stress in subcutaneous tissue was 25% to 35% of applied external stress. Guyton et al. (1971) suggested that there exists a difference between the normal tissue stress and the intersti-

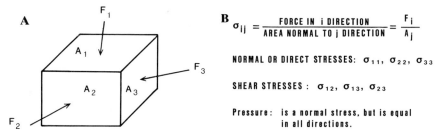

**Figure 11.13.** The concept of stress. **A:** Stress is force divided by area. Force can be decomposed into three components along three directions ($F_1$, $F_2$ and $F_3$). Similarly, there are three planes normal to the three directions. Let these surfaces have areas $A_1$, $A_2$ and $A_3$ normal to directions 1, 2 and 3, respectively. Force $F_1$ acting in direction 1, on a surface normal to direction 1 with area $A_1$ generates a direct stress (normal stress), $\sigma_{11} = F_1/A_1$. **B:** Similarly, force components $F_2$ and $F_3$ acting respectively on planes normal to second and third directions with area $A_2$ and $A_3$, result in direct (normal) stresses, $\sigma_{22} = F_2/A_2$ and $\sigma_{33} = F_3/A_3$. Force component $F_1$ can also act on surface normal to second direction with area $A_2$. This would generate a shear stress $\sigma_{12} = F_1/A_2$. Similarly we can have shear stresses $\sigma_{13}$ and $\sigma_{23}$ with force components $F_1$ and $F_2$ acting on surfaces $A_3$. Therefore, we can generalize that $\sigma_{ij}$ is force in i direction divided by area normal to j direction. For a solid $\sigma_{11}$, $\sigma_{22}$ and $\sigma_{33}$ need not be equal. Hydrostatic pressure is a stress that is equal in all directions. For a fluid, in a static state, $-P = \sigma_{11} = \sigma_{22} = \sigma_{33}$. For a solid, pressure is equal to one third of the sum of the three normal stresses, $(\sigma_{11} + \sigma_{22} + \sigma_{33})/3$. The difference between normal stress $\sigma_{11}$ and the hydrostatic pressure $-P$ is the extranormal stress $\tau_{ii}$.

tial fluid pressure, and conceived the extranormal stress as a solid tissue pressure. We suggest that total normal stress is the sum of interstitial fluid pressure and an extranormal stress:

$$\sigma_{ii} = -P + \tau_{ii}. \qquad (5)$$

The extranormal stress depends on the state of tissue deformation and stress-strain characteristics of the elastic matrix elements. Our results suggest that in normally hydrated tissue, 65% to 75% of external load is transmitted to interstitial fluid. In normal individuals the external load is shared by solid matrix elements and by interstitial fluids and ground substance. Only a fraction of external load is transmitted to interstitial fluid pressure. The remainder is supported by the solid matrix elements of the tissue as extranormal stress or as shear stress. Due to the loss of collagen integrity in patients with spinal cord injuries, 100% of the external load may be transmitted to interstitial fluid pressure, and the contribution of solid elements ($\tau_{ii}$) may be negligible.

With application of external load, tissue deforms as the result of the response of the connective tissue matrix. Some blood vessels are immediately occluded whereas others are occluded within the next few minutes as the load is transferred to deeper strata. Blood flow in a loaded region reaches steady state in minutes (Daly et al., 1976).

In addition, there is a slow viscous flow of interstitial fluid and ground substance out of the region under pressure (Guyton et al., 1966). The characteristic time for ground substance flow is in the order of a few hours (Kenyon, 1979). During indentation experiments on skin and subcutaneous tissues in anesthetized pigs (Reddy et al., unpublished observations, 1981), we observed a continual increase of the indentation depth even after 6 h of constant load (Fig. 11.14). Similarly, Vogel (1977) conducted creep tests using rabbit skin in vitro and found a similar tail-end effect which he attributed to viscous flow of interstitial ground substance.

The inverse relationship between pressure intensity and load duration for interstitial fluid volume to reach a given portion of its initial volume is similar to the threshold intensity and duration relationship in external pressure experimentally observed in studies of ulceration. The similarity between pressure-duration relationships in experimental production of ulceration and interstitial fluid flow suggests that slow viscous flow of interstitial fluid and ground substance may play a significant role in the mechanisms responsible for observed threshold pressure–time relationships, and therefore tissue breakdown. The fluid flow results are consistent with the external pressure data observed by Reswick and Rogers (1976) in human subjects. For an applied pressure of 150 mm Hg, load duration required to produce damage was 2 h in the experiments (see Fig. 11.6).

Although our simple linear model predicts that interstitial fluid volume approaches zero as time tends to infinity, this volume approaches a finite non-zero value and cannot be reduced indefinitely with time. More complex models are necessary for accurate prediction. However, the actual relationships between interstitial fluid pressure, stresses in solid tissue and external pressure still are not clear. As noted earlier, soft tissue contains networks of elastic elements (collagen and elastin) that are interspersed with blood, lymphatic capillaries and interstitial fluid. In normal

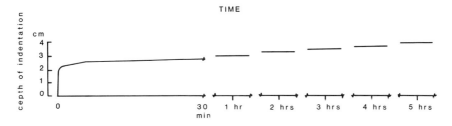

**Figure 11.14.** Indentation depth-time characteristics observed during constant load application through a 2-cm diameter hemispherical indentor placed over skin and subcutaneous tissue of an anesthetized Yorkshire pig.

individuals, stresses distribute themselves so that collagen network supports a substantial fraction of the load and protects the microvasculature from pressure-induced damage. However, in patients with spinal cord injuries, collagen in the soft tissue may be catabolized (Claus-Walker et al., 1982) leading to increased loading on the microvasculature, interstitial fluid and ground substance. Thus patients with spinal cord injuries may be more susceptible to decubitus ulcers.

The following damage mechanism is proposed. When interstitial fluid is squeezed out of a tissue region, direct contact of the cells induces contact stresses. These stresses on the fibroblasts cause rupture or perhaps interrupt collagen synthesis by contact inhibition. This inhibition and collagen breakdown continue even after the load is removed. After interstitial fluid loss and load release, interstitial fluid loss pressure becomes small (negative) enough to cause cavitation and capillary bursting in the area previously affected by external load. Dinsdale (1974) found increased vacuoles in cells after prolonged loading. This occurs because the characteristic time for interstitial fluid flow is long compared to the characteristic time for blood flow. The interstitium is flooded and subsequently protein is transferred into the surrounding tissues. At this point, any loss of function in the lymphatics due to prolonged pressure and hypoxia of smooth muscle also contributes to the process of tissue necrosis.

A summary of the proposed damage mechanism involves cell-to-cell contact stresses, capillary bursting, edema and damage to the microcirculation (Fig. 11.15). Nonfunctional lymphatics cause accumulation of metabolic waste products in a tissue already subject to degeneration and the tissue region is further poisoned from within. It should be emphasized that these are hypotheses, and therefore require experimental validation.

Soft tissue consists of several components: the microvasculature, lymphatics, interstitial fluids, ground substance, cells, fibrous network and nerves. At present very little is known about the responses of the lymphatic system and interstitial fluid to external pressure application. Also, further studies on skin microcirculation during prolonged loading are needed. The normal functioning of all major tissue components is probably essential for maintenance of tissue viability. Thus, the study of mechanical stresses on skin and subcutaneous tissue presents a fruitful domain for microcirculatory and biomechanical research.

## Summary

Prolonged or excessive external mechanical stress on tissue leads to decubitus ulceration of skin and subcutaneous tissues. Underlying damage mechanisms are poorly understood but may include external load induced

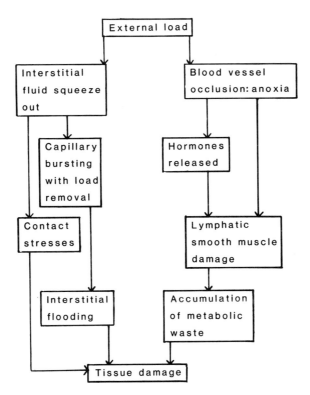

**Figure 11.15.** Proposed damage mechanisms for mechanical stress-induced tissue necrosis: application of external load on tissue causes occlusion of blood and lymph circulation. Prolonged occlusion leads to anoxia (hypoxia) which in turn leads to lymphatic smooth muscle damage. Hormones released during hypoxia (e.g., prostaglandin E, and serotonin) further inhibit lymph propulsion. Loss of lymphatic motility leads to accumulation of metabolic waste products and enzymes in the tissue which subsequently may result in tissue necrosis. Also, with prolonged external loads, interstitial fluid is squeezed out, inducing cell–cell contact stresses with possible contact inhibition of fibroblasts. After a sufficient amount of interstitial fluid is squeezed out and if the external load is removed, interstitial fluid pressure becomes sufficiently small (negative), instantaneously, to cause capillary bursting, interstitial flooding and edema. Damage to microcirculation and lymph circulation coupled with interstitial fluid flux may lead to tissue damage or tissue necrosis.

disturbances in microcirculation, lymphatic circulation, and interstitial fluid fluxes. Interstitial fluid flow during external load application may play an important role in ulcer formation. The flow responses of interstitial fluid and peripheral lymphatics during external load application are important and deserve further study.

## APPENDIX

### Model Calculations of Interstitial Fluid Flow

Consider a cylindrical slice of tissue of radius $a$. Let interstitial fluid pressure $P_a$ in this tissue be uniform. Now consider a concentric cylindrical slice of tissue comprising the surrounding region. For mathematical simplicity, assume that interstitial fluid pressure in this region varies with the radius only. In reality, interstitial fluid pressure may vary in more than one direction. At a radius $R$ from the center, let the pressure be $P_s$ (see Fig. 11.5).

The type of flow that can be assumed to exist in a complex medium such as connective tissue is percolative motion described by Darcy's law. In a one-dimensional case, Darcy's law states that flow per unit area $q$ is proportional to the product of hydraulic conductivity within the medium $K$ and the pressure gradient in the fluid $dP/dr$:

$$q = -K \left( \frac{dP}{dr} \right). \tag{1A}$$

Under steady-state conditions, the continuity equation can be expressed as:

$$\frac{1}{r} \frac{d}{dr} (rq) = 0. \tag{2A}$$

Substituting Eq. (1A) in Eq. (2A):

$$\frac{d}{dr} \left( -r \frac{dP}{dr} \right) = 0. \tag{3A}$$

The pressure gradient in steady state can be obtained by integrating Eq. (3A):

$$\frac{dP}{dr} = \frac{C_1}{r}, \tag{4A}$$

where $C_1$ is an integration constant.
Integrating again gives:

$$P = C_1 \ln (r) + C_2, \tag{5A}$$

where ln represents the natural logarithm and $C_2$ is another integration constant.
However,

$$P = P_s \text{ at } r = R. \tag{6A}$$

Substituting boundary condition (6A) in Eq. (5A):

$$C_2 = P_s - C_1 \ln R. \tag{7A}$$

Substituting Eq. (7A) in Eq. (5A):

$$P = C_1 \ln \frac{r}{R} + P_s.$$

(8A)

The second boundary condition is:

$$P = P_a \text{ at } r = a.$$

(9A)

Substituting the boundary condition in Eq. (8A):

$$P_a = C_1 \ln \left(\frac{a}{R}\right) + P_s \text{ and}$$

(10A)

$$C_1 = \frac{P_a - P_s}{\ln (a/R)}.$$

(11A)

Substituting Eq. (11A) in Eq. (8A):

$$P = \frac{P_a - P_s}{\ln (a/R)} \ln \left(\frac{r}{R}\right) + P_s.$$

(12A)

Finally, differentiating Eq. (12A) gives the pressure gradient in steady state:

$$\frac{dP}{dr} = \frac{1}{r} \frac{P_a - P_s}{\ln (a/R)}.$$

(13A)

Substituting Eq. (13A) in Eq. (1A) the radial velocity component outward from the region of pressure application $\dot{q}$ becomes:

$$\dot{q} = \frac{K\sigma}{r \ln (R/a)} (P_a - P_s),$$

(14A)

where $\sigma$, the pore fraction, is a ratio of interstitial volume to total tissue volume.

Upon integration of Eq. (14A) the total rate of flow out per unit length of cylinder $Q$ is:

$$Q = 2\pi r \dot{q} = \frac{(2K\sigma\pi)(P_a - P_s)}{\ln (R/a)},$$

(15A)

The rate of change of interstitial fluid volume in the pressurized region $\frac{dV}{dt}$ would be equal to negative of the rate of outflow per unit length of the cylinder:

$$\frac{dV}{dt} = -Q = -2K\sigma\pi \frac{(P_a - P_s)}{\ln (R/a)}.$$

(16A)

If $P_a > P_s$, fluid flows radially outward from interstitial spaces of the pressurized region to interstitial spaces of the unloaded region. If $K\sigma$ is a constant, then on integration:

$$V = V_0 - \frac{(2K\sigma\pi(P_a - P_s)t)}{\ln (R/a)}. \tag{17A}$$

If $K$ is a linear function of volume increase, (probably a more realistic assumption) then:

$$V = \frac{V_0 \exp(-2c(P_a - P_s)t)}{\ln (R/a)}, \tag{18A}$$

where $c = K\sigma\pi$.
In either case, Eq. (17A) or (18A), for a given ratio of $V/V_0$, the expression reduces to:

$$(P_a - P_s)t = \text{constant}. \tag{19A}$$

Then, if interstitial fluid pressure in the surrounding region is negligible ($P_s = 0$ at $r = R$), Eq. (19A) reduces to:

$$P_a \times t = \text{constant}. \tag{20A}$$

There are very little reliable data available for the hydraulic conductivity of tissue. Winters and Kruger (1968) reported a value of $0.45 \times 10^{-10}$ $cm^4 \cdot dyne^{-1} \cdot s^{-1}$ for the hydraulic conductivity of mesenteric tissue. Intaglietta and De Plomb (1973) reported a range of $1$–$9 \times 10^{-10}$ $cm^4 \cdot dyne^{-1} \cdot s^{-1}$ for subcutaneous tissue in a dog measured by following the fluid transfer between implanted capsules. In contrast Swabb and co-workers (1974) reported a value of around $5 \times 10^{-12}$ $cm^4 \cdot dyne^{-1} \cdot s^{-1}$ (Aukland and Nicolaysen, 1981). Since hydraulic conductivity increases with increasing fluid volume, Guyton's value may be an overestimation of $K$. It appears then that a value for hydraulic conductivity of $10^{-11}$ $cm^4 \cdot dyne^{-1} \cdot s^{-1}$ is reasonable to use for estimating interstitial fluid flow in the present calculations. For the purpose of present illustrative calculations, let interstitial fluid pressure be negligible at radii equal to or greater than $4a$, and let interstitial fluid volume $V_0$ per positive 1 cm length of cylinder be equal to 0.1 ml. For example, at an interstitial fluid pressure of $P_a = 150$ mm Hg ($2 \times 10^5$ dynes $\cdot$ cm$^{-2}$) in the loaded region, the time required for interstitial fluid volume to reach half of its initial value is:

$$t = \left(\frac{V}{V_0}\right) \frac{2\pi\sigma K}{P_a} \ln \frac{R}{a},$$

$$= 1.77 \text{ h} \tag{21A}$$

The values used in these calculations are approximations only. The calculated time required for interstitial fluid volume to reach half of its initial volume is about equal to the threshold duration of external pressure required for tissue breakdown observed in the experiments of Reswick and Rogers (1976). The general shapes of the two curves are similar (Fig. 11.6).

## References

Aukland K and Nicolaysen G (1981). Interstitial fluid volume: local regulatory mechanisms. *Physiol Rev* 61:556–643.

Bennett L, Kavner D, Lee BK and Trainor FA (1979). Shear vs pressure as causative factors in skin blood flow occlusion. *Arch Phys Med Rehab* 60:309–314.

Bennett L, Kavner D, Lee BY, Trainor FA and Lewis JM (1981). Skin blood flow in seated geriatric patients. *Arch Phys Med Rehab* 52:392–398.

Brand PW (1976). Pressure sores—the problem. In: *Bedsore Biomechanics*. Kennedi RM and Cowden JM (eds.). London: Macmillan, pp. 19–23.

Brand P and Mooney V (1977). *The Effects of Pressure on Human Tissue*. Carvill, LA: RSA Workshop Report, USPHS Hospital.

Cattell M (1936). Physiological effects of pressure. *Biol Rev* 11:441–476.

Claus-Walker J, DiFerrante N, Halstead LS and Tavella D (1982). Connective tissue turnover in quadriplagia. *Am J Physiol Med* 61:130–140.

Cochran GVB, Reddy NP, Brunski JB and Palmieri V (1980). Identification and control of biophysical factors responsible for soft tissue breakdown. In: *Proceedings of International Conference on Rehabilitation Engineering*, Toronto, June 13–18, 1980, pp. 163–166.

Daly CH, Chimoskey JE, Holloway GA and Kennedy D (1976). Effects of pressure loading on blood flow rate in human skin. In: *Bedsore Biomechanics*. Kennedi RM and Cowden JM (eds.). London: Macmillan, pp. 69–78.

Daniel RK and Wheatley DD (1981). Etiologic factors in production of pressure sores: experimental model. *Arch Phys Med Rehab* 62:492–498.

Dinsdale S (1974). *Mechanical Factors in the Pathogenesis of Ischemic Skin Ulcers in Swine*. Ph.D. Thesis, University of Minnesota.

Garber SL, Campion LJ and Krouskop TA (1982). Trochanteric Pressure in Spinal Cord Injury. *Arch Phys Med Rehab* 63:549–552.

Garber SL and Krouskop TA (1982). Body build and its relationship to pressure distribution in a seated wheelchair patient. *Arch Phys Med Rehab* 63:17–20.

Garfin SR, Pye SA, Hargens AR and Akeson WH (1980). Surface pressure distribution of the human body in the recumbent position. *Arch Phys Med Rehab* 61:409–413.

Groth KE (1942). Kinische beobachtungen und experimentelle studien uber entstehung des dekubitus. *Acta Chir Scand.* 87:198–200.

Guyton AC, Granger HJ and Taylor AE (1971). Interstitial fluid pressure. *Physiol Rev* 51:527–563.

Guyton AC, Scheel K and Murphee D (1966). Interstitial fluid pressure III. Its effects on resistance to tissue fluid mobility. *Circ Res* 19:412–419.

Hall JG, Morris B and Wolley G (1965). Intrinsic rhythmic propulsion of lymph in the anesthetized sheep. *J Physiol (Lond)* 180:336–349.

Halloway GA Jr, Daly CH, Kennedy D and Chimoskey J (1976). Effects of external pressure loading on human skin blood flow measured by [133]Xe clearance. *J Appl Physiol* 40:597–600.

Hargens AR (1981). *Tissue Fluid Pressure and Composition*. Baltimore: Williams & Wilkins, 275 pp.

Hargens AR, Sejersted OM, Kardel KR, Blom P and Hermansen L (1982). Intramuscular fluid pressure: a function of contraction force and tissue depth. Trans, 28th Orthop Res Soc 7:371.

Hargens AR and Zweifach BW (1977). Contractile stimuli in collecting lymph vessels. *Am J Physiol* 233:H57–H65.

Huch R, Huch A and Lübbers DW (1973). Transcutaneous measurement of blood $Po_2$-method and application in perinatal medicine. *J Perinat Med* 1:183–191.

Hussain, T (1953). Experimental study of some pressure effects on tissue with reference to bedsore problem. *J Pathol Bacteriol* 66:347–358.

Intaglietta M and De Plomb EP (1973). Fluid exchange in tunnel and tube capillaries. *Microvasc Res* 6:153–168.

Kenyon D (1979). A mathematical model of waterflux through aortic tissue. *Bull Math Biol* 40:62–69.

Kinmouth JB and Taylor GW (1956). Spontaneous rhythmic contractility in human lymphatics. *J Physiol (Lond)* 133:3P.

Kosiak M (1959). Etiology and pathophysiology of decubitus ulcers. *Arch Phys Med Rehab* 40:62–69.

Kosiak M (1961). Etiology of debucitus ulcers. *Arch Phys Med Rehab* 42:19–29.

Kosiak M, Kubicek WG, Olson M, Danz JN and Kottke FJ (1958). Evaluation of pressure as a factor in the production of ischial ulcers. *Arch Phys Med Rehab* 39:623–629.

Krouskop TA, Noble PC, Garber SL and Spencer WA (1983). The effectiveness of preventive management in reducing the occurrence of pressure sores. *J Rehab Res and Development* 20:74–83.

Krouskop TA, Reddy NP, Spencer W and Secor J (1978). Mechanisms of decubitus ulcer formation. *Med Hypotheses* 4:37–39.

Lindan O (1961). Etiology of decubitus ulcers; an experimental study. *Arch Phys Med Rehab* 42:774–783.

Manley MT and Darby T (1980). Repetitive mechanical stress and denervation in plantar ulcer pathogenesis in rats. *Arch Phys Med Rehab* 61:171–177.

McHale NG and Roddie IC (1976). The effect of transmural pressure on pumping activity in isolated bovine lymphatic vessels. *J Physiol (Lond)* 261:255–269.

Miller GE and Seale J (1981). Lymphatic clearance during compressive loading. *Lymphology* 14:161–166.

Milton SH (1972). Experimental studies on island flaps II. Ischemia and delay. *Plast Reconstr Surg* 49:444–447.

Mislin H and Schipp H (1967). Structural and functional relations of the mesenteric lymph vessels. In: *Progress in Lymphology*. Ruttiman A (ed.). Stuttgart: Theime, pp. 360–365.

National Academy of Sciences (1977). Compendium on U.S. Estimates of Disability.

Newson TP, Pearch MJ and Rolfe P (1981). Skin surface $Po_2$ measurement and the effect of externally applied pressure. *Arch Phys Med Rehab* 62:390–392.

Newson TP and Rolfe P (1982). Skin surface $Po_2$ and blood flow measurements over the ischial tuberosity. *Arch Phys Med Rehab* 63:553–556.

Nola GT and Vistnes LM (1980). Differential response of skin and muscle in experimental production of pressure sores. *Plast Reconstr Surg* 66:728–734.

Ohhashi T, Azuma T and Sakaguchi M (1980). Active and passive mechanical characteristics of bovine mesenteric lymphatics. *Am J Physiol* 239:H88–H95.

Ohhashi T, Kawai Y and Azuma T (1978). The responses of lymphatic smooth muscles to vasoactive substances. *Pfluegers Arch* 375:183–188.

Reddy NP (1974). *A Discrete Model of the Lymphatic System*. Ph.D. Dissertation, Texas A & M University, College Station, Texas.

Reddy NP and Cochran GVB (1979). Phenomenological theory underlying pressure-time relationships in decubitus ulcer formation. *Fed Proc* 38:1153.

Reddy NP, Cochran GVB and Krouskop TA (1981a). Interstitial fluid flow as a factor in decubitus ulcer formation. *J Biomech* 14:879–881.

Reddy NP, Krouskop TA and Newell PH Jr (1975). Biomechanics of a lymphatic system. *Blood Vessels* 12:261–278.

Reddy NP, Krouskop TA and Newell PH, Jr (1977). A computer model of the lymphatic system. *Comput Biol Med* 17:181–197.

Reddy NP, Palmieri V and Cochran GVB (1981b). Subcutaneous interstitial fluid pressure during external loading. *Am J Physiol* 240:R327–R329.

Reddy NP, Patel H, Cochran GVB and Brunski JB (1982). Model experiments to study the stress distribution in seated buttock. *J Biomech* 15:493–504.

Reddy NP and Staub NC (1981). Intrinsic propulsive activity of thoracic duct perfused in anesthetized dogs. *Microvasc Res* 21:183–192.

Reichel SM (1958). Shear force as a factor in decubitus ulcers in paraplegics. *JAMA* 166:762–763.

Reswick, JB and Rogers JE (1976). Experience at Rancho Los Amigos Hospital with devices and techniques to prevent pressure sores. In: *Bedsore Biomechanics*. Kennedi RM and Cowden JM (eds.). London: Macmillan, pp. 301–310.

Scholander PF, Hargens AR and Miller SL (1968). Negative pressure in the interstitial fluid of animals. *Science* 161:321–328.

Shields, JW (1980). Central lymph propulsion. *Lymphology* 13:9–17.

Snashall PD, Lucas J, Guz A and Floyer MA (1971). Measurement of interstitial "fluid" pressure by means of a cotton wick in man and animals: an analysis of the origin of the pressure. *Clin Sci* 41:35–52.

Swabb EA, Wei J and Gullino PM (1974). Diffusion and convection in normal and neoplastic tissues. *Cancer Res* 34:2814–2822.

Tirone P, Schiantarelli P and Rosati G (1973). Pharmacological activity of some neurotransmitters in isolated thoracic duct of dogs. *Lymphology* 6:65–68.

Vogel HG (1977). Strain of rat skin at constant load (creep experiments): influence of age and desmotropic agents. *Gerontology* 23:77–86.

Winters AD and Kruger S (1968). Drug effects on bulk flow through mesenteric membrane. *Arch Int Pharmacol* 173:213.

CHAPTER 12

# Lymph Transport in Skeletal Muscle

Thomas C. Skalak, Geert W. Schmid-Schönbein, and Benjamin W. Zweifach

## Introduction

The terminal lymphatic system represents an important mechanism for drainage of fluid from the interstitium, endowing the lymphatics with functions related to transport of tissue metabolites and immunological control. The lymphatic vessels originate as a separate vascular tree with the terminals deeply embedded in the tissue parenchyma at the level of the blood capillary network. Flow appears to be unidirectional from the lymphatic terminals into the collecting ducts. The ducts join into lymph nodes and eventually return most of the lymph fluid into the venous vasculature via the thoracic duct. Although these features are well recognized, important questions pertaining to the formation and transport of lymph fluid at the level of the terminal lymphatics remain unresolved.

The forces responsible for lymph fluid formation have generally been attributed to hydrostatic and osmotic pressure gradients that drive fluid through the tissue interstitium and across the capillary and lymphatic endothelial barriers. The precise mechanism responsible for setting up such gradients across the lymphatic endothelium, however, has not been identified, particularly for important organs such as skeletal muscle (Zweifach and Silberberg, 1979).

In this communication we will examine current proposals for the mechanism of lymph formation, with particular emphasis on skeletal muscle. The lymphatics referred to in this report are those deployed at the level of the microcirculation. Recent evidence from our laboratory indicates that the lymphatic system in muscle differs in several respects from those in other organs (Skalak et al., 1984). Therefore, a comparison will be made with lymphatics in the mesentery, which have been studied more extensively. We will summarize recent experiments that suggest that in two skeletal muscles of the rat, the lymph formation is, to a certain degree, the result of both active contraction and pulsatile elastic distention of arterioles and muscular venules. Since this hypothesis is new and relatively unexplored, we will point out several directions of future research. A number of general reviews concerning lymph formation have been published previously (Guyton, 1976; Casley-Smith, 1977; Zweifach and Silberberg, 1979).

## Background

Spontaneous contractions of lymph vessels are readily demonstrated in several organs, including the mesentery in mammalian species (Mislin and Schipp, 1967; Zweifach and Prather, 1975), the intestinal villi (Florey, 1927; Lee, 1965), and the bat wing (Webb and Nicoll, 1944; Wiederhielm and Weston, 1973; Nicoll, 1973, 1975).

### Mesenteric Lymphatic Network Structure

The network of lymphatics in the cat mesentery is shown in Figure 12.1A, which was obtained by sequential filling of the lymphatics using microinjections of carbon ink (Schmid-Schönbein et al., 1977). The overlay copy in Figure 12.1B shows, for reasons of clarity, the arterioles and lymphatics of the same mesentery area. The arterioles may be classified into those forming arcades and enclosing individual microvascular modules (Frasher and Wayland, 1972) and those branching from the arcades and feeding into the capillary network inside the modules. Arcade arterioles are usually paired with venules. The lymphatics originate in the capillary network with about one lymphatic terminal per microvascular module (Fig. 12.1). At this level the vessels are not contractile; they have lateral dimensions 5 to 10 times larger than those of adjacent capillaries and are quite permeable to macromolecules. If the lymphatic terminals are followed for several hundred micrometers downstream, one observes valves that prevent retrograde flow. They are typically located along those segments where the lymphatics tend to follow the arcade arterioles. At the sites where the first valves are located, the first smooth muscle cells in the lymphatic wall occur. The smooth muscle cells initially form a discontinuous layer and gradually become a single continuous layer (Fig. 12.2 and Fig. 12.3). The lymphatics then form a compartmental structure with narrowings of the vessel lumen at the valves and widening between valves (Fig. 12.1B). The major lymphatic vessel draining the area of the mesentery is not usually deployed in association with any arterioles or venules (Fig. 12.1B and 12.2).

### Mesenteric Lymphatic Vasomotion

Lymphatic terminals in mesenteric interstitium (Fig. 12.1B) have not been observed to contract, whereas those lymphatic compartments between valves show spontaneous vasomotion in some species. This lymphatic

A

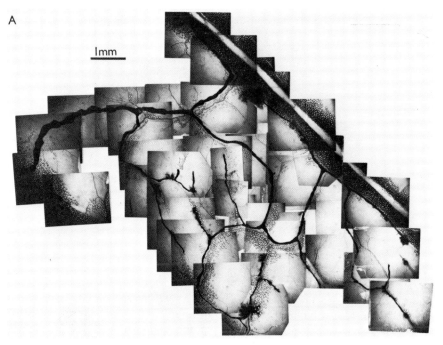

B

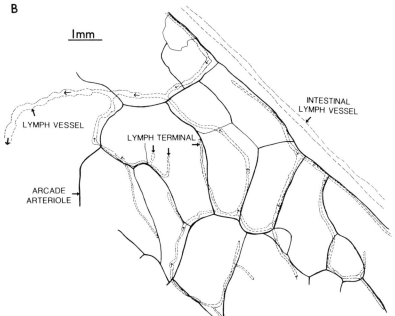

**Figure 12.1.** Lymphatic vessels in cat mesentery. **A:** A photo montage with lymphatics that have been injected with carbon solution. Paired arterioles and venules can be recognized but the magnification is too low to visualize the capillaries clearly. **B:** A hand drawing of the same area with only arterioles (*solid lines*) and lymphatics (*dashed lines*) shown. Flow directions are indicated by the *arrows* inside lymphatics. The lymph vessel on the left, which drains this terminal lymphatic network, is not associated with any blood vessel.

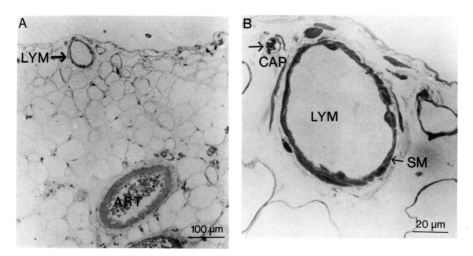

**Figure 12.2.** Cross-section of rat mesentery. **A:** An overview with mesenteric surface at the top, a lymphatic (LYM), an artery (ART) and several venules below. The magnified view in **(B)** shows that this same lymphatic has an almost circular cross-section and a discontinuous smooth muscle coat (SM). A neighboring capillary (CAP) is significantly smaller than the lymphatic.

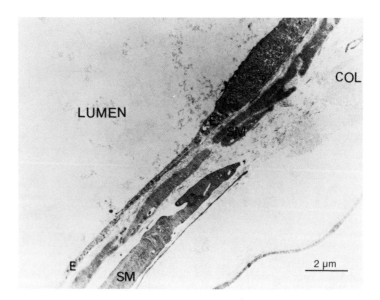

**Figure 12.3.** Electron microscopic view of lymphatic wall in rat mesentery. The endothelium (E) is strongly attenuated; the smooth muscle cells (SM) form a discontinuous coat and are lying adjacent to collagen fibers (COL).

vasomotion consists of rhythmic contractions that travel as peristaltic waves downstream along the vessel, leading to compression of the individual compartments, elevation of the hydrostatic pressure and forward propulsion of the lymph fluid. Retrograde fluid motion is prevented by the valves (Smith, 1949; Mislin and Schipp, 1967; Zweifach and Prather, 1975). Hargens and Zweifach (1977) demonstrated that in addition to rhythmic contractions, the lymphatic smooth muscle may also exhibit a myogenic response when intralymphatic pressure is raised by obstruction of the lumen downstream.

## Mesenteric Lymph Fluid Formation

What causes the flow of interstitial fluid across the walls of the lymphatic terminals? There is currently no agreement on this question. Using simultaneous measurements of interstitial fluid pressure with wick catheters and intralymphatic pressure by micropuncture, Clough and Smaje (1978) concluded that the existing pressure gradient is insufficient to account for a fluid flux across the lymphatic wall. They therefore suggest that the pressure gradient is provided by expansion of the lymphatics caused by the action of external forces on the mesentery, i.e., during intestinal peristalsis. Reddy et al. (1975) suggested that the spontaneous contraction of lymphatics in the presence of unidirectional flow through the valves should lead, by retrograde action, to an intralymphatic hydrostatic pressure reduction in the lymph terminals. This reduction may then be sufficient to set up a pressure drop from the interstitium toward the terminal. Casley-Smith (1977) suggested that osmotic forces play an important role. He presents evidence for the generation of an osmotic pressure gradient as a result of lymphatic ultrafiltration across endothelial junctions during compression of the lymphatics. None of these three hypotheses, however, has yet received general acceptance.

A key problem concerning the lymphatic filling question is the mechanism responsible for the expansion of the lymphatic terminals. These thin-walled vessels are readily collapsed so that lymph formation is possible only if they are expanded by some force. In the absence of a well-documented hydrostatic or osmotic pressure gradient in the exposed and resting mesentery preparation, the solution to the problem may be found by considering external forces that act on the mesentery sheet as a whole (Clough and Smaje, 1978). In the face of the thinness of the mesentery sheet and the high deformability of the lymphatic terminals, it is possible that if the forces on the two surfaces of the mesentery are equal and both directed outward, the lymphatic origins will be expanded. The fluid entering the lymphatics under these conditions will come from the interstitium. In view of their compartmental structure and peristaltic smooth muscle contractions, the collecting lymphatics may serve primarily as a transport mechanism for fluid leaving the mesentery. The forces acting on the mesentery during motion of the diaphragm, intestinal peristalsis, walking or other physical perturbations may contribute to the expansion of the lymphatic terminals.

The types of forces that are responsible for lymphatic filling are dependent on the natural unstressed shape of the lymphatic origins. If their unstressed shape is a collapsed one, then tensile normal stresses in the tissue are required to open them. If, on the other hand, their unstressed shape has a finite volume, then compressive pressures will lead to emptying and an elastic recoil of the tissue may account for filling. The mechanical support of the walls of the terminals due to neighboring cells, collagen fibers, etc., should be sufficient to restore the filled-lymphatic shape, allowing fluid to percolate into the lumen. Our observations, however, suggest that in the cat mesentery the unstressed shape is usually a collapsed one (Schmid-Schönbein et al., 1977).

## Recent Observations in Skeletal Muscle

The situation in skeletal muscle is different in several respects. Skeletal muscle lymphatics have no smooth muscle in their walls, and there exists a close relationship between the lymphatics and the accompanying arterioles and muscular venules. No lymphatics are observed in the capillary space of skeletal muscle (Skalak et al., 1984). This discussion will refer exclusively to lymphatics inside the skeletal muscle; no reference will be made to those in the outer perimysial sheet.

### Skeletal Muscle Lymphatic Network Structure

To describe the situation in more detail it is helpful to review some aspects of the vascular and interstitial spaces in skeletal muscle. Our observations are limited to the spinotrapezius muscle of the rat but similar observations were also recorded in the cremaster muscle of the same species. The spinotrapezius muscle is supplied with blood from four to five arterioles that originate in the brachial artery and several dorsal branches of the intercostal arteries. On entering the muscle they branch into an interconnected (arcading) arteriolar network that extends throughout the entire muscle. Vessel diameters range from about 40 to 100 $\mu$m. At regular intervals the arcading arterioles distribute branches designated as transverse arterioles, which feed directly into the capillary network. The capillaries primarily run longitudinally along the muscle fibers, forming a large oblong meshwork within a given muscle fiber bundle. Most capillaries are tightly fitted in the space between three adjacent skeletal muscle cells (Skalak et al., 1982). Electron microscopic studies performed in our laboratory show that the interstitial space around the capillaries is extraordinarily small, comprising <3% of the muscle volume.

Microinjections of a contrast medium indicate that the lymphatics lie in close juxtaposition to the arcade arterioles and some transverse arterioles. They follow the arteriolar course closely, even along undulations (Fig. 12.4). Lymphatic terminals in skeletal muscle have a different shape than those in the mesentery. They consist of short lateral extensions that are often coincident with transverse arterioles. Some lymphatic segments have no such outpocketings that could be construed as terminals. Some of the larger draining venules in the spinotrapezius muscle are also occasionally accompanied by lymphatics. A number of arterioles have no accompanying lymphatic and at large feeder arteries, several lymphatics are usually present (Fig. 12.5). The close physical alignment of these vessels has been reported by several authors (Aagaard, 1913; Nadezhdin, 1957; Kozma and Gellért, 1958; Stingl and Štembera, 1974). The microinjection experiments suggested the existence of valves in the large lymphatics, and histological sections showed that double-leaflet valves were present (Skalak et al., 1984).

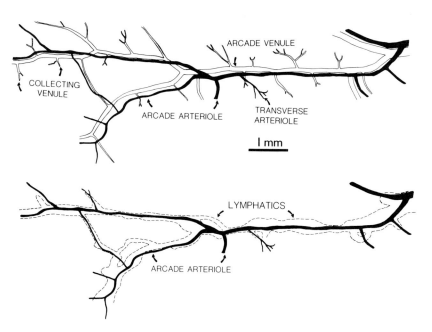

**Figure 12.4.** Arterioles, venules and lymphatics in spinotrapezius muscle of the rat. The drawings are direct copies from color Polaroid micrographs of lymphatics filled with Evans Blue (Skalak et al., 1984). At the **top** an arcade arteriole with transverse arteriole and adjacent venules are shown. At the **bottom** the same arteriole is reproduced with the adjacent lymphatic. The lymphatic closely follows the course of the arteriole. Occasionally short extensions of the lymphatics along the transverse arterioles are present.

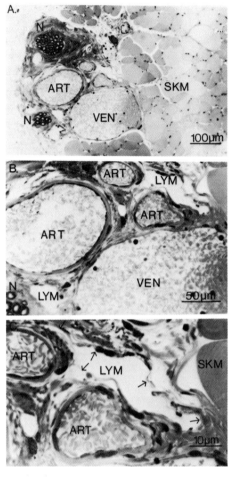

**Figure 12.5. A:** Light microscopic cross-sections of arterioles (ART), venules (VEN), nerves (N) and lymphatic at the level of one of the larger feeder arterioles to the skeletal muscle fibers (SKM) of the spinotrapezius muscle. These vessels are positioned on the surface of the muscle (*left side in* **A**). **B:** Lymphatics (LYM) that are partially open. Adjacent arterioles are dilated. **C:** One lymphatic (LYM). It has a single endothelial coat (*arrows*) and irregular cross-sectional shape.

## Skeletal Muscle Lymphatic Histology

Light and electron microscopic cross-sections (Figs. 12.6–12.8) confirm the close proximity of the lymphatics to the arterioles. Cross-sections of the lymphatics are noncircular and a portion of the lymphatic endothelium is often in direct contact with the arteriolar smooth muscle layer. The lymphatics have no smooth muscle of their own (Fig. 12.9) and the wall consists of a highly attenuated endothelium. When the lymphatic endothelial cells are mechanically sheared and pulled in vivo with micropipettes, it can be seen that they are firmly attached to their substrate of interstitial collagen fibers, arteriolar smooth muscle and even skeletal muscle fibers. The basement membrane is discontinuous and the endothe-

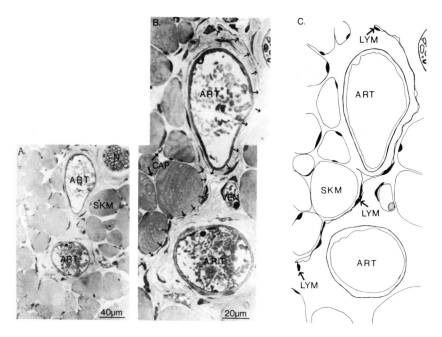

**Figure 12.6.** Light microscopic cross-section **(A)** of two arterioles (ART) in rat spinotrapezius muscle with adjacent lymphatic (LYM) that is almost completely collapsed. The arteriole-lymphatic pairs are deeply embedded in the skeletal muscle fibers (SKM) and are accompanied by a nerve (N) and a venule (VEN) **(B).** Lymphatics are not readily identifiable at this magnification. The lymphatic stretches across both blood vessels (**B,** *arrows*; **C**) and its endothelium (*arrows* in **B**) is highly attenuated, similarly to the endothelium in distended lymphatics.

lium has large numbers of vesicles, the majority of which are attached to either the luminal or abluminal endothelial membrane. In the cross-sections, the endothelial cells show regions with tight junctions and regions with open junctions. This organization of the lymphatic wall is uniform over the extent of the muscle, suggesting that the exchange area extends to all lymphatics (Skalak et al., 1984). In this case all lymphatics in the organ may be regarded as terminals.

## Skeletal Muscle Lymphatic Filling

An important and consistent finding in this study is the following observation (Figs. 12.7 and 12.8): when arterioles are dilated, as indicated by a stretched-out vascular endothelium, the adjacent lymphatics are completely (Fig. 12.6) or partially (Fig. 12.7) collapsed. On the other hand, when arterioles are contracted, as indicated by the deformation of the

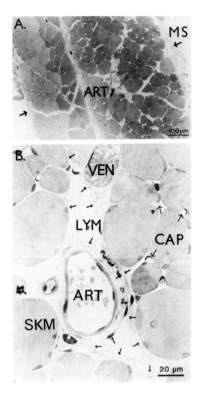

**Figure 12.7.** Light microscopic cross-section of skeletal muscle with an arteriole (ART), venule (VEN) and lymphatic (LYM) in partially occluded state. The vessels are embedded in the muscle fibers **(A)** midway between the perimysial muscle surfaces (MS). Capillaries (CAP) are small in comparison to the lymphatic vessel **(B)**. The lymphatic endothelium (*arrows*) is highly attenuated and is tightly molded between skeletal muscle fibers (SKM) and the vascular smooth muscle.

vascular endothelium and its intrusion of the vessel lumen, the adjacent lymphatics are open (Fig. 12.8). Arcading arterioles and the accompanying lymphatics are deeply embedded in the muscle proper, usually between several muscle fiber bundles. Vascular distensibility studies in our laboratory indicate that the blood vessels in this skeletal muscle are comparatively stiff. Most of the mechanical support for these vessels is provided by the adjacent skeletal muscle fibers, much like a tunnel in a gel (Fung, 1966). Thus the arteriole-lymphatic pairs are located in a space that is relatively constant in a resting muscle. The volume displacements associated with arteriolar vasomotion or with pulsatile elastic vessel distensions may therefore be accommodated by a simultaneous lymphatic volume displacement. Contraction of the arterioles leads to expansion of the adjacent lymphatics and dilation of the arterioles leads to compression of the lymphatics. In the presence of the valves, only unidirectional flow is possible. Thus, expansion of the lymphatics requires fluid to enter across the endothelial wall, and during compression this fluid flows along the path of least resistance which, according to the micropipette injection experiments, is clearly along the lymphatic channels rather than backward into the interstitium.

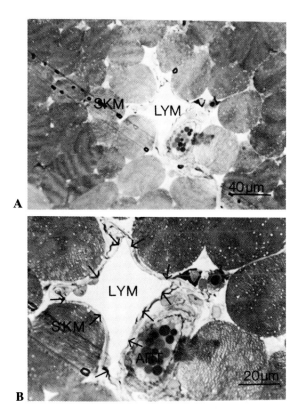

**Figure 12.8.** Light microscopic cross-section of skeletal muscle with a contracted arteriole (ART) and adjacent open lymphatic vessel (LYM). The vessels are deeply embedded in skeletal muscle fibers (SKM) **(A)**. The lymphatic endothelium is highly attenuated (**B**, *arrows*).

## Theoretical Considerations of Lymph Transport in Skeletal Muscle

The mechanism of lymph formation suggested by these observations is not directly dependent on the presence of an osmotic pressure gradient, although it is possible that molecular concentration gradients may exist in the interstitium and affect fluid flow. There may also exist a hydrostatic pressure gradient from capillaries to the lymphatics. Both will be neglected in the following analysis.

Consider an arteriole-lymphatic pair embedded in collagen fibers and bundles of skeletal muscle fibers as seen in the histological sections (Fig. 12.7). A tissue volume $V_T$ consists of the skeletal muscle fibers with

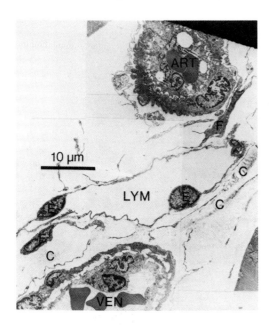

**Figure 12.9.** Transmission electron micrograph of an open lymphatic vessel (LYM) adjacent to a contracted arteriole (ART) and a venule (VEN) in rat spinotrapezius muscle. The lymphatic endothelium (E) is attenuated and attached abluminally to collagen fiber bundles (C) which are intermingled with fibroblast cells (F). Due to a short period of fixation with $OsO_4$, the collagen fibers appear as light structures at this magnification.

volume $V_M$, the arteriole volume $V_A$, lymphatic volume $V_L$, interstitial volume $V_I$, and capillary volume $V_C$ such that:

$$V_T = V_M + V_I + V_A + V_L + V_C. \tag{1}$$

All of these volumes are time-dependent and if there is no net tissue volume gain due to the blood flow then $dV_T/dt = 0$ and

$$0 = \frac{dV_M}{dt} + \frac{dV_I}{dt} + \frac{dV_A}{dt} + \frac{dV_L}{dt} + \frac{dV_C}{dt}. \tag{2}$$

Current experiments in our laboratory indicate that capillaries in skeletal muscle are relatively rigid at their normal distending pressure (Skalak et al., 1983), so that $V_C$ = constant. In the absence of muscle fiber contraction and swelling of the interstitium, Eq. (2) reduces to

$$0 = \frac{dV_A}{dt} + \frac{dV_L}{dt} \tag{3}$$

or $V_A + V_L$ = constant. Equation (3) reflects the arteriole-lymphatic relationship that we observed. In the presence of lymphatic valves that prevent retrograde flow the resultant flow $J_L$ out of the lymphatic is

$$J_L = \frac{dV_L}{dt} \text{ for } \frac{dV_L}{dt} \leq 0 \tag{4a}$$

and filling of single lymphatics with interstitial fluid occurs when

$$J_L = 0 \text{ for } \frac{dV_L}{dt} > 0. \tag{4b}$$

A number of investigators have indicated that passive compression or active contraction of skeletal muscle leads to an enhancement of lymphatic flow (Jacobsson and Kjellmer, 1964; Garlick and Renkin, 1970; Lewis and Yates, 1972; Szabó et al., 1972). Nonetheless, the lymph flow is still finite in a resting muscle (Paldino and Hyman, 1966). To assess the influence of muscle contraction versus that of arteriolar volume expansion, consider the skeletal muscle fibers with volume $V_M$. Let their cross-sectional area and length before and after contraction be designated as $A_{Mo}$, $l_o$ and $A_M$, $l$, respectively; then assuming constant fiber volume

$$A_{Mo}l_o = A_M l \tag{5a}$$

or

$$\frac{l}{l_o} = \frac{A_{Mo}}{A_M}. \tag{5b}$$

On shortening, the muscle fiber cross-sectional area $A_M$ increases. The question arises as to the degree to which this increase is accompanied by a corresponding increase in vascular, interstitial and lymphatic cross-sectional area. For uniform strain field the lateral expansions are linearly proportional. Because of the presence of cell membranes, collagen fibers and basement membranes, which have nonuniform mechanical properties, and the complex nature of the muscle fiber attachment, a more detailed analysis of this strain field during muscle shortening is needed. In any case, if muscle shortening leads to a change of lymphatic volume it serves as a mechanism of lymph formation. Thus the frequency and magnitude of volume changes caused by vasomotion, pressure pulsation and muscle contraction will determine their relative influence on the resultant lymph flow. In an exercising muscle shortening and lengthening may be the dominant mechanism; in a resting muscle it may be vasomotion. Arteriolar volumetric expansions caused by the pulse pressure may also be a contributing factor. In the spinotrapezius muscle arteriolar pulse pressure variations of 20 to 30 mm Hg are not unusual and are accompanied by arteriolar diameter changes of the order of about 0.5 $\mu$m.

The mechanism for lymph formation proposed here is independent of whether the interstitial hydrostatic pressure is positive or negative, a question that has been debated previously (Guyton, 1963; Scholander et al., 1968; Wiederhielm and Weston, 1973). Assuming that the arterial wall is impermeable and predominantly supports a membrane tension $T_A$, equilibrium of forces requires

$$T_A = R_A(P_A - P_L), \tag{6}$$

where $R_A$ is the radius of the artery; $P_A$ and $P_L$ are the intraarterial and lymphatic hydrostatic pressures, respectively. The relationship between $T_A$ and $R_A$ depends on the mechanical properties of the smooth muscle and other elements in the wall. Our electron microscopic investigation of the lymphatic wall shows, throughout the muscle, a highly attenuated endothelium with many open junctions and large numbers of cytoplasmic vesicles, suggesting that exchange is possible across all lymphatics. In addition, the thinness of the endothelial sheet and many points of high radii of curvature suggest that the lymphatic wall does not support large bending stresses. During the filling phase of the lymphatic

$$\frac{dV_L}{dt} = - K_L(P_L - P_I),$$    (7)

where $P_L$ and $P_I$ are the hydrostatic pressures of lymph and interstitial fluid; both are time-dependent. $K_L$ is the lymphatic permeability coefficient. Solving Eq. (6) for $P_L$ and substituting into Eq. (7), we find

$$\frac{dV_L}{dt} = K_L\left(\frac{T_A}{R_A} + P_I - P_A\right).$$    (8)

Thus, filling of the lymphatics is possible if

$$\frac{T_A}{R_A} > P_A - P_I.$$    (9)

Typical values of $P_A$ in the arcade and transverse arterioles may have a range of 50 to 100 mm Hg, and in exercise or in animals with hypertension $P_A$ may be larger (Zweifach et al., 1981). Observations indicate that the smooth muscle in this organ can generate sufficient tension to contract against these high pressures. At rest, interstitial fluid pressures $P_I$ are of relatively small magnitude ($< \pm 7$ mm Hg) and probably have an insignificant effect on the arteriolar pulsations or vasomotion regardless of whether they are positive or negative. However, in a strongly dehydrated tissue with lower values of $P_I$, lymph formation may be limited because of the inability of smooth muscle to generate sufficient tension.

## Synopsis and Future Research

### Vasomotion

Vasomotion has been observed in the arteriolar vessels of the spinotrapezius muscle in the resting state (Borders and Zweifach, 1983). It consists of irregularly periodic changes in the diameters of arcading and transverse arterioles and is caused by the action of smooth muscle. Vasomotion appears to be an essential mechanism for preservation of tissue homeostasis (Intaglietta, 1981; Intaglietta and Gross, 1982) and may provide a regular driving force for convective fluid transport through the interstitium. The transport of large molecular substances, such as albumin, is also influenced by the presence of convective flow.

Vasomotion is easily modified by anesthetic or vasodilatory agents. In this context, it is interesting to note that lymph flow from many organs of intact animals is depressed by anesthetic agents (Quin and Shannon, 1975). In humans, it has been observed that administration of vasodilatory drugs such as nifedipine, which is a $Ca^{2+}$ blocking agent in smooth muscle, leads to swelling of the skeletal muscle in the legs (Guazzi et al., 1980; Johnson et al., 1981). If future studies on human skeletal muscle reveal a similar picture of arteriole-lymphatic pairs, then these indirect observations of tissue edema may be explained by the depressant action of anesthetics and vasodilators on arteriolar vasomotion and lymphatic pumping.

## Interstitial Fluid Flow

In mesentery and skeletal muscle, the density of the lymphatics is low in comparison to the capillary density. Thus, it is possible that a capillary may be several hundred micrometers away from the nearest lymphatic terminal. The question arises then: How far from a lymphatic will the pressure reduction during arteriolar contraction still have an influence on interstitial flow? It is probable, because of the incompressibility of the fluid medium, that the local pressure reduction at the lymphatics may be transmitted for considerable distances. The rate at which the pressure falls off as a function of the distance from the lymphatic depends on the interstitial compressibility, the geometry of the muscle and the conditions governing flow at the perimysium (Blake and Intaglietta, 1982).

The flow of interstitial fluid may be facilitated by the presence of pre-formed tissue clefts that are devoid of membranes. In the mesentery, tissue clefts extend from lymphatic terminals into the tissue (Hauck, 1972). The relatively large volume of collagen fibers around arteriole-lymphatic pairs in skeletal muscle may be the origin of lymph fluid. The collagen fibers form a potentially large space for interstitial fluid, whereas the space between capillaries and muscle fibers is smaller. Collagen fibers may also serve as guidewires for low resistance water pathways in the interstitium (Kihara, 1956; Witte, 1957).

## Skeletal Muscle Lymphatic Valves

The exact distribution of valves in skeletal muscle lymphatics is currently unknown. We observed that most, but not all, arcading arterioles are accompanied by lymphatics; some lymphatics form interconnected arcades. The arterioles do not contract simultaneously over the extent of the arcading system, and phase and amplitude changes of the vasomotor diameter excursions frequently occur at the vascular bifurcations. Thus, it is possible that to prevent retrograde flow, lymphatic valves are located at strategically important points in the network determined by the lymphatic network geometry and the exact phasic relationship of arteriolar vasomotor cycles.

## Vascular Smooth Muscle

Since lymphatic endothelium is often in contact with the abluminal side of the vascular smooth muscle, tissue metabolites, which are carried in the lymph fluid, may have direct influence on smooth muscle contraction. This metabolic influence may be exerted on arteriolar as well as venous smooth muscles. It has long been known that the arteriolar vascular smooth muscle is an important determinant of hemodynamic parameters in the capillary bed. Contraction and dilation of arterioles have a pronounced effect on capillary velocity, red cell distribution and other hemodynamic parameters. The observations in the resting spinotrapezius muscle suggest that the same vascular smooth muscle perturbations also have an important influence on lymphatic flow and therefore on the tissue fluid balance at rest.

Blood flow and tissue fluid transport may thus be closely coupled processes in which rhythmic time dependent variations are fundamental conditions for preservation of tissue homeostasis.

## Summary

A review of the terminal lymphatic system in the mesentery and the spinotrapezius muscle is provided. Whereas the mesentery lymphatics have terminals in the capillary bed and have collecting vessels with valves and peristaltic smooth muscle contraction, the lymphatics in skeletal muscle exhibit different features. In skeletal muscle, none of the lymphatics is contractile. Histological cross-sections of the wall show an attenuated endothelium with many vesicles, discontinuous basement membrane and cell junctions without zonula occludens. The lymphatic cross-sections are noncircular and lymphatics are generally wrapped around or in immediate proximity to the arterioles. When the arterioles are dilated, the adjacent lymphatics are partially or completely collapsed, whereas when the arterioles are contracted the lymphatics are open. This suggests that periodic arteriolar diameter changes, such as those that occur during arteriolar vasomotion, are responsible for opening and closing lymphatics, and therefore contribute to lymph fluid formation. This is the first suggestion that vascular smooth muscle not only influences hemodynamic parameters in the microcirculation but simultaneously influences interstitial fluid filtration and lymph formation.

## Acknowledgment

This work is supported by USPHS HL-10881 and NSF Award PCM-82-15607.

# References

Aagaard OC (1913). Über die Lymphgefässe der Zunge, des quergestreiften Muskelgewebes und Speicheldrüsen des Menschen. *Anat Heft* 47:493–648.

Blake TR and Intaglietta M (1982). Hydrodynamic considerations in the transport of fluid in the interstitium as a consequence of spontaneous arteriolar vasomotion. *Microvasc Res* 23:243.

Borders JL and Zweifach BW (1983). Vasomotion: a mechanism for resistive change in hypertension. *Am J Physiol* (in press).

Casley-Smith JR (1977). Lymph and lymphatics. In: *Microcirculation, Vol. 1.* Kaley G and Altura BM (eds.). Baltimore: University Park Press, pp. 423–502.

Clough G and Smaje LH (1978). Simultaneous measurement of pressure in the interstitium and the terminal lymphatics of the cat mesentery. *J Physiol* 283:457–468.

Florey H (1927). Observations on the contractility of lacteals. Part 1 and 2. *J Physiol (Lond)* 62:267–272, 63:1–18.

Frasher WA and Wayland H (1972). Repeating modular organization of the microcirculation of cat mesentery. *Microvasc Res* 4:62–76.

Fung YC (1966). Microscopic blood vessels in the mesentery. In: *Biomechanics. Proceedings of Symposium of Applied Mechanics Division,* American Society of Mechanical Engineers, pp. 151–166.

Garlick DG and Renkin EM (1970). Transport of large molecules from plasma to interstitial fluid and lymph in dogs. *Am J Physiol* 219:1595–1605.

Gauzzia MD, Fiorentini C, Olivari MT, Bartorelli A, Necchi G and Polese A (1980). Short- and long-term efficacy of a calcium-antagonistic agent (nifedipine) combined by Methyldopa in the treatment of severe hypertension. *Circulation* 61:913–919.

Guyton AC (1963). Concept of negative interstitial pressure based on pressures in implanted capsules. *Circ Res* 12:399–414.

Guyton AC (1976). Interstitital fluid pressure and dynamics of lymph formation. *Fed Proc* 35:1861–1862.

Hargens AR and Zweifach BW (1977). Contractile stimuli in collecting lymph vessels. *Am J Physiol* 223:H57–H65.

Hauck G (1972). Pathways between capillaries and lymphatics. *Pflügers Arch* 336 (*Suppl.* 17):S55–S57.

Intaglietta M (1981). Vasomotor activity, time dependent fluid exchange and tissue pressure. *Microvasc Res* 21:153–164.

Intaglietta M and Gross JF (1982). Vasomotion, tissue fluid flow and formation of lymph. *Int J Microcirc Clin Exp* 1:55–65.

Jacobsson S and Kjellmer I (1964). Flow and protein content of lymph in resting and exercising skeletal muscle. *Acta Physiol Scand* 60:278–285.

Johnson SM, Mauritson DR, Willerson JT and Hillis LD (1981). Comparison of verapamil and nifedipine in the treatment of variant angina pectoris: Preliminary observations in 10 patients. *Am J Cardiol* 47:1295–1300.

Kihara T (1956). Das extravaskuläre Saftbahnsystem. *Okajimas Folia Anat Jpn* 28:601–621.

Kozma M and Gellért A (1958). Mikroskopische Beiträge zu Frage der Lymphgefässe in der Skeletmuskulatur. *Acta Morphol Acad Sci Hung* 8:15–20.

Lee JS (1965). Motility, lymphatic contractility and distension pressure in intestinal absorption. *Am J Physiol* 208:621–627.

Lewis GP and Yates C (1972). Flow and composition of lymph collected from the skeletal muscle of the rabbit hind limb. *J Physiol (Lond)* 226:57.

Mislin H and Schipp R (1967). Structural and functional relations of the mesenteric lymph vessels. In: *Progress in Lymphology*. Rüttiman A. (ed.). New York: Hafner, pp. 360–365.

Nadezhdin VN (1957). The lymph-vessel architectonics in the interior of the muscles, tendons, and fascia. *Arkh Anat Gist Embriol* 34:90–100.

Nicoll PA (1973). Formation and flow of lymph and lymphatic permeability. In: *Regulation and Control in Physiological Systems, Vol. 15*. Iberall AS and Guyton AC (eds.). Philadelphia: WB Saunders, pp. 122–126.

Nicoll PA (1975). Excitation-contraction of single vascular smooth muscle cells and lymphatics in-vivo. *Immunochemistry* 12:511–515.

Paldino RL and Hyman C (1966). Removal of small and large molecules from microinjection sites in rat skeletal muscle. *Am J Physiol* 210:576–578.

Quin JW and Shannon AD (1975). The effect of anesthesia and surgery on lymph flow, protein and leucocyte concentration in lymph of the sheep. *Lymphology* 8:126–135.

Reddy NP, Krouskop TA and Newell PH (1975). A note on the mechanisms of lymph flow through the terminal lymphatics. *Microvasc Res* 10:214–216.

Schmid-Schönbein GW, Zweifach BW and Kovalcheck S (1977). The application of stereological principles to morphometry of the microcirculation in different tissues. *Microvasc Res* 14:303–317.

Scholander PF, Hargens AR and Miller SL (1968). Negative pressure in the interstitial fluid of animals. *Science* 161:321–328.

Skalak TC, Schmid-Schönbein GW and Zweifach BW (1982). Topological and morphological studies of the microvascular network in rat spinotrapezius muscle. *Int J Microcirc Clin Exp* 1:321–322.

Skalak TC, Schmid-Schönbein GW and Zweifach BW (1983). Viscoelastic properties of small blood vessels in skeletal muscle. *Microvasc Res* 25:258 (Abstract 89).

Skalak TC, Schmid-Schönbein GW and Zweifach BW (1984). New morphological evidence for a mechanism of lymph formation in skeletal muscle. *Microvasc Res* 28:95–112.

Smith RO (1949). Lymphatic contractility—A possible intrinsic mechanism of lymphatic vessels for the transport of lymph. *J Exp Med* 90:497–509.

Stingl J and Štembera O (1974). Distribution and ultrastructure of the initial lymphatics of some skeletal muscles in the rat. *Lymphology* 7:160–168.

Szabó G, Anda E and Vándor E (1972). The effect of muscle activity on the lymphatic and venous transport of lactate dehydrogenase. *Lymphology* 5:111–114.

Webb RL and Nicoll PA (1944). Behavior of lymphatic vessels in the living bat. *Anat Rec* 88:351–367.

Wiederhielm CA and Weston BV (1973). Microvascular, lymphatic and tissue pressures in the unanesthetized mammal. *Am J Physiol* 225:992–996.

Witte S (1957). Fluoroszenzmikroskopische Untersuchungen über die Capillarpermeabilität. *Z Ges Exp Med* 129:358–367.

Zweifach BW, Kovalcheck S, DeLano F and Chen P (1981). Micropressure-flow relationships in a skeletal muscle of spontaneously hypertensive rats. *Hypertension* 3:601–614.

Zweifach BW and Prather JW (1975). Micromanipulation of pressure in terminal lymphatics in the mesentery. *Am J Physiol* 228:1326–1335.

Zweifach BW and Silberberg A (1979). The interstitial-lymphatic flow system. In: *International Review of Physiology, Vol. 18.* Guyton AC and Young DB (eds.). Baltimore: University Park Press, pp. 215–260.

CHAPTER 13

# Regional Pressure and Nutrition of Skeletal Muscle during Isometric Contraction

Ole M. Sejersted and Alan R. Hargens

## Introduction

Skeletal muscle constitutes about 40% of human body weight and is highly adaptable to short-term and long-term activity levels with respect to its metabolism and performance (Saltin and Gollnick, 1983). As a response to the increase in power output in short-term adaptation, exercising skeletal muscle can increase its metabolic rate 50 times that at rest. On the other hand, with continued long-term overloading, enlargement of cross-sectional area of individual fiber exemplifies another type of metabolic adaptation. It is generally agreed that increased physical activity raises muscle mass by increased fiber areas rather than increased fiber numbers (Gollnick et al., 1981). On the other hand, disuse reduces areas of individual fibers as opposed to a reduction of fiber number.

For any type of adaptation it is important that the metabolic needs of the muscle are met by proper supply of nutrients. In this respect short-term regulation includes a high vasodilatory capacity, whereas on a long-term basis the number of capillaries surrounding each fiber can be changed (Ingjer, 1979; Hudlicka, 1980). Little is known about mechanical factors that might affect blood supply to the working muscle. Some mechanical factors may be subject to alterations, for instance, in relation to changes in muscle geometry, fiber stress and muscle mass both during short-term and long-term adaptations. Since vessels are squeezed and blood flow is reduced during contraction (Sadamoto et al., 1983), it is generally agreed that isometric work is mostly dependent on anaerobic ATP production (Tønnesen, 1964; Lassen and Kampp, 1965; Mortimer et al., 1971). This is clearly an oversimplification since tolerance to isometric work is highly variable between individuals and between different muscles. On the other hand, dynamic exercise allows blood to flow intermittently during each relaxation phase. Because transmural pressure is one important determinant of vessel diameter and resistance to flow, knowledge of the tissue fluid pressure at rest (Guyton et al., 1971) and during contraction is fundamental for proper analysis of the regional flow patterns. In this chapter we examine some recent measurements of intramuscular fluid pressure in the human vastus lateralis muscle (Sejersted et al., 1984). These measurements allow some predictions of pressure development during muscle contraction as a function of fiber geometry. Fiber geometry will change with acute, muscle-length shortening and with chronic hypertrophy or atrophy. Hence, profiles of intramuscular fluid pressure are probably modified by both short-term and long-term adaptation of skeletal muscle. Since regional intramuscular fluid pressure and blood supply vary considerably within a muscle during contraction, the use of muscle biopsies for metabolic studies of exercising muscle might give more variable results than previously expected, especially during isometric work.

Another important consideration is whether intramuscular fluid pressure can be used as a parameter of local function (force generation). Classically, two indirect techniques have been used to quantitate contraction force of human muscles. Electromyographic (EMG) activity, measured by needle electrodes in the muscle under study, rises in proportion to contraction strength. However, a recent report by Andriacchi and coworkers (1982) indicates that EMG activity is not a linear function of contraction force at high isometric loads. Training also reduces the integrated EMG/tension at submaximal levels of isometric contraction (Komi et al., 1978), and muscle temperature and fatigue influence the EMG waveform (Petrofsky, 1979). Alternatively, measurement of isometric torque across a joint is even less reliable than EMG studies because more than one muscle contributes to the generation of torque. By interpreting intramuscular fluid pressure with the law of Laplace, we recently evaluated intramuscular fluid pressure as a measure of local fiber stress or contraction force (Sejersted et al., 1984).

Previous studies demonstrated that intramuscular fluid pressure increases linearly with submaximal isometric contraction force (Mazzella, 1954; Hargens et al., 1981; Saltin et al., 1981; Kirkebø and Wisnes, 1982; Sadamoto et al., 1983). Although Hill (1948) was among the first to note that internal stress or pressure increases with muscle contraction, subsequent studies revealed great variability in this pressure development within a given muscle and between muscles at a given force of muscle contraction (Saltin et al., 1981; Kirkebø and Wisnes, 1982). This variability is explicable in terms of the relationship between fiber geometry and local fluid pressure, and might have important consequences for short-term and long-term muscle nutrition and for development of fatigue due to inadequate perfusion.

## Intramuscular Pressures with Contraction

Our recent studies of intramuscular fluid pressure during isometric contraction (Sejersted et al., 1984) were performed on seven normal male volunteers. Human subjects are best for these experiments because they cooperate well and various levels of contraction can be maintained constant over extended periods of time. Our subjects' ages ranged between 18 and 34 years, and both sedentary and well-trained individuals were included. Each subject was informed of the details of all experimental procedures and written, informed consent was obtained. This study was previously approved by the Ethics Committee of the Institute of Muscle Physiology, Oslo, Norway.

Each subject generated isometric contraction of his quadriceps muscles while sitting in a chair apparatus (Fig. 13.1). Symmetrical and equal contraction of the quadriceps muscles of both legs was elicited by attaching a force transducer (positioned below and behind each subject) to the axle of a wheel, over which a wire was connected to cuffs secured to each ankle. The force transducer was connected to a four-channel Gould recorder and separately to a Tarkan recorder that was visible to each subject, allowing him to maintain a predetermined level of isometric force.

Intramuscular fluid pressure was continuously recorded in the vastus medialis muscle by one or more polyethylene catheters (Fig. 13.2). After injection of 1 ml lidocaine anesthesia in skin and fascia overlying the muscle, an intravenous placement unit was inserted into the muscle. The placement unit was inserted at about a 45° angle and advanced 5 to 6 cm toward the patella and parallel with muscle fibers within the vastus medialis. After fully retracting the inner steel trocar, the pressure-measuring

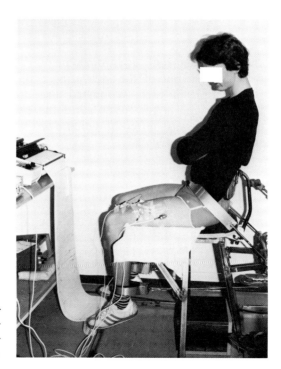

**Figure 13.1.** Position of subject for studies of intramuscular fluid pressure during isometric extension of the knee.

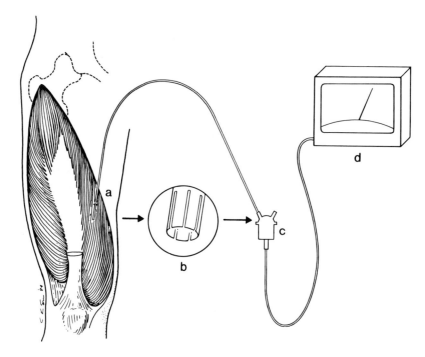

**Figure 13.2.** Measurement of intramuscular fluid pressure: (a) insertion of plastic catheter into midportion of vastus medialis; (b) close-up view of slit catheter tip; (c) low-volume displacement pressure transducer, and (d) recorder.

catheter was introduced through the outer plastic shield. Then air bubbles were flushed out of the measuring catheter prior to retraction of the shielding plastic tube. We tested three types of catheters (PE-50 wick, PE-50 slit and larger PE-60 slit catheters) and three different pressure transducers with different volume-displacement and frequency of response characteristics.

## Catheter-Transducer Optimization

In vitro studies demonstrated that the larger PE-60 slit catheter had the best frequency response to a 15 mm Hg step increase in hydrostatic pressure (Fig. 13.3). However, either slit catheter (PE-50 or PE-60) is suitable for studies of MVC in which maximum force is developed in about 1 s and is maintained for 2 to 3 s. However, wick catheters are unsuitable for studies of MVC and for any muscular contraction that lasts for less than 1 min. This latter result supports an earlier study by Baumann and associates (1979).

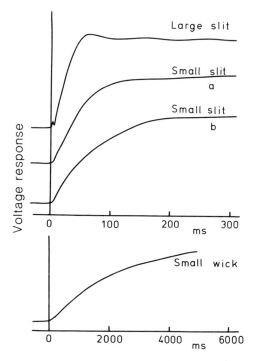

**Figure 13.3.** Responses to a 15 mm Hg pressure step with three different catheters about 20 cm long connected to a low-volume displacement AE 840 pressure transducer. The large-slit catheter (PE 60, inner diameter 0.76 mm) had four or five slits 2 to 3 mm long at the tip. The delay time to reach 50% of maximal response ($t_{delay}$) was 23 ms, and the rise time ($t_{rise}$) from 10% to 90% of maximal response was about 35 ms. Two curves are shown for the small-slit catheter (PE 50, inner diameter 0.53 mm) with four or five slits about 1.5 mm long at the tip. The values for $t_{delay}$ and $t_{rise}$ were 20 and 90 ms, respectively, after filling the dome and catheter with $CO_2$ before flushing with gas-free water (curve a). After ordinary flush of an air-filled system, $t_{rise}$ is 50 ms longer (curve b) due to presence of small invisible air bubbles. The wick catheter contains a small Dexon wick at the tip and $t_{rise}$ is very long. (From OM Sejersted et al., 1984.)

## In Vivo Tests

Catheters were checked for free movement of fluid between the muscle tissue and saline-filled catheter line (Fig. 13.4). To test if clots or kinks obstructed fluid movements during in vivo recordings, several tests were performed. Figure 13.4A indicates the build-up of resting pressures after closure of the three-way stopcock positioned on the outlet opposite to the catheter on the transducer dome. When contraction was started before closure of the stopcock, intramuscular fluid leaks out. When the stopcock

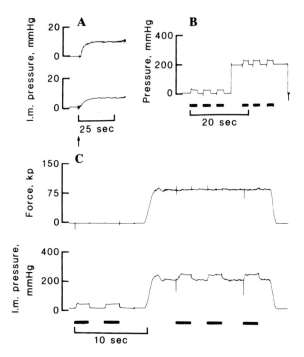

**Figure 13.4.** In vivo tests of catheter performance. **A:** Pressure recording by two slit catheters from a *resting* muscle. After insertion of the catheters, the stopcock on the transducer dome, connected to the outlet opposite to the catheters, was left open so that fluid could leak out freely from the muscle through the catheters and the dome. After closure of the stopcock, pressure builds up in the course of 5 to 12 s. **B, C:** Comparison of pressure responses to infusion of isotonic saline at a rate of 70 μl/s through a PE 60 slit catheter in vitro **(B)** and in vivo **(C)**. Infusion (noted by *dark underlines*) was performed by a syringe pump against zero or resting pressures and against 200 mm Hg obtained by a water column or by muscular contraction. (From OM Sejersted et al., 1984.)

was subsequently closed, pressure rose slowly, but in contrast to the resting conditions never reached plateau before the subject was exhausted. This fluid was only slowly replaced within the muscle. A further test for free fluid communication was easily carried out by compressing and decompressing the catheter. If, during compression, fluid was squeezed into the muscle, a pressure drop and slow return to precompression levels was registered on removing the clamp.

Infusion of sterile saline to a rate of 70 μl/s through the pressure transducer in vitro raised the recorded pressure by about 25 mm Hg. With the catheter tip inside the muscle, the recorded increment in pressure by identical injections was about the same as in vitro both at rest and during contraction (Fig. 13.4C). Thus, the compliance of the intramuscular fluid compartment is so high that the resistance of the catheters dominates the pressure response to continuous infusions. To obtain a true estimate of the pressure rise within the muscle, the experiment was therefore repeated, but isotonic saline was now injected through a separate channel (Fig. 13.5). An infusion rate of 120 μl/s raised resting pressure by <5 mm Hg, but at 30% of MVC (125 mm Hg), the pressure rise was five times greater. Pressure response closely followed infusion rate (Fig. 13.5). Even the injection of several milliliters of fluid did not cause long-lasting elevations of either apparent resting pressures or contraction pressures. Finally, fluid communication was also tested by gentle digital compression of the thigh.

Leakage of fluid along the outside of the catheters did not occur during contraction, since initial peaks or pressure decline during constant force was rarely seen. Such recordings were omitted. However, injected fluid accumulated subcutaneously during rest in some cases.

## Intramuscular Fluid Pressure-Contraction Force

Contractions were performed with 2 to 3 min rest periods between decreasing and subsequently increasing force (Fig. 13.6). The coefficient of variation for repetitive pressure recordings at unchanged force was <7%.

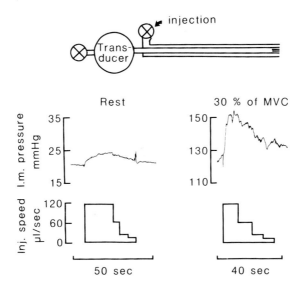

**Figure 13.5.** Responses of intramuscular fluid pressure to graded injection of isotonic fluid through a catheter separate from the pressure recording catheter as shown at top. Injection rate was reduced in steps and the pressure responses at rest and during contraction (30% MVC) are depicted. The opening of the outer plastic sheath was sealed with epoxy glue. MVC is maximum voluntary contraction. (From OM Sejersted et al., 1984.)

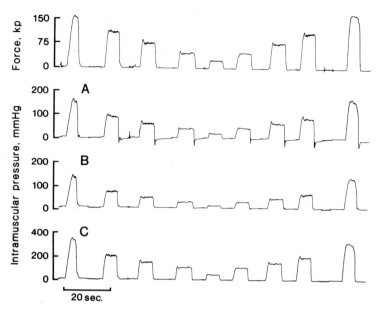

**Figure 13.6.** Original tracings of force and three intramuscular pressure recordings in the right human vastus medialis muscle (representative recordings). With subject sitting in the chair apparatus, extension force was recorded at the ankle. The first and last contractions represent MVC, and 3- to 5-min rest periods intervened between each contraction. The lower contraction forces were predetermined at 70%, 50%, 30% and 15% of MVC. Pressure was recorded by: **(A)** Millar Mikrotip pressure transducer, **(B)** Bentley Trantec transducer and **(C)** AE 840 transducer. (From OM Sejersted et al., 1984.)

Figure 13.6 also illustrates the pressure variations within the muscle during contraction. On relaxation, resting pressures were rapidly obtained. Even during very rapid contractions, force and pressure rose in parallel.

The relationship between relative contraction force and intramuscular fluid pressure measured with three different recording systems was linear, but the slope varied greatly (Fig. 13.7). Varying slopes were also present when pressures were plotted against the absolute force. It seemed that catheters positioned close to the femur gave the highest pressures, whereas very low or almost no responses were obtained just beneath the fascia. The highest pressure obtained equalled 570 mm Hg at MVC in tissue near the femur.

All pressure recording systems performed equally well, but insertion of the Millar Mikro-tip catheter was somewhat painful. Further, this pressure transducer could not be zeroed during the experiment and often drifted slightly. Therefore, the slit catheters connected to extracorporeal transducers were preferred.

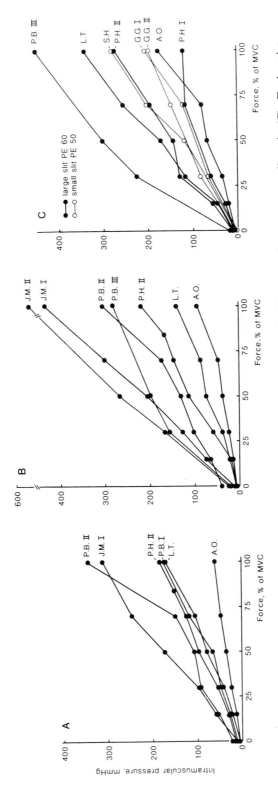

**Figure 13.7.** Relationships between relative contraction force and intramuscular fluid pressure as recorded by: **(A)** Millar Mikro-tip transducer, **(B)** Bentley Trantec transducer and **(C)** AE 840 transducer. Two transducers (**B** and **C**) were connected to large-slit catheters (PE 60) except for some recordings in (**C**). Each point represents the mean of four or five contractions. Initials for the subjects are indicated, and some of them (e.g., PB I and PB II) participated more than once. (From OM Sejersted et al., 1984.)

271

The reason for the great variation in the pressure/force relationship was more systematically explored by measuring resting and contraction pressures at different depths in the muscle. No attempt was made to estimate the exact perpendicular depth from the fascia to the catheter tip. Nevertheless, Figure 13.8 demonstrates that contraction pressures declined linearly with decreasing distance from the point where the catheters penetrated the muscle fascia. Resting pressures did not vary systematically.

Another factor contributing to intramuscular pressure variability could be unequal recruitment of different parts of the muscle. According to Figures 13.6 and 13.8, this was probably not the case during contractions lasting up to 5 s. However, Figure 13.9 indicates that during prolonged contraction, local fluid pressure at one point in the muscle indeed varied greatly. There was no definite trend in average intramuscular pressure. The actual fluid pressure varied with at least two frequencies. There were rapid oscillations (<5 mm Hg) which seemed to parallel variations in contraction force. In addition, there were large pressure variations (15–20 mm Hg or 50–60% of the highest recorded pressure) with a frequency of about 1/min. This latter variation was not parallel to any variation in contraction force.

Another subject was asked to maintain one of the pressure recordings at a constant level (Fig. 13.10). His contraction lasted 2 min before exhaustion. The contraction force fell steadily by almost 30%, and the other pressure recording showed great variability which was unrelated to force.

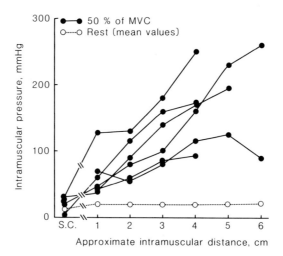

**Figure 13.8.** Relationship between intramuscular distance and intramuscular fluid pressure recorded at rest and during contraction at 50% of MVC. The slit catheters were withdrawn in steps of 1 cm and gently flushed with 0.05 to 0.10 ml sterile, isotonic saline before each new recording. S.C. represents pressure measured in subcutaneous tissue. (From OM Sejersted et al., 1984.)

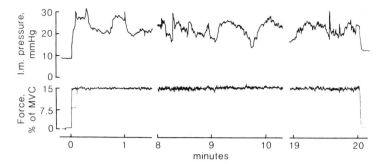

**Figure 13.9.** Intramuscular fluid pressure at constant force of 15% of MVC. Pressure was recorded with a slit catheter and contraction maintained for 20 min until exhaustion. (From OM Sejersted et al., 1984.)

At this contraction force, the slow oscillations observed in Figure 13.9 were almost absent.

## Anatomy of Vastus Medialis Muscle

Muscle fibers of the distal part of the muscle arise from a tendon sheet attached to the linea aspera. The same tendon sheet serves as an attachment for the adductor magnus muscle. The outermost fibers arise from the superficial fascia. Fibers run in a parallel fashion at an angle of about 45° to the axis of the femur and are organized in layers parallel to the muscle surface. The layers are interspaced by loose connective tissue. The fibers

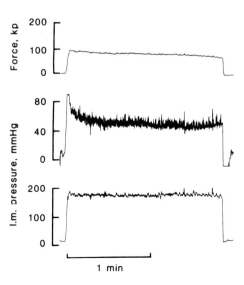

**Figure 13.10.** Force and one intramuscular (i.m.) fluid pressure recording **(upper two panels)** while the other pressure recorded **(lower panel)** was intentionally kept constant by the subject. Contraction was maintained until exhaustion (about 2 min). (From OM Sejersted et al., 1984.)

are attached to the medial retinaculum of the patella. The outer muscle layers are curved, whereas the deeper fibers follow a straight course. However, during contraction the fibers will be forced to adapt to the curvature of the femur. The radius of curvature during contraction can be roughly estimated as 15 to 20 cm.

## Relationship of Intramuscular Fluid Pressure and EMG to Isometric Contraction Force

Recent studies of the biceps brachii muscle indicate that both intramuscular fluid pressure and EMG increase linearly with contraction force (Körner et al., 1984*a*). Although no attempt was made to study the effects of muscle depth on pressure and EMG, very high correlation coefficients (r > 0.96) were obtained for both intramuscular fluid pressure (Fig. 13.11) and EMG (Fig. 13.12) as a function of isometric load in a given subject. Parker and associates (1984) find that intramuscular pressure correlates well with varying isometric loads even during fatigue (Figs. 13.13 and 13.14). On the other hand, the correlation between EMG and load deteriorates with fatigue (Fig. 13.14). Finally, recovery of the mean frequency of EMG signal is poor at pressure levels exceeding 20 mm Hg (Körner et al., 1984*b*). Körner and collaborators conclude that localized muscle fatigue may occur in muscle regions with pressures exceeding 20 mm Hg during contraction.

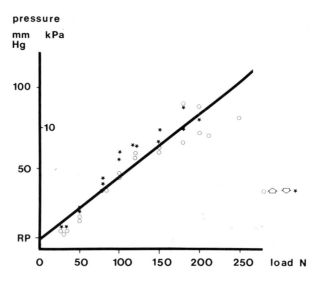

**Figure 13.11.** Relationship between intramuscular fluid pressure and forearm load in a given subject. *Circles* represent increasing loads; *stars* represent decreasing loads. RP, resting pressure. (From L Körner et al., 1984*a*.)

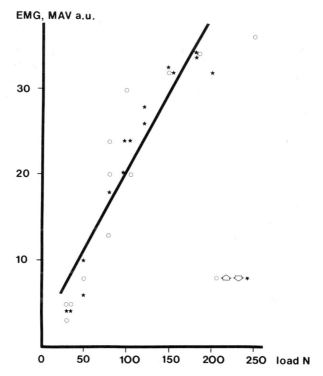

**Figure 13.12.** Relationship between EMG and forelimb load in same subject as Figure 13.11. *Circles* represent increasing loads; *stars* represent decreasing loads. (From L Körner et al., 1984*a*.)

The loads and corresponding pressures were higher in our study of the vastus medialis (Sejersted et al., 1984) than in the study of biceps brachii (Körner et al., 1984*a*). However, the loads in the former were placed on all four quadricep muscles. In addition, as outlined below, differences in fiber geometry could explain why intramuscular pressures may differ widely even if fiber stresses are equal.

## Mechanisms of Muscle Pressure Generation

Local intramuscular pressure is thus a linear function of isometric contraction force at submaximal as well as maximal levels of voluntary contraction. The great variability of intramuscular pressures at a given level of isometric contraction is primarily due to the depth dependence of tissue fluid pressure in skeletal muscle. The general applicability of our data depends on whether they can be extrapolated to other muscles.

In the normal vastus medialis the steep pressure gradient from deep to

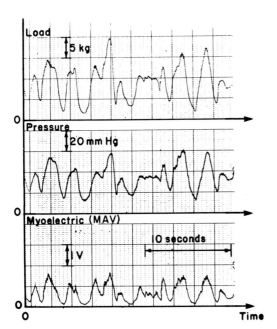

**Figure 13.13.** Typical tracking experiment to evaluate correlations of intramuscular pressure and myoelectric signals with isometric load of the biceps brachii. (From P Parker et al., 1984.)

peripheral tissues and the low pressures beneath the fascia during contraction suggest that fasciae contribute little to pressure development. In contrast, in the tibialis anterior muscle the tense fascia may be responsible for pressures during contraction (Garfin et al., 1981) and the homogenously elevated intramuscular fluid pressure in the compartment syndrome (Hargens et al., 1977, 1979; Mubarak and Hargens, 1981). Thus, in

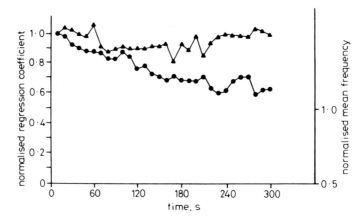

**Figure 13.14.** During fatigue, regression coefficient for intramuscular pressure as an estimate of load (▲) remains near unity whereas regression coefficient for myoelectric signal (●) deteriorates with time. Data are averaged for biceps brachii of nine human subjects. (From P Parker et al., 1984.)

general the depth dependence of pressure presently found is restricted to muscles that are not confined to an inexpandable compartment.

However, even when taking into account the depth dependence of pressure one gets the impression that pressures at the same depth and at about the same relative force are not the same in different muscles. High pressures have been reported by several authors in the vastus medialis during contraction (Sylvest and Hvid, 1959; Edwards et al., 1972; Sejersted et al., 1984), whereas in the biceps muscle, pressures are lower by a factor of 10 (Körner et al., 1984a). None of these studies gives exact information on recording depth. Nevertheless, it seems to be another factor than muscle thickness and fiber stress which also determines contraction pressure at a given depth.

To approach this problem the relationship between pressure and fiber stress was interpreted in terms of the law of Laplace. The consequence of the application of this law is that the radius of fiber curvature is an important determinant of pressure. This was in fact stated by Hill (1948), who suggested that high fluid pressure is caused by the curved muscle fibers exerting an inward pressure during contraction. Hence, the pressure at any position in a muscle with one distinct fiber direction will be:

$$P = P_o + n \cdot \Delta h \cdot s/r,$$

where $P_o$ is the pressure under the fascia, $n$ is the number of muscle layers with definite thickness $\Delta h$, $s$ is the fiber stress and $r$ is the radius of the fiber curvature. Thus, another factor that would explain differences in absolute pressures is the curving of the fibers (Sejersted et al., 1984).

In resting muscle the fiber curvature in general is not very prominent. However, when the muscle is shortened, the muscle volume is maintained and consequently the muscle circumference will increase. Due to the inelasticity of tendons and skeleton, the fibers cannot be separated at their outspring or insertion. Hence, the increased circumference must be accompanied by increased curving of the fibers (Fig. 13.15A). For an idealized spindle-shaped muscle, the curvature of the fibers is delineated as a function of muscle length in Figure 13.15B. Independent of the initial fiber curvature, muscle shortening of 20% (probably close to the working range for human muscles) will decrease the radius of fiber curvature by 50%. Even though this is a theoretical construct, fiber curvature will decrease relatively more than the degree of shortening. The vastus medialis muscle must, in addition, comply to the curvature of the femur. The prediction made from these calculations on a muscle model is that pressure during contraction at any point in the muscle will be higher by a factor close to two when the muscle is shortened by 20%.

The theoretical relationship between radius of curvature and intramuscular fluid pressure at different radii is shown in Figure 13.15C. For isometric contractions, pressures will follow one of the straight lines; whereas during muscle shortening, the radius will decrease and the slope

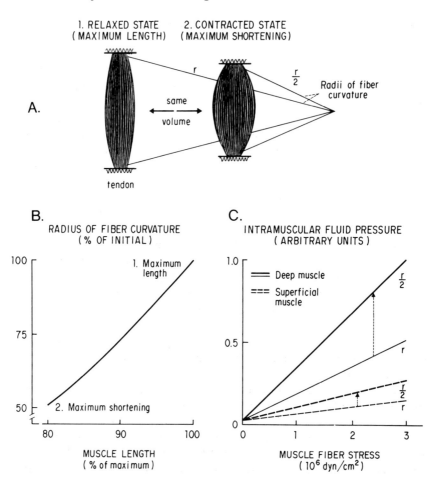

**Figure 13.15.** During contraction, muscle shortening could cause greater fiber curvature, at least in outermost muscular layers **(A)**. For an idealized spindle-shaped muscle with one fiber direction and similar curvature for all fibers, the radius of fiber curvature is reduced by one-half with a 20% shortening of the skeletal muscle **(B)**, assuming isovolumetric conditions during the contraction (shortening). This relationship is independent of the absolute radius of fiber curvature or muscle length. Therefore, there is a linear relationship between intramuscular fluid pressure and fiber stress at different radii of curvature, and hence different muscular depths **(C)**. *Dashed arrows* indicate the maximum rise of intramuscular fluid pressure if a muscle is allowed to shorten by 20% during an isotonic contraction (constant fiber stress).

of the pressure-stress relationship will be steeper as indicated. In some muscles the radius of fiber curvature may approach infinity and muscle fibers may also be parallel during contraction so that very little pressure develops. Clearly, detailed analysis of fiber geometry and intramuscular pressures might reveal differences between muscles with consequences for their function and endurance.

One important outgrowth of our studies concerns predicting which muscles or which part of a muscle can maintain blood perfusion during contraction. Wisnes and Kirkebø (1976) demonstrated that blood flow to inner muscle zones was decreased more than that in superficial regions during sustained contraction. Petrofsky and associates (1981) noted that in cat soleus muscle, as opposed to the gastrocnemius muscle, blood flow was well maintained during isometric contraction. Different blood flow patterns may exist during dynamic exercise (Laughlin and Armstrong, 1982). In a later study, Petrofsky and Hendershot (1984) demonstrated that pressures in the cat gastrocnemius in general are twice as high as those in the soleus. This observation also coincides with longer endurance times of the soleus during isometric contractions. It is generally recognized that the microcirculation is compromized at an intramuscular pressure of about 30 mm Hg (Hargens et al., 1978; Hargens, 1981; Mubarak and Hargens, 1981). This pressure might not be reached even at maximum force in some muscles, but it is clearly reached deep in the vastus medialis at 10% to 15% of MVC in some subjects. Anaerobic conditions lead to accumulation of both lactate and potassium (Vyskočil et al., 1983) in the interstitial space. Their accumulation may activate free nerve endings and represent the afferent signal to sympathetic stimulation (Rybicki et al., 1984) and pain sensations. In accordance with this concept of local accumulation of lactate and potassium, the results of Parker and co-workers (1984) indicate that regional recovery of sarcolemnal electrical properties is prevented at maintained high pressures. Even though localized fatigue might not be sufficient to affect the power output of a whole muscle, we propose that fatigue can be experienced even though it is present in only a small region of muscle.

On the basis of the above arguments, we hypothesize that isometric work is endured for a longer time with a slender than with a bulging muscle, and that isometric work is better performed with the muscle stretched than shortened. Maximum fiber stress is, of course, dependent on the length–force relationship which should also be taken into consideration. Thus the same fiber stress is only achieved at a higher relative force when the muscle is stretched.

Another important finding of our recent results, which modifies the above predictions, is that local tissue fluid pressure oscillates considerably at prolonged low-percentage MVC despite the fact that isometric force is maintained constant. Such oscillations may provide a mechanism whereby one low-pressure region of the muscle receives relatively high microcirculatory flow while a neighboring high-pressure zone is ischemic.

The great variability in pressure and the pressure gradient within the muscle has important consequences also for the experimentalist. Muscle biopsies obtained during isometric contractions may originate from a perfused or a nonperfused region within the muscle, depending on the depth from which the biopsy was taken. Hence, the high variability in lactate accumulation during isometric contraction as reported by Karlsson (1971) may be explained in terms of the pressure-flow relationship. Further, fluid pressure gradients within the muscle will cause local fluid transfer. Hence, washout techniques for measuring blood flow must take into account this phenomenon. The low flow estimates obtained by the Xe-133 washout technique (Cerettelli et al., 1984) might be caused by fluid movements in the interstitium.

Finally we would like to comment on intramuscular pressure as a measure of local fiber stress. With knowledge of recording depth and fiber geometry and fiber curvature, the law of Laplace would allow calculation of local fiber stress on the basis of pressure measurements. Such information is rarely available. However, changes in pressure during one recording certainly reflect local fiber stress and this observation explains the good relationship between EMG and pressure observed by Körner and co-workers (1984a). Further, repetitive measurements in one subject at the same depth in the same muscle probably also allow conclusions about changes in local fiber stress, for example, as a consequence of training.

## Summary

This chapter evaluates intramuscular fluid pressure as a function of contraction force and examines the implications of these pressures in light of nutritional blood-flow patterns during exercise in normal human subjects. Intramuscular fluid pressure was continuously recorded at various percentages of maximum voluntary contraction (percent MVC) using various tissue catheters at various tissue depths within the vastus medialis. Slit catheters yielded the highest frequency response. Mean maximum, isometric-contraction force was simultaneously recorded in a chair apparatus with ankle connected to a calibrated force transducer. Intramuscular pressure (range 0–600 mm Hg) correlated well with percent MVC at low, medium and high isometric contraction states but the slope of the pressure-force relationship was highly variable. Much of the variability of intramuscular pressure, both within the same muscle and between subjects at all percent MVC, was related to catheter depth. Pressure was a direct function of intramuscular depth. During long-term isometric contraction of low percent MVC, intramuscular pressure remained constant initially but oscillatory pressures were observed in several subjects just prior to fatigue. Other investigators find that pressure is more representative of muscle load than EMG during fatigue. The highest recorded pressure at MVC was 570 mm Hg near the femur surface. Intramuscular fluid pressure obeys the Laplace law and regional microcirculatory blood flow is probably lower in deeper tissues than in superficial muscle during isometric contraction. Assuming isovolumetric contraction effects a maximal 20% shortening of muscle fibers, the radius of fiber curvature may decrease by 50% and intramuscular pressure will consequently increase more in deeper than in superficial tissues. These considerations have broad application to: (1) overall muscle nutrition during exercise, (2) occurrence of and adaptations to fatigue in local tissue regions, (3) variability of metabolites in biopsy specimens and (4) use of intramuscular pressure as an index of local muscle function.

## Acknowledgments

The study was supported by the Council for Working Environment, Ministry of Local Government and Labor, Oslo, Norway and by the Veterans Administration and by USPHS/NIH grants AM-25501 and AM 26344 and a Research Career Development Award AM-00602 to ARH.

## References

Andriacchi TP, Anderson GBJ, Bjork R and Ortengren R (1982). A study of the relationship between external moments and myoelectric activity about the knee. *Trans Orthop Res Soc* 7:exhibit 255.
Baumann JU, Sutherland DH and Hanggi A (1979). Intramuscular pressure during walking: an experimental study using the wick catheter technique. *Clin Orthop* 145:292–299.
Cerettelli P, Marconi C, Pendergast D, Meyer M, Heisler N and Piiper J (1984). Blood flow in exercising muscles by xenon clearance and by microspheric trapping. *J Appl Physiol Respir Environ Exercise Physiol* 56:24–30.
Edwards RHT, Hill DK and McDonnell M (1972). Myothermal and intramuscular pressure measurements during isometric contractions of the human quadriceps muscle (abstr). *J Physiol (Lond)* 224:58P–59P.
Garfin SR, Tipton CM, Mubarak SJ, Woo S.L-Y, Hargens AR and Akeson WH (1981). Role of fascia in maintainance of muscle tension and pressure. *J Appl Physiol Respir Environ Exercise Physiol* 51(2):317–320.
Gollnick PD, Timson BF, Moore RL and Riedy M (1981). Muscular enlargement and the number of fibers in the skeletal muscle of rats. *J Appl Physiol Respir Environ Exercise Physiol* 50:936–943.
Guyton AC, Granger HJ and Taylor AE (1971). Interstitial fluid pressure. *Physiol Rev* 51:527–563.
Hargens AR (ed.) (1981). *Tissue Fluid Pressure and Composition.* Baltimore: Williams & Wilkins, 275 pp.

Hargens AR, Akeson WH, Mubarak SJ, Owen CA, Evans KL, Garetto LP, Gonsalves MR and Schmidt DA (1978). Fluid balance within canine anterolateral compartments and its relationship to compartment syndromes. *J Bone Joint Surg* 60A:499–505.

Hargens AR, Gomez MA, Evans KL, Tipton CM and Akeson WH (1981). Correlation of interstitial fluid pressure and contraction force in canine skeletal muscle. *Bibl Anat* 20:260–262.

Hargens AR, Mubarak SJ, Owen CA, Garetto LP and Akeson WH (1977). Interstitial fluid pressure in muscle and compartment syndromes in man. *Microvasc Res* 14:1–10.

Hargens AR, Romine JS, Sipe JC, Evans KL, Mubarak SJ and Akeson WH (1979). Peripheral nerve-conduction block by high muscle-compartment pressure. *J Bone Joint Surg* 61A:192–200.

Hargens AR, Schmidt DA, Evans KL, Gonsalves MR, Cologne JB, Garfin SR, Mubarak SJ, Hagen PL and Akeson WH (1981). Quantitation of skeletal-muscle necrosis in a model compartment syndrome. *J Bone Joint Surg* 63A:631–636.

Hill AV (1948). The pressure developed in muscle during contraction. *J Physiol (Lond)* 107:518–556.

Hudlicka O (1980). Effect of training on macro- and microcirculation changes in exercise. *Exercise Sport Sci Rev* 6:181–230.

Ingjer F (1979). Effects of endurance training on muscle fiber ATPase activity, capillary supply, and mitochondrial content in man. *J Physiol (Lond)* 294:419–422.

Karlsson J (1971). Lactate and phosphage concentrations in working muscle of man with special reference to oxygen deficit at the onset of work. *Acta Physiol Scand Suppl* 358:25–30.

Kirkebø A and Wisnes A (1982). Regional tissue fluid pressure in rat calf muscle during sustained contraction or stretch. *Acta Physiol Scand* 114:551–556.

Komi PV, Viitasalo JT, Rauramaa R and Vihko V (1978). Effect of isometric strength training on mechanical, electrical, and metabolic aspects of muscle function. *Eur J Appl Physiol* 40:45–55.

Körner L, Parker P, Almström C, Andersson GBJ, Herberts P, Kadefors R, Palmerud G and Zetterberg C (1984a). Relation of intramuscular pressure to the force output and myoelectric signal of skeletal muscle. *J Orthop Res* 2:289–296.

Körner L, Parker P, Almstrom C, Herberts P and Kadefors R (1984b). The relation between spectral changes of the myoelectric signal and the intramuscular pressure of human skeletal muscle. *Eur J Appl Physiol* 52:202–206.

Lassen NA and Kampp M (1965). Calf muscle blood flow studied during walking studied by the $Xe^{133}$ method in normals and in patients with intermittent claudication. *Scand J Clin Lab Invest* 17:447–453.

Laughlin MH and Armstrong RB (1982). Muscular blood flow distribution patterns as a function of running speed in rats. *Am J Physiol* 243:H296–H306.

Mazzella H (1954). On the pressure developed by the contraction of striated muscle and its influence on muscular circulation. *Arch Int Physiol* 63:334–347.

Mortimer JT, Kerstein MD, Magnusson R and Petersen I (1971). Muscle blood flow in the human biceps as a function of developed muscle force. *Arch Surg* 103:376–377.

Mubarak SJ and Hargens AR (1981). *Compartment Syndromes and Volkmann's Contracture*. Philadelphia: WB Saunders, pp. 1–232.

Parker P, Körner L and Kadefors R (1984). Estimator of muscle force from transducer total pressure. *Med Biol Eng Comput* 22:453–457.

Petrofsky JS (1979). Frequency and amplitude analysis of the EMG during exercise on the bicycle ergometer. *Eur J Appl Physiol* 41:1–15.

Petrofsky JS and Hendershot DM (1984). The interrelationship between blood pressure, intramuscular pressure, and isometric endurance in fast and slow twitch skeletal muscle in the cat. *Eur J Appl Physiol* 53:106–111.

Petrofsky JS, Phillips CA, Sawka MN, Hanpeter D and Stafford D (1981). Blood flow and metabolism during isometric contraction in cat skeletal muscle. *J Appl Physiol Respir Environ Exercise Physiol* 50:493–502.

Rybicki KJ, Kaufman MP, Kenyon JL and Mitchell JH (1984). Arterial pressure responses to increasing interstitial potassium in hindlimb muscle of dogs. *Am J Physiol* 247:R717–R721.

Sadamoto T, Bonde-Petersen F and Suzuki Y (1983). Skeletal muscle tension, flow, pressure, and EMG during sustained isometric contractions in humans. *Eur J Appl Physiol* 51:395–408.

Saltin B and Gollnick PD (1983). Skeletal muscle adaptability: significance for metabolism and performance. In: *Handbook of Physiology, Section 10: Skeletal Muscle*. Peachey LD, Adrian RH and Geiger SR. Bethesda, Maryland: American Physiological Society, pp. 555–631.

Saltin B, Sjøgaard G, Gaffny FA and Rowell LB (1981). Potassium, lactate, and water fluxes in human quadriceps muscle during static contractions. *Circ Res* 48 (*Suppl I*) 18–24.

Sejersted OM, Hargens AR, Kardel KR, Blom P, Jensen O, and Hermansen L (1984). Intramuscular fluid pressure during isometric contraction of human skeletal muscle. *J Appl Physiol Respir Environ Exercise Physiol* 56:287–295.

Skalak R (1982). Approximate formulas for myocardial fiber stresses. *J Biomech Eng* 104:162–163.

Sylvest O and Hvid N (1959). Pressure measurements in human striated muscles during contraction. *Acta Rheum Scand* 5:216–222.

Tønnesen KH (1964). Blood flow through muscle during rhythmic contraction measured by $^{133}$Xenon. *Scand J Clin Lab Invest* 16:646–654.

Vyskočil F, Hnik P, Rehfeldt H, Vejsada R and Ujec E (1983). The measurement of $K_e^+$ concentration changes in human muscles during volitional contractions. *Pflügers Arch* 399:235–237.

Wisnes A and Kirkebø A (1976). Regional distribution of blood flow in calf muscles of rat during passive stretch and sustained contraction. *Acta Physiol Scand* 96:256–266.

Wisnes A and Kirkebø A (1982). Regional tissue fluid pressure in rat calf muscle during sustained contraction or stretch. *Acta Physiol Scand* 114:551–556.

# CHAPTER 14

# Hyperbaric Oxygen and Tissue Viability

## Michael B. Strauss and George B. Hart

## Introduction

Hyperbaric oxygen (HBO) is a therapy that has recognized effects on blood flow and the viability of ischemic tissue. A pressurized vessel of the monoplace or multiplace variety is required to administer HBO. The monoplace chamber is pressurized with oxygen and the patient breathes the pure gas directly. In the multiplace chamber the vessel is pressurized with air and the patient breathes pure oxygen through a mask. HBO treatment regimens vary depending on the mode of treatment, the disorder, the intended goals and the age of the patient. Treatment pressures are usually between 1.5 and 3 atmospheres absolute (ATA) pressure. Treatment durations are from 1 to 2 h. They may be repeated as frequently as every 4 h or as infrequently as once per day.

During the past decade, clinical use of HBO increased rapidly. Relief of tissue hypoxia and reduction in swelling are the common denominators in its use. Unfortunately, until recently the justification for using HBO to improve tissue viability was based on the clinical observations that it seemed to work. Refinements in methods to measure oxygen tensions and intracompartmental fluid pressures make it possible to document the value of HBO. This chapter discusses the physiology and physics of HBO and the role of HBO in clinical situations where tissue viability is threatened because of hypoxia.

## Background

Hyperbaric therapy has a history of longer than 300 years. Henshaw in 1662 was the first to use hyperbaric therapy (Jacobson et al., 1965). He believed elevated barometric pressures alleviated acute diseases. By the middle of the 19th century hyperbaric chambers had become very popular in Europe. "Compressed air baths," considered an item of luxury, flourished. Unfortunately, little attention was given to documenting the benefits or understanding the mechanisms. In the 1920s Cunningham (1927) believed that elevated partial pressures of oxygen were useful in treating hypoxic conditions. Unfortunately, his work was censured by the American Medical Association because he believed conditions such as cancer, syphilis and diabetes mellitus were caused by anaerobic organisms.

Hyperbaric therapy remained in a state of dormancy until 1960 when Boerema and his associates (1960) verified that physically dissolved oxygen achieved through hyperbaric exposures could sustain life in the absence of hemoglobin-borne oxygen. This discovery initiated the renaissance of HBO therapy and kindled much interest in this field. Even though no guidelines at that time existed for its use, research into the mechanisms of HBO was stimulated. International congresses on HBO, begun in 1963 and held every 4 years, became a format for the exchange of ideas between clinicians and scientists in this field. However, university-based medical centers showed little interest in HBO, perhaps because of lack of familiarity with the equipment, its multidisciplinary uses and the lack of conclusive studies to prove its effectiveness. Conversely, interest was maintained by military physicians who found HBO to be useful for many conditions other than dysbarism.

Subsequently the uses and mechanisms of HBO have become further elaborated while the equipment to deliver HBO improved. The monoplace chamber has been refined to the degree that it can be easily adapted to the hospital setting while maintaining all necessary life support measures for the critically ill patient. Current usage is based on recommendations of the Hyperbaric Oxygen Committee of the Undersea Medical Society (1983). Use of HBO is based on clinical diagnoses and verified effects of HBO (Table 14.1). Accepted uses include those disorders where the benefits of HBO have been proven conclusively. Twelve conditions are included in this category. If this modality is not used, there may be loss of life or limb, or morbidity may be prolonged. Two disorders, thermal burns and exceptional blood loss anemia, are placed in a special consideration category. The benefits of HBO are well-defined, but other methods of handling these two conditions may obviate the need for this modality. Seventeen conditions are placed in an investigational category. Theoretical and laboratory information demonstrate the value of HBO, but clinical experience is insufficient to justify placing these conditions in the accepted uses category. The common denominator in virtually all the conditions for which HBO is used is tissue ischemia, infection or combinations of the two.

Delivery of oxygen and substrates is essential for tissue viability. Oxygen is more flow-limited than other nutrients. Guyton and associates (1964) summarized this concisely: "of the elements of normal tissue metabolism, oxygen is the most flow limited, i.e., the supply of oxygen is directly dependent on blood flow." This is because ordinarily 97.5% of the blood oxygen content is attached to the hemoglobin molecule whereas

**Table 14.1.** Hyperbaric oxygen therapy usage*

| Acute | Subacute | Chronic |
|---|---|---|
| **Accepted usage** | | |
| Gas embolism | Soft tissue infections (mixed) | Radiation necrosis |
| Carbon monoxide | | Refractory osteomyelitis |
| poisoning | | Refractory mycoses |
| Cyanide poisoning | | |
| Decompression sickness | | |
| Cerebral edema | | |
| Crush injury | | |
| Gas gangrene | | |
| Compromised skin grafts | | |
| **Special considerations for use** | | |
| Thermal burns | | |
| Exceptional blood loss | | |
| anemia | | |
| **Investigational uses** | | |
| Head trauma | Intraabdominal abscess | Radiation myelitis, cystitis |
| Hydrogen sulfide poisoning | Intracranial abscess | enteritis, proctitis |
| Carbon tetrachloride | Fracture healing | Multiple sclerosis |
| poisoning | Pseudomembranous colitis | Lepromatous leprosy |
| Spinal cord injury | Pyoderma gangrenosum | |
| Cerebrovascular accident | Refractory anaerobic | |
| Retinal artery occlusion | infections/actinomycosis | |
| Meningitis | | |
| Sickle cell crisis/retino- | | |
| pathy | | |

* Current recommendations of the HBO Committee of the Undersea Medical Society.

substrates are physically dissolved in the plasma. There is no additional attachment of oxygen to the hemoglobin molecule after the oxygen partial pressure reaches 100 mm Hg pressure in the normal alveolus (Fig. 14.1). Flow impedance in the microcirculation first limits movements of cellular elements of blood. Plasma continues to stream by regions of stasis so substrate delivery to the tissues ordinarily is less affected in low-flow states than oxygen delivery.

The other 2.5% of the blood oxygen content is carried by physically dissolved oxygen in the plasma. This small amount of oxygen is insufficient to meet mammalian tissue oxygen requirements. However, in contrast to hemoglobin-borne oxygen the amount of physically dissolved oxygen increases directly as the partial pressure of the alveolar oxygen increases (Fig. 14.1). The solubility of oxygen in whole blood at 37°C is approximately 0.0236 ml of oxygen/ml of blood/mm Hg of alveolar oxygen pressure. Henry's Law summarizes this effect and states that the amount of gas that physically dissolves in a liquid is directly proportional to its partial pressure.

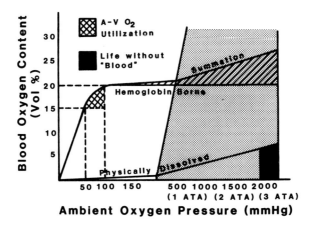

**Figure 14.1.** Oxygenation of blood. Whereas physically dissolved oxygen in the plasma increases in a linear fashion as ambient oxygen pressure is increased, the oxygen-carrying capacity of hemoglobin is not increased after the hemoglobin molecule becomes fully saturated at approximately 100 mm Hg pressure.

When a pressure of 3 ATA (2280 mm Hg) is reached, over 6 vol% of oxygen is physically dissolved in the plasma. The normal arterial-venous oxygen difference is 5 vol%. Thus, sufficient oxygen is physically dissolved in the plasma with HBO to meet the body's oxygen requirements even in the absence of hemoglobin-borne oxygen (Fig. 14.1). This effect was verified by Boerema and co-workers (1960) when they kept piglets without red blood cells alive with HBO. Thus, under hyperbaric oxygen conditions, oxygen delivery becomes no more flow-limited than substrate delivery. The hyperoxygenation effect is a purely physical effect of hyperbaric oxygen.

Bubble reduction is another physical effect of hyperbaric oxygen. Intravascular bubbles affect tissue viability when they impede blood flow. In conditions where gas emboli occur as listed in Table 14.2, reduction in bubble size improves flow states. Bubble reduction occurs in direct response to increased ambient pressure as described by Robert Boyle. Boyle's Law states that the volume of a gas varies inversely with the pressure. At pressures used in clinical exposures bubble volume is reduced two- to threefold. The reduction in bubble is proportionally less (Fig. 14.2) with each succeeding atmosphere increment in pressure. For example, if the pressure is doubled, the bubble volume is reduced by 50%. However, if the pressure is increased from 3 to 4 atm the bubble volume is reduced by only 8.3%.

HBO also affects blood flow. HBO reduces blood flow by approximately 20% through the mechanism of vasoconstriction (Bird and Tefler, 1965). In contrast to the mechanical effects of hyperoxygenation and

**Table 14.2.** Conditions in which intravascular bubbles may occur

| Condition | Cause | Ambient pressure of gas emboli genesis | Comments |
|---|---|---|---|
| Dysbaric air embolism | Diving | Hyperbaric | Brain is the primary target organ. Arterial gas emboli occlude circulation. |
| Serious (type 2) decompression sickness of spinal cord, brain or lung | Diving | Hyperbaric | Spinal cord most frequently affected. Venous gas emboli occlude circulation. |
| Open heart surgery Neurosurgery Gynecological surgery Carotid artery surgery | Accidental entry of air into cardiovascular system during surgery | Normobaric | Diagnosis is easily delayed or missed. The patient's deficit may be attributed to the "post-anesthesia" syndrome or hypoperfusion of the brain during surgery. |
| Hemodialysis | Accidental inflow of air during dialysis | Normobaric | Neurological deficits are usually immediately recognized and treatment results with HBO are uniformly good if started early. |
| Criminal abortions, Oral-genital intercourse, Criminal injections of air (intravenous, intraarterial) | Air entry is into dilated vessels of the pelvis | Normobaric | Death may be attributed to other causes. Documentation of intravascular gas emboli is difficult post-mortem. |

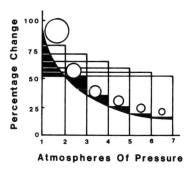

**Figure 14.2.** The volume of a gas bubble is reduced (*shaded areas*) proportionally less with each atmosphere increase in pressure.

bubble reduction, vasoconstriction is a physiological effect of high partial pressures of oxygen on the blood vessel. Vasoconstriction is useful in reducing vasogenic edema associated with hyperemic states. Once flow and blood pressure are reduced, the gradient for interstitial fluid resorption is shifted to favor movement of fluid from the interstitium to the microcirculation. This is the mechanism postulated for the 20% to 30% reductions in intracranial pressures observed in patients treated with HBO for traumatic cerebral edema (Sukoff and Ragatz, 1982). Reductions of similar size in edema have been measured in experimentally induced anterior compartment syndromes in dogs treated with HBO (Strauss et al., 1983).

On first impression, the vasoconstrictive effect of HBO would seem undesirable since hemoglobin-borne oxygen delivery to the tissues is lowered secondary to reduced blood flow. Hyperoxygenation compensates for the reduced flow so that the net effect is maintenance of or even an elevation of tissue oxygenation in the presence of reduced flow (Lambertsen et al., 1953, Bird and Tefler, 1965). Consequently, when tissue oxygenation is compromised directly by interference with blood flow through the microcirculation as well as indirectly by swelling and increased tissue pressure, hyperbaric oxygen is useful.

## The Use of Hyperbaric Oxygen to Improve Tissue Oxygenation

HBO appears to be particularly beneficial in situations where tissue oxygenation is compromised at the microcirculation level. Anemia; increased diffusion distance (edema fluid); frank interruptions of blood vessels, or low-flow states from vasoconstriction, arteriosclerosis, or vasculitis are conditions where tissue oxygenation is compromised and tissue viability can become threatened (Fig. 14.3). In acute blood loss anemias, HBO supplements hemoglobin-borne oxygen delivery. When blood is not immediately available for transfusions of patients in hypovolemic shock or the patient refuses to accept blood products because of religious convictions, HBO therapy should be considered. Intermittent HBO treatments can sustain life and reduce morbidity until the patient compensates for the acute blood loss or transfusions are available. This use is a direct application of hyperoxygenation of plasma.

HBO provides an improved gradient for oxygen to diffuse from the capillary to the cell in situations where partial barriers exist (Fig. 14.4). Edema is a partial barrier, increasing the distance oxygen must diffuse from the capillary to the cell. Other barriers include scar, necrotic tissue, osteomyelitic bone, foreign material, autologous grafts and noncirculating blood. Oxygen tensions in blood increase 10-fold under hyperbaric conditions at 2 ATA (Bassett and Bennett, 1977). According to Peirce (1969)

**Figure 14.3.** Use of HBO to improve tissue oxygenation. Conditions such as anemias, partial barriers, blood vessel interruptions and low blood flow states reduce tissue oxygenation. HBO exposures may augment tissue oxygenation enough to maintain viability of the ischemic tissues.

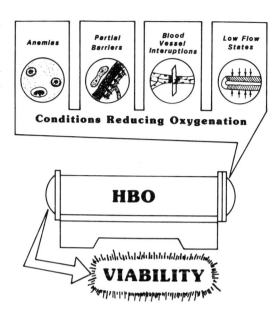

the effective penetration of oxygen into nonperfused tissue is directly proportional to the square root of the oxygen tension. Thus, effective diffusion is increased by a factor of the square root of 10 (i.e., 3.16) under HBO at 2 ATA (Fig. 14.4). This corresponds well to clinical observations of halving the rate of flap necrosis in patients in whom HBO is initiated immediately when signs of compromised flap circulation appear (Perrins, 1975).

The experience with HBO in the presence of frank interruptions of

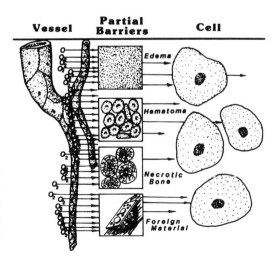

**Figure 14.4.** HBO enhancement of diffusion through partial barriers. The diffusing capacity of oxygen is increased approximately threefold at a HBO treatment pressure of 2 ATA.

major blood vessels is limited. HBO is expected to enhance tissue survival only if collateral circulation exists. If none exists, HBO accelerates demarcation of living from dead tissues. Stalker and co-workers (1973) confirmed this in dogs. Wang and associates (1966) found that if collateral circulation was present, HBO enhances tissue survival. Gorman and associates (1965) observed that HBO is beneficial in patients with advanced chronic arterial disease with major vessel occlusions during the immediate treatment period only.

HBO is frequently used in low-flow states to augment tissue oxygenation. Low-flow states in the microcirculation may be due to cardiac insufficiency, shock, direct trauma to the vasculature, arteriosclerosis, radiation vasculitis or profound vasoconstriction. Oxygen is required for metabolic processes (Fig. 14.5) associated with wound healing, neovascularization and oxidative leucocyte killing (Hunt et al., 1969; Hohn, 1977; Mader et al., 1980). If oxygen tensions in the interstitial fluids are not 30 to 40 mm Hg, these processes will not occur. The consequences are nonhealing wounds, uncontrolled infections or combinations of the two in the low-flow-state regions. HBO augments tissue oxygenation in these regions so that wound healing and infection control are promoted.

The hyperoxygenation effect is not observed when air is pressurized to

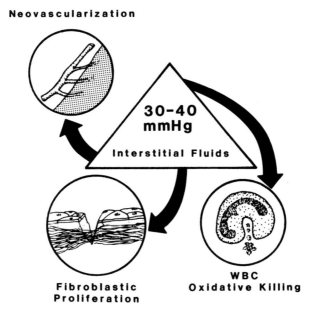

**Neovascularization**

**30-40 mmHg**

**Interstitial Fluids**

**Fibroblastic Proliferation**

**WBC Oxidative Killing**

**Figure 14.5.** Oxygen tension for wound healing. If intermittent oxygen tensions of 30 to 40 mm Hg are not present at the margins of a wound, reparative processes such as neovascularization, fibroblastic proliferation and white blood cell (WBC) oxidative killing will not occur.

the depths used for HBO treatments or when topical oxygen exposures are used (Bassett and Bennett, 1977). While a patient is breathing air at 2 ATA, the amount of dissolved oxygen is increased only twofold. With topical exposures Gruber, Heitkamp and associates (1970) found that oxygen does not diffuse through the intact skin. Fischer (1975) measured oxygen diffusion with topical exposures through an open wound and recorded penetrations to only 1 mm.

Strauss (1981) summarized the experiences reported with HBO in crush injuries and acute ischemias. It was found that the success of HBO in acute ischemias was proportional to the frequency of treatments and that HBO was beneficial in salvaging limbs that would have otherwise been amputated. Gruber and co-workers (1970a) demonstrated in rats that HBO exposures normalized tissue oxygen tensions observed in ischemia pedicle flaps, composite skin grafts and third-degree burns. HBO was also reported to be useful in ergotamine-induced ischemias (Merrick et al., 1978; Bakker, 1979), purpura gangrenosa (Waddell et al., 1965) and allergic vasculitis (Monies-Chass et al., 1976). Okuboye and Ferguson (1968) demonstrated that HBO lessened the amount of tissue loss in experimentally induced frost bite injuries in rabbits.

## Recent Studies Dealing with HBO and Tissue Viability

It is known that under HBO conditions at 2 ATA, blood oxygen tensions immediately rise 10-fold from about 150 mm Hg to 1500 mm Hg (Fig. 14.6). Blood oxygen tensions rapidly fall when the pressure returns to normal. Our studies with mass spectrometer probes show that oxygen tensions in muscle and subcutaneous tissue respond differently than oxygen tensions in the blood (Fig. 14.6). Oxygen tensions in muscle and subcutaneous tissues increase from a baseline of 30 to 40 mm Hg to 250 to 300 mm Hg under HBO exposures at 2 ATA (Wells et al., 1977). In contrast to plasma, it takes about 60 min to achieve peak oxygen tensions. After the HBO exposure is completed, the tensions return to normal over a 2- to 3-h period. This information suggests that HBO behaves as a drug in the interstitial fluids of muscles and subcutaneous tissues in terms of its dose-duration response.

Preliminary studies with the mass spectrometer demonstrate differences in tissue oxygenation with HBO between men and women, between parous and nulliparous women, and between athletes and nonathletes. Women have more ability to take up oxygen in their tissues than men (Fig. 14.7). The muscle and subcutaneous tissues of parous women take up significantly ($p < 0.05$) more oxygen than these tissues do in nulliparous women. Athletes at rest do not take up as much oxygen as the nonathletes. During HBO exposures nonsmokers did not improve their tissue oxygenation as compared to smokers. Conclusions cannot yet be drawn

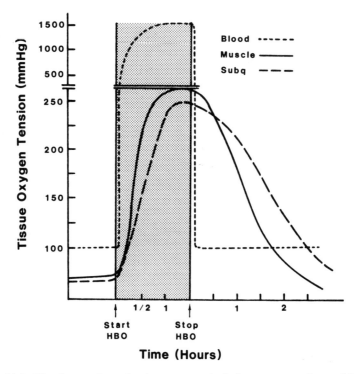

**Figure 14.6.** Blood, muscle and subcutaneous (subq) oxygen tensions with HBO. As predicted from the gas laws and solubility laws, tissue oxygen tensions increase 10-fold with HBO from their baseline levels. After HBO is stopped, the oxygen tensions in muscle and subcutaneous tissues remain elevated for 1 to 3 h.

from these observations, but it appears that hormonal as well as conditioning factors influence tissue oxygenation during HBO exposures.

In collaboration with Hargens and his associates at the University of California, San Diego we studied the effect of HBO exposures on a model compartment syndrome in skeletal muscle (Strauss et al., 1983). Because the insult on a compartment syndrome is primarily at the microcirculation level and the pathophysiology is twofold (ischemia and edema), HBO seemed a logical intervention. Muscle damage was studied by three techniques. To quantitate muscle damage, technetium-99m stannous pyrophosphate ($^{99m}$Tc-PYP) uptake was measured in the leg with compartment syndrome (induced by infusion of autologous plasma) and compared to the opposite control leg. Wet muscle weights from the experimental and control legs were compared to measure edema. Finally, the muscles of both legs were examined histologically.

In all three of the parameters studied, intermittent HBO exposures

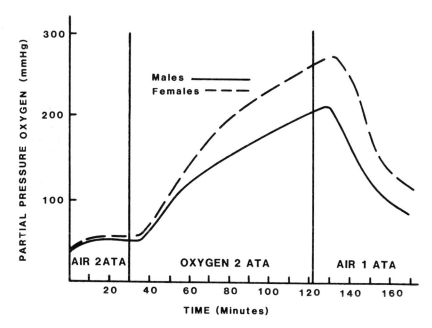

**Figure 14.7.** Subcutaneous oxygen uptake under HBO conditions in men and women. Subcutaneous tissue oxygen uptake is approximately 30% greater in women (260 mm Hg) than in men (200 mm Hg).

proved beneficial (Strauss et al., 1983). Muscle necrosis quantified by uptake of $^{99m}$Tc-PYP was significantly reduced (p < 0.01) after HBO exposure as compared to a series of control animals that did not receive HBO treatments (Fig. 14.8). At the highest intracompartmental pressures studied, 100 mm Hg, the muscle weight ratios (experimental compartment to the weight of the muscle from control compartment of the opposite limb) were significantly less (p < 0.05) than in the dogs not receiving HBO (Table 14.3). Histological evaluation of muscle damage closely correlated with the pyrophosphate uptake and edema measurements and showed that normal muscle architecture was preserved in the HBO-treated group (Fig. 14.9). The relative benefits of HBO became greater as the intracompartmental pressure was raised in the experimental limb.

Our clinical observations of patients with threatened amputations because of nonhealing wounds complicated by infection, ischemia or both reveal that HBO is a useful adjunct to the wound management program. For example, over a 12-month period, 50 patients were referred to us for HBO treatments because healing was insufficient using usual treatment methods and major amputations were felt to be inevitable. The underlying problem in this group of patients was ischemia at the microcirculatory level. Intermittent HBO exposures were added to a comprehensive

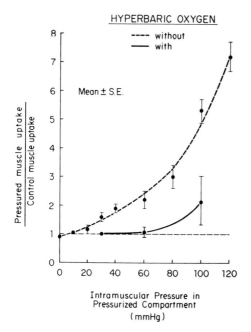

HYPERBARIC OXYGEN

---- without
— with

Mean ± S.E.

Pressured muscle uptake / Control muscle uptake

Intramuscular Pressure in
Pressurized Compartment
(mmHg)

**Figure 14.8.** Ratios (pressurized/ opposite control limb) of uptake of technetium-99m-stannous pyrophosphate in muscles from animals receiving HBO (*solid line*) and from animals not receiving hyperbaric oxygen (*broken line*). The *horizontal broken line* represents a ratio of unity. At the pressurization levels of 60 and 100 mm Hg the differences in muscle injury were significantly different ($p < 0.02$ and $p < 0.01$, respectively). (From MB Strauss et al., 1983.)

wound care program. These combined measures resolved 88% of the wound problems. Six percent of the patients died. Six percent required major amputations. The clinical responses observed in this group of patients correlate well with theoretical benefits and laboratory studies that document the usefulness of HBO in improving survival and wound healing in ischemic tissues (Gruber et al., 1970*b*, Bassett and Bennett, 1977).

**Table 14.3.** Comparison of weights of anterolateral compartment muscles of HBO-treated and untreated dogs

| Compartment syndrome | Weight ratio in HBO-treated dogs (means ± SEM) | Weight ratio in untreated dogs (means ± SEM) |
|---|---|---|
| 30 mm Hg for 8 h | 0.99 ± 0.01 (n = 2) | 1.06 ± 0.03 (n = 11) |
| 60 mm Hg for 8 h | 1.01 ± 0.01 (n = 4) | 1.04 ± 0.02 (n = 6) |
| 100 mm Hg for 8 h | 0.98 ± 0.02[a] (n = 6) | 1.18 ± 0.04 (n = 8) |

Results are expressed as weight ratios (experimental anterolateral compartment/contralateral, control anterolateral compartment). All weights were measured 48 h after initiation of the compartment syndrome.
[a] Significantly different from untreated dogs at $p < 0.05$.
From MB Strauss et al. (1983).

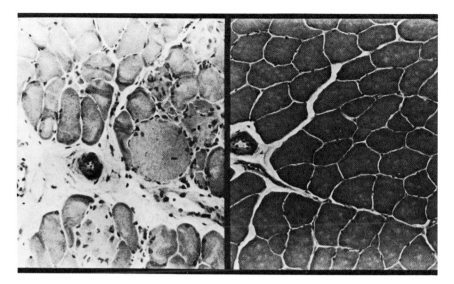

**Figure 14.9.** Effects of HBO in preventing muscle damage in compartment syndromes of dogs. Note the absence of injury in skeletal muscle **(right)** of the dogs treated with intermittent hyperbaric oxygen exposures after generation of muscle compartment syndromes (8-h pressurizations at 100 mm Hg pressure) by infusion of autologous plasma. Muscle damage in an untreated animal **(left)** includes perivascular edema, hyalinization, cellular infiltration, central migration of nuclei and variation in fiber size. (×100). (From MB Strauss et al., 1983.)

## Discussion

Notable advances are anticipated in the near future with regard to use of HBO. As methods to measure tissue oxygenation are refined and the importance of interstitial fluid oxygen tensions appreciated, HBO therapy will probably become a standard of practice. It is anticipated that the indications for HBO will become based on tissue oxygen tensions rather than on current methods of diagnosis (Strauss and Hart, 1984). In the future an anticipated scenario would be as follows: A patient is admitted with a crush injury. After surgical intervention, tissue oxygen levels are measured at the injury site. If the tissue oxygen tensions are below the critical level of 30 to 40 mm Hg, HBO is started. If tissue gas tensions normalize during HBO treatment, HBO treatments are continued until the tissue oxygen tensions stabilize at a level that will allow continued wound healing. If the viability of a region is not established, the measurement of tissue oxygen tensions in the injured region will show whether or not the tissues will survive. If survival is not possible, the tissue oxygen measurements offer objective indications for debridement or early amputation.

HBO may be used with low-molecular-weight dextran, sympathetic blocks, vasodilators or other measures that enhance flow in the microcirculation. Even though the vasoconstrictive effect of HBO seems counterproductive in situations where improved flow in the microcirculation is required, the quantity of oxygen delivered to the tissues is usually increased due to hyperoxygenation. As vasogenic edema decreases from the vasoconstrictive effect, blood flow characteristics and tissue oxygenation improve. It is ironic that most of the studies confirming the effects of HBO on tissue oxygenation, blood flow and wound healing were done only after clinical observations suggested its usefulness.

## Summary

The use of HBO to benefit problems of tissue viability is at a crucial period of time. The physiological effects of HBO are well understood. Its three most important mechanisms are hyperoxygenation, bubble reduction and vasoconstriction. These mechanisms complement each other. Sufficient clinical data exist to justify using HBO for problems where tissue viability is threatened because of hypoxia, edema or combinations of the two. It is an adjunct to the other medical and surgical care a patient receives. Unfortunately, such basic information as the monitoring of tissue oxygen tensions in disease states, optimal HBO treatment schedules and objective criteria for ending HBO treatment are not yet available.

It is anticipated that HBO will be used more frequently in the future. For example, the efficacy of HBO in patients with multiple trauma where coexisting problems of shock, direct injury to tissues, stasis in the microcirculation and edema complicate tissue oxygenation has not been established. The information available at present suggests that HBO is a useful adjunct to the other care used for these patients. Consideration is already being given to require that HBO therapy be available in trauma centers. This is at present recommended in Michigan and a Hyperbaric Oxygen Advisory Committee has been appointed as part of New York's Emergency Medical Service.

In this complex medical era of cost-effectiveness on one hand and threat of litigation on the other, it is essential that the clinician be aware of the indications for use of and mechanisms of action of HBO. As research is generated, clinical experience is gained, and new equipment is developed; the use of HBO is expected to become a standard of practice for a spectrum of clinical disorders in which tissue viability is threatened because of hypoxia.

## References

Bakker DJ (1979). Experience in the treatment with HBO of acute vascular insufficiency of the extremities caused by ergotamine intoxication. In: *Fourth Annual Conference on the Clinical Application of Hyperbaric Oxygen,* Long Beach, California, June 7–9.

Bassett BE and Bennett PB (1977). Introduction to the physical and physiological bases of hyperbaric therapy. In: *Hyperbaric Oxygen Therapy*. (Davis JC and Hunt TK (eds.): Bethesda, Maryland: Undersea Medical Society, pp. 11–24.

Bird AD and Tefler ABM (1965). Effect of hyperbaric oxygen on limb circulation. *Lancet* i:355.

Boerema I, Meyne NG, Brummelkamp WK, Brouma S, Mensch MH, Kamermans F, Stern Hauf M and Van Aalderen W (1960). Life without blood: a study of the influence of high atmospheric pressure and hypothermia on dilution of the blood. *J Cardiovasc Surg* 1:133–146.

Cunningham OJ (1927). Oxygen therapy by means of compressed air. *Anesth Analg* 6:64–66.

Fischer BH (1975). Treatment of ulcers on the legs with hyperbaric oxygen. *J Dermatol Surg* 1:55–58.

Gorman JF, Stansell GB and Douglass FM (1965). Limitations of hyperbaric oxygen in occlusive arterial disease. *Circulation* 32:936–939.

Gruber RP, Brinkley FB, Amato JJ and Mendelson JA (1970a). Hyperbaric oxygen and pedicle flaps, skin grafts, and burns. *Plast Reconstr Surg* 45:24–30.

Gruber RP, Heitkamp DH, Billy LJ and Amato JJ (1970b.). Skin permeability to oxygen and hyperbaric oxygen. *Arch Surg* 101:69–70.

Guyton AC, Ross JM, Carrier O and Walker JR (1964). Evidence for tissue oxygen demand as the major factor causing autoregulations. *Circ Res* XV, Suppl 1 to XIV and XV, 1-60–1-69.

Hohn DC (1977). Oxygen and leucocyte microbial killing. In: *Hyperbaric Oxygen Therapy*. Davis JC and Hunt TK (eds.): Bethesda, Maryland: Undersea Medical Society, pp. 101–110.

Hunt TK, Zederfeldt B and Goldstick TK (1969). Oxygen and healing. *Am J Surg* 118:521–525.

Jacobson JH II, Morsch JHC and Rendall-Baker L (1965). The historical perspective of hyperbaric therapy. *Ann NY Acad Sci* 117:651–670.

Kindwall EP (Chairman) (1979). *Hyperbaric Oxygen Therapy. A Committee Report*. Bethesda, Maryland: Undersea Medical Society, UMS Publ. No. 30CR(HBO).

Lambertsen CJ, Kough RH, Cooper DY, Emmel GL, Loeschcke HH and Schmidt CF (1953). Oxygen toxicity. Effects in man of oxygen inhalation at 1 and 3.5 atmospheres upon blood gas transport, cerebral circulation and cerebral metabolism. *J Appl Physiol* 5:471–485.

Mader JT, Brown GL, Guckian JC, Wells CH, and Reinarz JA (1980). A mechanism for the amelioration by hyperbaric oxygen of experimental staphylococcus osteomyelitis in rabbits. *J Infect Dis* 142:915–922.

Merrick J, Gufler K and Jacobsen E (1978). Ergotism treated with hyperbaric oxygen and continuous epidural analgesia. *Acta Anaesthesiol Scand (Suppl)* 67:87–90.

Monies-Chass I, Herer D, Alon U and Birkhahn HJ (1976). Hyperbaric oxygen in acute ischaemia due to allergic vasculitis. *Anaesthesia* 31:1221–1224.

Okuboye JA and Ferguson CC (1968). The use of hyperbaric oxygen in the treatment of experimental frostbite. *Can J Surg* 11:78–84.

Peirce EC (1969). *Extracorporeal Circulation for Open-Heart Surgey*. Peirce EC (ed.): Springfield, Illinois: Charles C Thomas, pp. 83–84.

Perrins DJ (1975). The effect of hyperbaric oxygen on skin flaps. In: *Skin Flaps*.

Grabb WC and Myers MB (eds.): Boston: Little, Brown and Company, pp. 53–63.

Stalker CG, McEwan AJ and Ledingham I McA. (1973). The effect of increased oxygen in acute limb ischaemia. *Br J Surg* 60:144–148.

Strauss MB (1981). Role of hyperbaric oxygen therapy in acute ischemias and crush injuries—an orthopaedic perspective. *HBO Rev* 2:87–106.

Strauss MB, Hargens AR, Gershuni DH, Greenberg DA, Crenshaw AG, Hart GB and Akeson WH (1983). Reduction of skeletal muscle necrosis using intermittent hyperbaric oxygen in a model compartment syndrome. *J Bone Joint Surg* 65A:656–662.

Strauss MB and Hart GB (1984). Crush injury and the role of hyperbaric oxygen. *Top Emerg Med* 6:9–24.

Sukoff MH and Ragatz RE (1982). Hyperbaric oxygenation for the treatment of acute cerebral edema. *Neurosurgery* 10:29–38.

Waddell WB, Saltzman HA, Fuson RL and Harris J (1965). Purpura gangrenosa treated with hyperbaric oxygenation. *JAMA* 191:971–974.

Wang MCH, Reich T, Lesko WS and Jacobson JH II. (1966). Hyperbaric oxygenation: oxygen exchange in an acutely ischemic vascular bed. *Surgery* 59:94–101.

Wells CH, Goodpasture JE, Horrigan DJ and Hart GB (1977). Tissue gas measurements during hyperbaric oxygen exposure. In: *Proceedings of the Sixth International Congress on Hyperbaric Medicine* Smith G (ed.): Aberdeen, Scotland: Aberdeen University Press, pp. 118–124.

# Index